WHAT'S WRONG WITH ME?

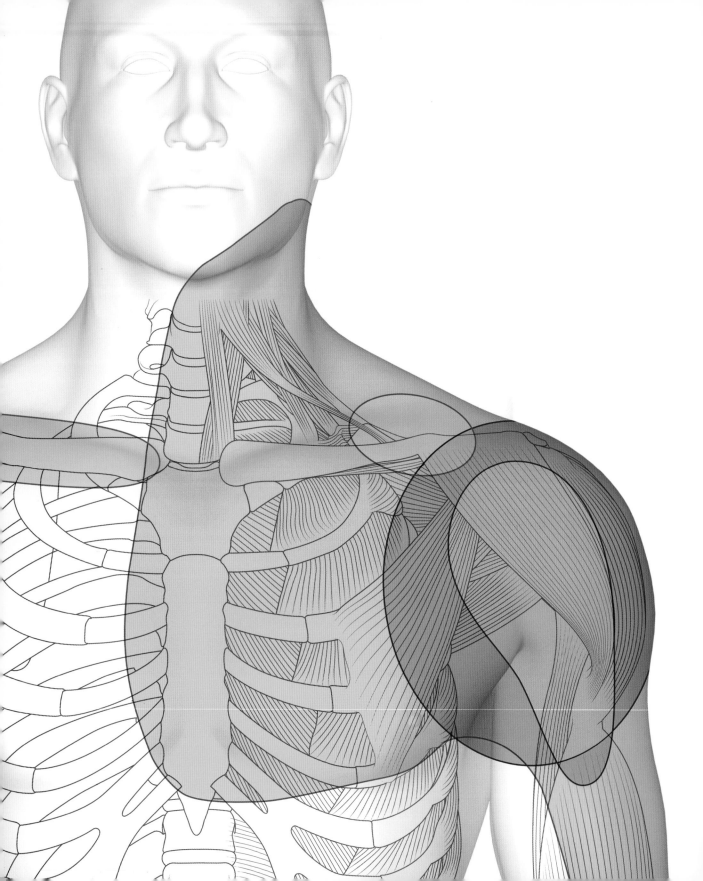

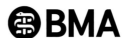

WHAT'S WRONG WITH ME?

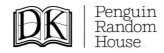

DK LONDON
Senior Editor Janet Mohun
Project Art Editor Duncan Turner
Project Editors Lili Bryant, Miezan van Zyl
Designer Gregory McCarthy
Senior Jacket Designer Mark Cavanagh
Jacket Editor Claire Gell
Jacket Design Development Manager Sophia MTT
Pre-Production Producer David Almond
Producer Anna Vallarino
Managing Editor Angeles Gavira
Managing Art Editor Michael Duffy
Art Director Karen Self
Associate Publishing Director Liz Wheeler
Publishing Director Jonathan Metcalf

BRITISH MEDICAL ASSOCIATION
Chair of the Council Dr Chaand Nagpaul
Treasurer Dr Andrew Dearden
Chairman of Representative Body Dr Anthea Mowat

DK DELHI
Senior editor Suefa Lee
Project art editor Rupanki Arora Kaushik
Art editor Anjali Sachar
Assistant art editors Sonakshi Singh,
Simar Dhamija
Jacket designer Juhi Sheth
Jackets editorial coordinator Priyanka Sharma
DTP designers Jaypal Chauhan,
Nand Kishor Acharya, Rakesh Kumar
Picture researcher Aditya Katyal
Senior managing editor Rohan Sinha
Managing art editor Sudakshina Basu
Managing jackets editor Saloni Singh
Pre-production manager Balwant Singh
Production manager Pankaj Sharma
Picture research manager Taiyaba Khatoon

BMA CONSULTING MEDICAL EDITOR
Dr Michael Peters MBBS

First published in Great Britain in 2018 by
Dorling Kindersley Limited 80 Strand, London, WC2R 0RL

Copyright © 2018 Dorling Kindersley Limited
A Penguin Random House Company
2 4 6 8 10 9 7 5 3 1
001–299745–Jan/2018

READER NOTICE

British Medical Association What's wrong with me? provides information on a wide range of medical topics, and
every effort has been made to ensure that the information in this book is accurate and up-to-date (as at the date
of publication). The book is not a substitute for expert medical advice, however, and is not to be relied on for
medical, healthcare, pharmaceutical, or other professional advice on specific circumstances and in specific
locations. You are advised always to consult a doctor or other health professional for specific information on
personal health matters. Please consult your GP before changing, stopping, or starting any medical treatment.
Never disregard expert medical advice or delay in seeking advice or treatment due to information obtained from
this book. The naming of any product, treatment, or organization in this book does not imply endorsement by
the BMA, BMA Consulting Medical Editor, other consultants or contributors, editor, or publisher, nor does the
omission of any such names indicate disapproval. The BMA, BMA Consulting Medical Editor, consultants,
contributors, editor, and publisher do not accept any legal responsibility for any personal injury or other damage
or loss arising directly or indirectly from any use or misuse of the information and advice in this book.

A CIP catalogue record for this book is available from the British Library.
ISBN: 978-0-2412-8724-8

Printed and bound in China

A WORLD OF IDEAS:
SEE ALL THERE IS TO KNOW

www.dk.com

CONTENTS

PART 1
WHOLE-BODY SYMPTOM GUIDE

PART 2
HEAD-TO-TOE
SYMPTOM GUIDE

PART 3
DIRECTORY OF CONDITIONS

CONTRIBUTORS

Dina Kaufman MBBS, MRCGP, DCH, DRCGP
Part-time GP in London with special interests in women's health and psychological medicine.

Michael Dawson MMedSc, FRCGP
Former Shropshire GP, now a national part-time educator and mentor.

Mike Wyndham MBBS, MRCGP
A GP for 35 years with special interests in postgraduate medical education in primary care, management of skin disease, and the application of photography to medical practice.

Martyn Page
Freelance editor and writer based in London.

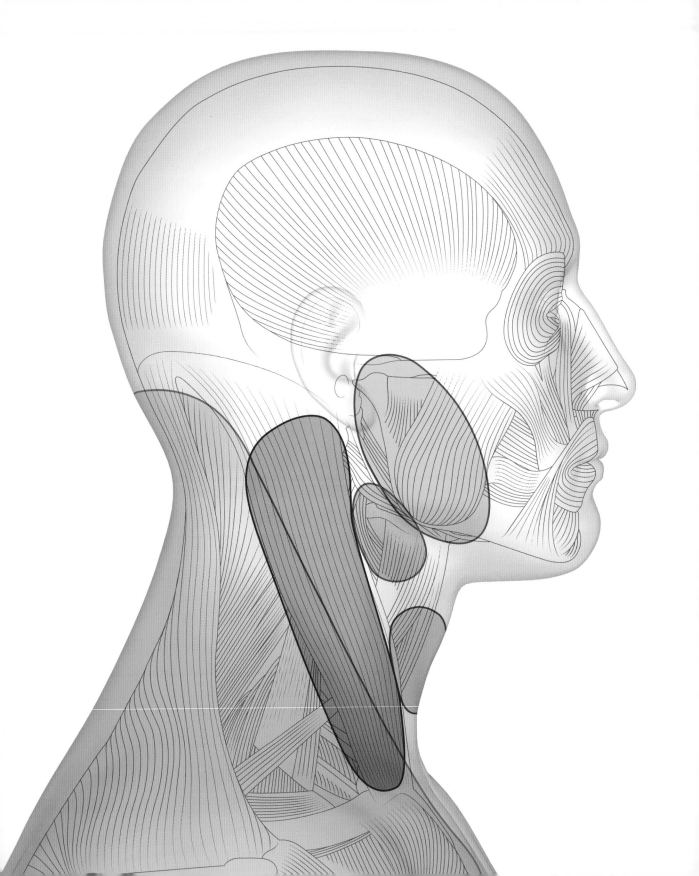

FOREWORD

People today are more aware of health issues than ever before, but they are frequently confronted with a bewildering array of advice with little guidance through this maze. This leaves many confused about who and when to ask for help, and sometimes suffering because they do not want to bother their doctor with "trivial complaints". You may have been struggling with a symptom for a while or you have had pain after a fall or some other injury. In either case, this book provides a clear, simple, visual guide to help you pinpoint the problem and make an informed decision on what to do.

The series of head-to-toe diagnostic guides provide a quick, easy way to check-out your symptoms and enable you to identify what the problem might be. It may also help you to decide when to see a doctor and how seriously to take certain symptoms so that you don't delay when something is potentially urgent or life-threatening.

Not only does the book tell you what the problem might be, it goes on to explain more about the condition and what it might mean for you.

However, a book can only give general guidance and is no substitute for professional advice. When you can't find an answer in the book, or are in any doubt about a medical condition, you should see your own doctor.

Michael Peters

Dr. Michael Peters
BMA Consulting Medical Editor

HOW TO USE THIS BOOK

This book is divided into three parts. Part 1 deals with general complaints, where the symptoms cannot be pinpointed to any particular part of the body. Part 2 is a series of head-to-toe visual diagnostic guides that help to identify conditions or injuries where symptoms occur in specific areas of the body. A cross-reference links to an easy-to-follow description of the condition in Part 3.

All conditions are given a rating to suggest the urgency with which treatment should be sought. Potentially life-threatening situations and ailments that need urgent medical advice are clearly flagged.

KEY TO SYMBOLS

A series of symbols indicate whether medical advice is needed and how speedily this should be sought.

✚ Symptoms usually resolve without specific treatment. Text may state to seek medical advice if condition persists, or in particular groups, such as children.

✚✚ See a doctor (or dentist if appropriate) for advice, diagnosis and potential treatment, within a few days. Text will say if medical attention is needed sooner.

✚✚✚ Get medical attention or advice as soon as possible, either by telephone or visiting the accident and emergency department. Additional text will tell you if the condition is a medical emergency.

✚ Seek urgent medical attention if you or the person affected has the symptoms listed. These usually need immediate treatment and may be life-threatening.

PART 1 WHOLE-BODY SYMPTOM GUIDE

This part of the book covers general unwellness and full-body symptoms grouped together under general symptoms, such as Nausea and Vomiting.

Symptoms are further grouped where possible to make identification easier

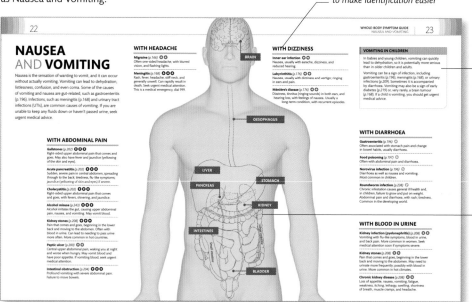

Special panels group conditions together under various criteria, for example by age-related or gender-specific complaints.

Relevant organs are shown, to aid in understanding the origin of the problem

PART 2 HEAD-TO-TOE SYMPTOM GUIDE

This section is organized from head to toe so that you can easily find the relevant page. The conditions are grouped and connected to the areas they affect, with colour-coding to help distinguish areas.

Symptoms that require urgent medical attention are clearly flagged

If symptoms can occur anywhere in the featured part of the body, the condition is not colour-coded

Cross-references lead to descriptions in Part 3; symbols indicate what action is needed (see opposite)

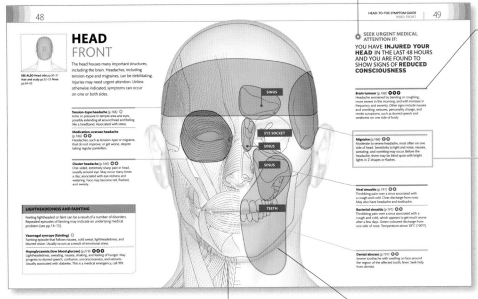

Migraine *(p.166)* ✚ ✚
Moderate to severe headache, side of head. Sensitivity to ligh sweating, and vomiting may o headache, there may be blind lights in Z-shapes or flashes.

Symptom checker
A list of possible conditions leads off each area. Clear and simple descriptions set out the major symptoms for each condition so that you can determine if they match yours.

Anatomical illustrations give enough detail to understand the structures involved

Coloured areas indicate where symptoms are experienced; unless otherwise indicated, symptoms may occur on both sides

PART 3 DIRECTORY OF CONDITIONS

Organized by body system, this section gives descriptions of each condition, including information on the known causes and possible treatments.

HEADACHE
Medication-overuse headache
Tension-type headache

Condition names
The names of conditions listed in Parts 1 and 2 appear as main headings or subheadings at the top of each description.

MIGRAINE

Migraine is a recurrent, often se headache that usually occurs or of the head and may be accomp symptoms such as nausea and v

Descriptions
Each condition is given a clear, concise description to give an overview of the problem.

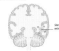

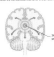

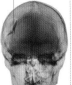

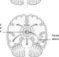

PART 1
WHOLE-BODY SYMPTOM GUIDE

DIZZINESS AND FAINTING

Occasionally feeling slightly unsteady is common and not usually a matter for concern. True dizziness, or vertigo, in which you feel that everything is spinning around, is not normal, but can result from certain medication or drinking too much alcohol. Isolated episodes of feeling faint are common and not usually significant. Repeated instances of faintness or passing out for no apparent reason may indicate an underlying medical problem.

⊕ **SEEK URGENT MEDICAL ATTENTION IF:**

YOU HAVE **SHORTNESS** OF **BREATH** OR **PERSISTENT CHEST PAIN**

A PERSON **LOSES CONSCIOUSNESS**

VERTIGO DISORDERS

Benign paroxysmal positional vertigo *(p.175)* ⊕ ⊕
Sudden onset of vertigo (sensation that your surroundings are moving or spinning around) when moving head. Usually no associated tinnitus (noises in ears) or hearing loss.

Labyrinthitis *(p.176)* ⊕ ⊕
Vertigo, worsened by change of head position; tinnitus; and hearing loss. Fever, and feeling of fullness or pressure in the ear may also be present.

Ménière's disease *(p.176)* ⊕ ⊕
Attacks of vertigo, hearing loss, and tinnitus. Lasts between a few minutes and several days. Attacks may recur over periods ranging from days to years.

Acoustic neuroma *(p.176)* ⊕ ⊕
One-sided, slowly developing hearing loss with tinnitus. Loss of balance may develop along with headaches and numbness or weakness of the face on the affected side.

DIZZINESS AND MEDICATION

Some types of medication, or combinations of medications, can cause dizziness (lightheadedness or faintness) as a side effect. Drugs that most commonly cause this problem include certain antidepressants, anticonvulsants, many antihypertensives (drugs to control high blood pressure), and sedatives.

FAINTNESS IN PREGNANCY

Feeling faint during pregnancy is fairly common and not usually a cause for concern. It is due to hormonal changes causing blood vessels to relax, lowering blood pressure. However, pregnant women who experience frequent attacks of faintness or pass out should see a doctor.

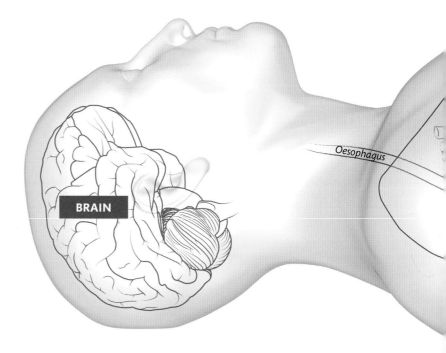

Oesophagus

BRAIN

DIZZINESS OR FAINTNESS DISORDERS

Anaemia (p.186) ➕➕
Tiredness or lack of energy with feeling faint, pale skin, rapid heart rate, and headaches.

Hypotension (low blood pressure) (p.183) ➕➕
Lightheadedness, blurred vision, feeling weak, nausea, heart palpitations (noticeable heartbeat), and fainting. Symptoms are short-lived and may be worse after standing up or prolonged standing. Seek urgent medical attention if in elderly person, if it is persists, or if person does not regain full consciousness.

Heart rhythm problems (arrhythmias) (p.181) ➕➕
Dizziness, with awareness of the heart beating, fast or slow, regular or irregular. May be associated with shortness of breath or chest pain. Seek medical advice if persistent. Seek urgent medical attention if with chest pain or shortness of breath.

Heart valve disorders (p.182) ➕➕
Dizziness, with fast and irregular heartbeats, shortness of breath, tiredness, and swelling of the ankles and feet. If any chest pain or shortness of breath, seek urgent medical help.

Hypoglycaemia (p.219) ➕➕➕
Lightheadedness, sweating, nausea, shaking, and feeling of hunger. May progress to slurred speech, confusion, unconsciousness, and seizures. Usually associated with diabetes. This is a medical emergency, dial 999.

Transient ischaemic attack (TIA) (p.169) ➕➕➕
Symptoms are the same as a stroke (see below), but are short-lived, clearing up completely within 24 hours. This is a medical emergency, dial 999.

Stroke (p.169) ➕➕➕
Dizziness and loss of balance and coordination associated with the sudden start of symptoms. These include drooping of face on one side, weakness or paralysis down one side of body, slurred speech, difficulty with swallowing, or double vision. This is a medical emergency, dial 999.

Minor head injury (p.167) ➕➕
Lump, bruise, or bleeding at the injury site; mild headache; nausea; and slight dizziness.

Serious head injury (p.167) ➕➕➕
Any high impact injury, loss of consciousness, amnesia, vomiting, seizure, or change in behaviour require urgent medical attention, dial 999.

Heat exhaustion (p.239) ➕➕
Feeling faint with headache, weakness, intense thirst, muscle cramps, nausea, and vomiting; fast pulse; small amounts of dark urine.

Cervical spondylosis (p.158) ➕➕
Dizziness, unsteadiness, or double vision brought on by moving the head quickly. Mild to moderate pain extending from the neck to back of head.

Epileptic seizure (p.167) ➕➕
Seizures with loss of consciousness and uncontrollable jerking of trunk and limbs. Seek urgent medical attention if it is the first attack, if consciousness does not return within 5 minutes, or if the person does not regain full consciousness.

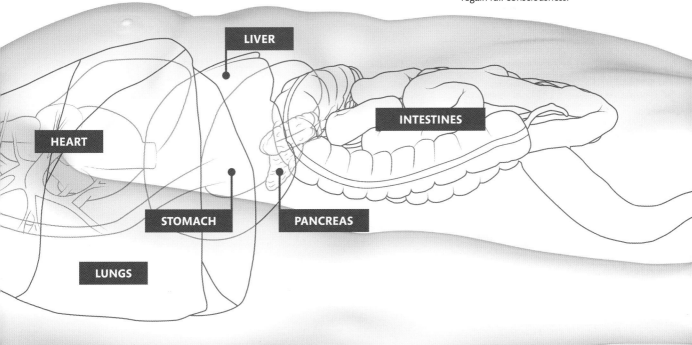

SEIZURES

Seizures are sudden episodes of abnormal electrical activity in the brain. These can cause dramatic, involuntary contraction of many muscles in the body and, if severe, result in convulsive movements of the limbs and trunk, and unconsciousness.

⊕ SEEK URGENT MEDICAL ATTENTION IF:

IT IS THE **FIRST TIME** THE PERSON HAS HAD A SEIZURE

THE SEIZURE LASTS FOR **MORE THAN 5 MINUTES**

THE PERSON **DOES NOT REGAIN FULL CONSCIOUSNESS** AFTER THE SEIZURE

MULTIPLE EPISODES

Epilepsy *(p.167)* ⊕ ⊕
Seizures may range from a short-lived loss of awareness in absence seizures, with twitching of the face or limb, to generalized seizures with loss of consciousness and uncontrollable jerking of trunk and limbs. Seek urgent medical attention if it is the first attack, if consciousness does not return within 5 minutes, or if the person does not regain full consciousness.

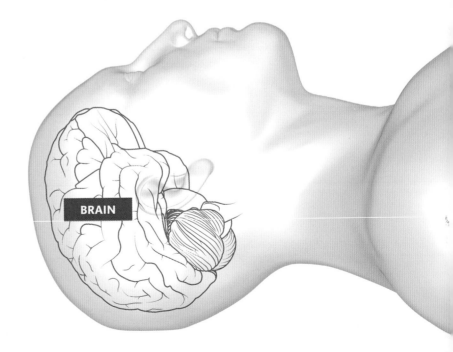

BRAIN

SINGLE EPISODE

Head injury *(p.167)* ✚✚✚
Seizures and unconsciousness. May be preceded by headache, drowsiness, confusion, nausea, and vomiting. There may also be a lump, bruise, or bleeding at the injury site; clear fluid or blood leaking from the ears; and no recollection of the injury. Symptoms may develop hours or days after the injury.

Stroke *(p.169)* ✚✚✚
Sudden start of symptoms include drooping of face on one side, weakness or paralysis on one side of body, slurred speech, difficulty with swallowing, and double vision. In older people, seizures are common in the weeks following a stroke. This is a medical emergency, dial 999.

High fever ✚✚✚
Seizures; temperature over 38°C (100.4°F) with chills, headache, weakness, poor concentration, sleepiness in the day, nausea, vomiting, and confusion.

Severe heatstroke *(p.239)* ✚✚✚
Confusion, disorientation, fast and shallow breathing, seizures, and unconsciousness.

Alcohol poisoning *(p.239)* ✚✚✚
Seizures and unconsciousness. May be preceded by confusion, slurred speech, loss of coordination, vomiting, and slow or irregular breathing. Medical emergency, dial 999.

Drug overdose *(p.239)* ✚✚✚
Seizures and unconsciousness. May be preceded by nausea, vomiting, abdominal pain, diarrhoea, rapid heart beat, chest pain, breathlessness, and confusion. May be fatal. This is a medical emergency, dial 999.

Abrupt drug or alcohol withdrawal ✚✚✚
Seizures, which may be preceded by restlessness, tremor of hands, sweating, abdominal cramps, diarrhoea, nausea, vomiting, hallucinations, and confusion. This is a medical emergency, dial 999.

Encephalitis *(p.168)* ✚✚✚
Usually flu-like symptoms, such as fever and headache, followed by confusion, drowsiness, seizures, and coma. This is a medical emergency, dial 999.

Hypoglycaemia *(p.219)* ✚✚✚
Lightheadedness, sweating, nausea, shaking, and feeling of hunger. May progress to slurred speech, confusion, and unconsciousness. Usually associated with diabetes. Severe or untreated hypoglycaemia may cause seizures. This is a medical emergency, dial 999.

Meningitis *(p.168)* ✚✚✚
General neck stiffness, fever, feeling very unwell, and light hurts eyes. May have a rash that doesn't fade after pressure is briefly applied. Seizures tend to occur in severe cases that do not receive prompt treatment. May rapidly result in death. This is a medical emergency, dial 999.

Brain tumour *(p.168)* ✚✚✚
Seizures associated with headache worsened by bending or coughing, more severe in the morning, and with increase in frequency and severity. Other signs include nausea and vomiting, personality change, and stroke symptoms, such as slurred speech and weakness or paralysis on one side of body.

GENERAL PAIN

Everyone will experience pain at some point in their lives. Pain can be constant or intermittent, and shooting, burning, stabbing or dull, depending on its cause and location. Pain is chronic once it has been present for over three months and can originate from any body part, namely the muscles, bones, joints, nerves, or an internal organ.

MUSCULAR AND JOINT PAIN

Arthritis *(p.157)* ➕ ➕
Pain, swelling, and limitation of movement in a joint may be due to various types of arthritis, including rheumatoid arthritis, septic arthritis, reactive arthritis, and psoriatic arthritis. Joint stiffness may be worse in the morning; skin may be red or hot if joint infected; and pain may cause trouble sleeping. Commonly affects hands, knees, hips, and spine.

Polymyalgia rheumatica *(p.161)* ➕ ➕
Painful, stiff muscles, especially after waking in the morning; fever; night sweats; extreme fatigue; sometimes severe headache and scalp tenderness.

Fibromyalgia *(p.162)* ➕ ➕
Deep, burning, aching pain that may move around body. Worse with activity, stress, and weather changes. Muscle stiffness, tingling, and tiredness.

Systemic lupus erythematosus *(p.189)* ➕ ➕
Swollen, painful joints, extreme tiredness, and skin rashes on the wrists, hands, and face (commonly a red, butterfly-shaped rash on the nose and cheeks). Rash may be painful or itchy and worsened by exposure to sunlight.

Lyme disease *(p.236)* ➕ ➕
Spreading circular rash that appears like a target where tick bite has occurred; flu-like symptoms; fatigue; headache; fever; stiff neck; muscle and joint pain.

PAIN AND CANCER

Cancer can cause pain in different parts of the body, depending on the site of the tumour. A tumour growing inside the kidney may press on other internal organs, causing pain in the lower back and side. Bowel cancer can cause a blockage to the passage of faeces, resulting in cramping abdominal pains. Bone cancers *(p.155)* result in dull aches, which may be worse at night. Pressure on the brain from a brain tumour *(p.168)* may cause severe headaches. Primary breast cancer *(p.216)* is not usually painful.

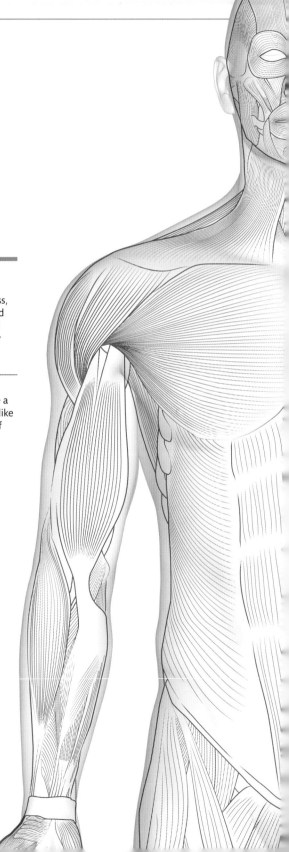

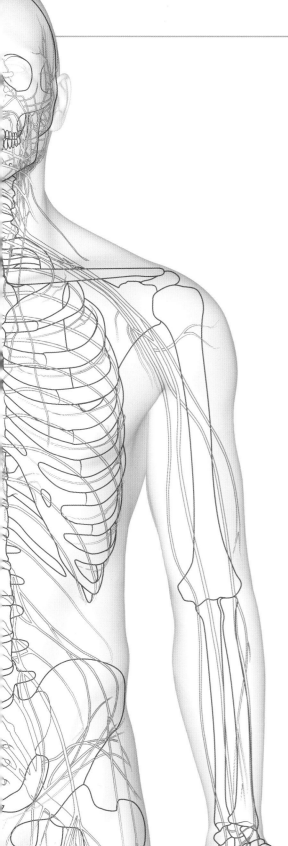

BONE DISORDERS

Paget's disease of bone *(p.155)* ✚✚
May affect any bone in the body, but most commonly affects the pelvis, collarbone, spine, skull, or leg bones. Bones are painful, weaker, and misshapen, with fractures and arthritis in the nearby joints. More common in men than women, and rare under 55 years of age.

NERVE PAIN

Diabetic neuropathy *(p.219)* ✚✚
Burning, shooting pains; tingling; numbness; loss of coordination, sometimes leading to falls. Commonly affects feet and legs, sometimes hands and arms. More common in those with poor control of their diabetes.

Peripheral neuropathy *(p.172)* ✚✚
Burning, shooting pains; tingling; numbness; loss of coordination, sometimes leading to falls. Commonly affects feet and legs, sometimes hands and arms.

Nutritional neuropathy *(p.172)* ✚✚
Burning, shooting pains; tingling; numbness. Symptoms often begin in the tips of fingers and toes and slowly progress along the limbs. Sore, red tongue; symptoms of anaemia, such as fatigue.

Complex regional pain syndrome *(p.172)* ✚✚
Severe, persistent pain triggered by an injury, usually affecting a single limb. Overlying skin may be extremely tender, red, swollen, or stiff.

MOBILITY

Problems with mobility may arise from long-term conditions affecting the muscles, nerves, and joints. However, some mobility problems may be short-lived. Also, any condition that causes pain may restrict a person's ability to move about. Falling over may be mainly a balance problem, but it is usually aggravated by difficulties with limb movements.

ONE-SIDED LIMP

Sciatica (p.173) ✚ ✚
Lower back pain associated with pain down leg to calf or big toe. If severe, may lead to numbness, weakness, or paralysis in buttock, leg, or foot on one side of body, causing hip to drop and the body to lean towards affected side.

Spinal polio (p.234) ✚ ✚
Usually a one-sided paralysis with body leaning towards affected side with each step; there is a compensatory body swing to other side. Affected leg is lifted high so that toes clear the ground.

Stroke (p.169) ✚ ✚ ✚
Sudden onset of facial weakness, associated with possible loss of speech and weakness or paralysis of one side of body. Also muscle stiffness in affected side, and balance and coordination problems. This is a medical emergency, dial 999.

GENERAL MUSCLE IMPAIRMENT

Muscle cramps (p.161) ✚
Sudden, involuntary, sustained (seconds to several minutes) contraction of a muscle, causing severe pain and temporary incapacity. Muscle soreness remains for a while once cramp has ceased. More likely in tired muscles and at night.

Restless legs syndrome (p.162) ✚
An unpleasant feeling in legs with urge to move them. Worse at rest. More likely if have anaemia, kidney failure, Parkinson's disease, diabetes, rheumatoid arthritis, or if pregnant.

Polymyalgia rheumatica (p.189) ✚ ✚
Stiffness, pain, and aching muscles, especially in the morning. Neck, shoulder, upper arm, and hips may be affected. May cause difficulty turning over, getting up, or raising arms above shoulder height.

Chronic fatigue syndrome (p.166) ✚
Severe fatigue unrelated to exertion, muscle pains, poor sleep, impaired memory or concentration, pain in multiple joints, and headaches. There are often dizziness and balance problems.

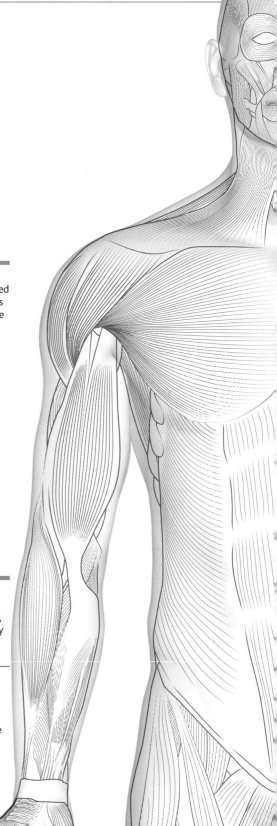

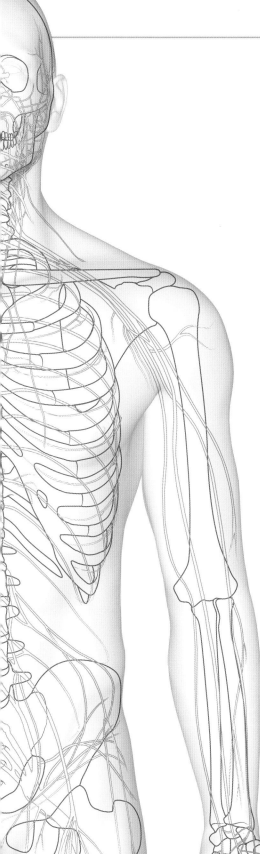

MEDICATION AND FALLS

Unsteadiness and falling over is more likely when taking four or more different medications. Medication side-effects and interactions can impair brain function, causing unsteadiness. Medication for conditions such as raised blood pressure, depression, nausea, and poor sleep are liable to have the side-effect of unsteadiness. Others drugs can cause a fall the levels of potassium in the blood, resulting in tiredness, weakness, and leg cramps. Many long-term illnesses (which usually require treatment with medication) are also more likely to cause falls.

GENERALIZED NERVE IMPAIRMENT

Alzheimer's disease *(p.170)* ➕ ➕
Cautious walking, slow and wide-based with arms away from body as if walking on ice. Associated with memory problems, poor judgement, mood changes, anxiety, agitation, confusion, delusions, and behavioural changes.

Multiple sclerosis *(p.171)* ➕ ➕
Uncoordinated walk with irregular steps, feet wide apart, stepping first onto heel then toes with a double tap. Difficulty walking one foot in front of the other. There may be double vision, fatigue, speech difficulties, and incontinence.

Parkinson's disease *(p.171)* ➕ ➕
Involuntary tremors that occur at rest (often in one hand), slow movements, muscle stiffness, shuffling walk, stooped posture, expressionless face, insomnia, depression.

Motor neuron disease *(p.171)* ➕ ➕
Rapidly progressive muscle weakness and wasting of mainly voluntary muscles, causing tripping or stumbling progressing to an inability to walk, grip, or even swallow properly. There may be dementia and crying/laughing for no apparent reason.

Spinal muscle atrophy *(p.162)* ➕ ➕
Muscle weakness, floppy limbs, twitching and variable (usually increasing) impairment of mobility. In infants, there may be weakness in ability to cough and cry when respiratory muscles affected.

Huntington's disease *(p.171)* ➕ ➕
Poorly coordinated jerky movements with hesitant leg raising and persistently bent knees. Often with uncontrolled arm and head movements.

GENERAL JOINT IMPAIRMENT

Arthritis *(p.157)* ➕ ➕
Pain, swelling, and limitation of movement in a joint may be due to various types of arthritis, including rheumatoid arthritis, septic arthritis, reactive arthritis, and psoriatic arthritis. Joint stiffness may be worse in the morning, skin may be red or hot if joint infected, and pain may cause trouble sleeping. Commonly affects hands, knees, hips, and spine.

Ankylosing spondylitis *(p.158)* ➕ ➕
Increasing and long-standing lower back pain, spinal stiffness, inflamed joints and tendons, and fatigue causing much reduced mobility. If long-term and severe, person may be hunched over. More common in men.

Systemic lupus erythematosus *(p.189)* ➕ ➕
Swollen, painful joints, extreme tiredness, and skin rashes on the wrist, hand, and face (commonly a red, butterfly-shaped rash on the nose and cheeks).

NAUSEA AND **VOMITING**

Nausea is the sensation of wanting to vomit, and it can occur without actually vomiting. Vomiting can lead to dehydration, listlessness, confusion, and even coma. Some of the causes of vomiting and nausea are gut-related, such as gastroenteritis (p.196). Infections, such as meningitis (p.168) and urinary tract infections (UTIs), are common causes of vomiting. If you are unable to keep any fluids down or haven't passed urine, seek urgent medical advice.

WITH ABDOMINAL PAIN

Gallstones *(p.202)* ✚✚✚
Right-sided upper abdominal pain that comes and goes. May also have fever and jaundice (yellowing of the skin and eyes).

Acute pancreatitis *(p.202)* ✚✚✚
Sudden, severe pain in central abdomen, spreading through to the back; tiredness, flu-like symptoms; jaundice (yellowing of skin and eyes) if severe.

Cholecystitis *(p.202)* ✚✚✚
Right-sided upper abdominal pain that comes and goes, with fevers, shivering, and jaundice.

Alcohol misuse *(p.243)* ✚✚✚
Alcohol irritates the gut, causing upper abdominal pain, nausea, and vomiting. May vomit blood.

Kidney stones *(p.208)* ✚✚✚
Pain that comes and goes, beginning in the lower back and moving to the abdomen. Often with blood in urine. Can lead to needing to pass urine more often. More common in hot countries.

Peptic ulcer *(p.200)* ✚✚
Central upper abdominal pain, waking you at night and worse when hungry. May vomit blood and have poor appetite. If vomiting blood, seek urgent medical attention.

Intestinal obstruction *(p.204)* ✚✚✚
Profound vomiting with severe abdominal pain. Failure to move bowels.

WITH HEADACHE

Migraine *(p.166)* ✚✚
Often one-sided headache, with blurred vision, and flashing lights.

Meningitis *(p.168)* ✚✚✚
Rash, fever, headache, stiff neck, and generally unwell. Can rapidly result in death. Seek urgent medical attention. This is a medical emergency, dial 999.

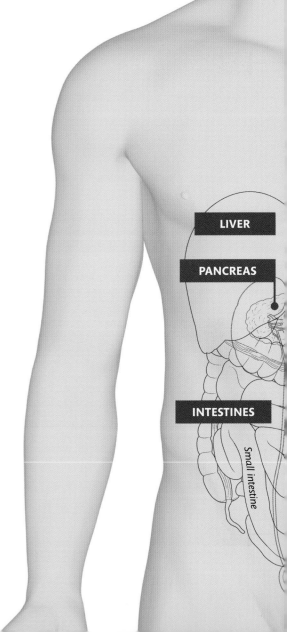

LIVER

PANCREAS

INTESTINES

Small intestine

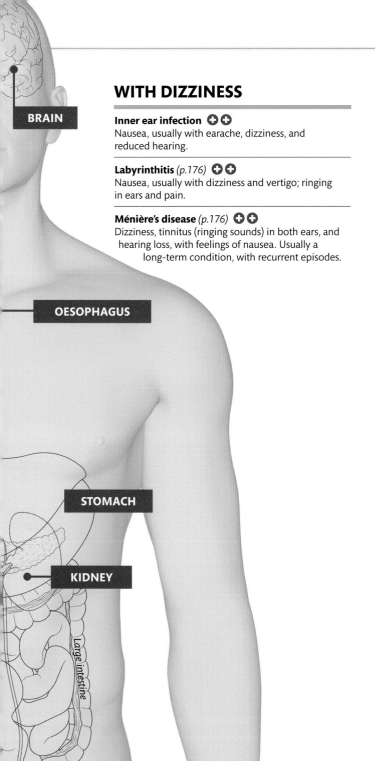

BRAIN

OESOPHAGUS

STOMACH

KIDNEY

Large intestine

BLADDER

WITH DIZZINESS

Inner ear infection ✚✚
Nausea, usually with earache, dizziness, and reduced hearing.

Labyrinthitis *(p.176)* ✚✚
Nausea, usually with dizziness and vertigo; ringing in ears and pain.

Ménière's disease *(p.176)* ✚✚
Dizziness, tinnitus (ringing sounds) in both ears, and hearing loss, with feelings of nausea. Usually a long-term condition, with recurrent episodes.

VOMITING IN CHILDREN

In babies and young children, vomiting can quickly lead to dehydration, so it is potentially more serious than in older children and adults.

Vomiting can be a sign of infection, including gastroenteritis (*p.196*), meningitis (*p.168*), or urinary infections (*p.209*). Sometimes it is accompanied by diarrhoea. Vomiting may also be a sign of early diabetes (*p.219*) or, very rarely, a brain tumour (*p.168*). If a child is vomiting, you should get urgent medical advice.

WITH DIARRHOEA

Gastroenteritis *(p.196)* ✚
Often associated with stomach pain and change in bowel habits, usually diarrhoea.

Food poisoning *(p.197)* ✚
Often with abdominal pain and diarrhoea.

Norovirus infection *(p.196)* ✚
Diarrhoea as well as nausea and vomiting. Most common in children.

Roundworm infection *(p.238)* ✚
Chronic infestation causes general ill health and, in children, failure to grow and put on weight. Abdominal pain and diarrhoea, with rash; tiredness. Common in the developing world.

WITH BLOOD IN URINE

Kidney infection (pyelonephritis) *(p.208)* ✚✚
Vomiting with flu-like symptoms, blood in urine, and back pain. More common in women. Seek medical attention soon if symptoms severe.

Kidney stones *(p.208)* ✚✚
Pain that comes and goes, beginning in the lower back and moving to the abdomen. May need to urinate more frequently; possibly with blood in urine. More common in hot climates.

Chronic kidney disease *(p.208)* ✚✚
Loss of appetite, nausea, vomiting, fatigue, weakness, itching, lethargy, swelling, shortness of breath, muscle cramps, and headache.

FATIGUE

It is normal to feel tired or lacking in energy after exercising strenuously, working hard for a long period, or a poor night's sleep. More persistent fatigue is also common during pregnancy or after a viral illness, such as influenza or a cold. However, prolonged, persistent, severe fatigue without an obvious cause may indicate an underlying health problem.

MEDICATION

Some medications, over-the-counter complementary remedies, and recreational drugs can cause fatigue, for example, some medications used to treat high blood pressure (such as beta blockers), or may cause drowsiness, for example, some antihistamines. Consult your doctor or pharmacist if you think your fatigue may be due to a medication or remedy.

Diabetes (p.219) ✚✚
Fatigue and muscle weakness, excessive thirst, and needing to urinate more often than usual. May also be recurrent infections and slow healing of wounds.

Anaemia (p.186) ✚✚
Tiredness or lack of energy with feeling faint, pale skin, rapid heart rate, and headaches.

Hypothyroidism (p.220) ✚✚
Extreme tiredness in association with other symptoms of an underactive thyroid gland, such as hair loss, dry skin, weight gain, constipation, and a hoarse voice.

Heart failure (p.181) ✚✚
Long-term breathlessness, after activity or at rest; fatigue; and swollen ankles. Less commonly there may be a persistent cough, wheezing, and loss of appetite.

Inflammatory bowel disease (p.203) ✚✚
Fatigue associated with, usually, longstanding and continuous bloody diarrhoea, abdominal pain, fever, and weight loss.

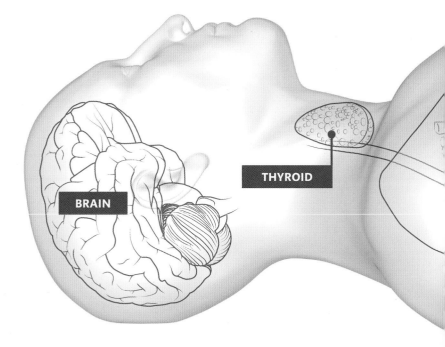

BRAIN

THYROID

Glandular fever (p.235) ⊕⊕
Extreme tiredness with fever, sore throat, and enlarged lymph nodes in neck, armpit, and groin. Associated with puffiness around the eyes and abdominal pain. If abdominal pain is severe, seek urgent medical attention.

Hepatitis (p.200) ⊕⊕
Fatigue with other symptoms, including jaundice and itchy skin. Feeling generally unwell and right-sided abdominal discomfort.

Tuberculosis (p.236) ⊕⊕
Extreme tiredness with chest pain, fever, night sweats, and weight loss. May be coughing up blood. Symptoms usually develop slowly, over several weeks.

Leukaemia (p.187) ⊕⊕
Tiredness, pale skin, breathlessness, dizziness, fever, night sweats, and swollen lymph nodes in the neck, armpits, or groin. May also have swelling of the abdomen, joint or bone pain, easy bruising and bleeding, and susceptibility to infections.

Multiple sclerosis (p.171) ⊕⊕
Fatigue, double vision or painful loss of vision in one eye, lack of bladder control, and muscle spasms. May also have altered sensation and numbness, often in the legs, balance and coordination problems, and pain in any body part.

Systemic lupus erythematosus (p.189) ⊕⊕
Extreme tiredness with swollen, painful joints; skin rashes on the wrist, hand, and face (commonly a red, butterfly-shaped rash on the nose and cheeks). Rash may be painful or itchy and worsened by exposure to sunlight.

Sickle-cell disease (p.186) ⊕⊕
Tiredness and general weakness. Severe crippling pain during a sickle-cell crisis can affect any body part. An increased susceptibility to major infections, and delayed puberty in adolescents.

Malnutrition (p.197) ⊕⊕
Persistent tiredness and weakness, listlessness, and increased susceptibility to illness, with slow recovery time. If due to eating too little, there may also be weight loss.

Depression (p.242) ⊕⊕
Persistent low mood, loss of enjoyment in leisure activities, and feelings of guilt, worthlessness, and despair. Also difficulty concentrating, remembering things, and making decisions.

Seasonal affective disorder (p.242) ⊕⊕
Similar symptoms to depression (see above), but usually starts in autumn or winter and improves in spring.

Insomnia (p.241) ⊕
Inadequate sleep due to difficulty in falling asleep or staying asleep for long enough; fatigue; poor concentration; and irritability. See doctor if persists and affects daily life.

Chronic fatigue syndrome (p.166) ⊕⊕
Overwhelming fatigue and joint pain, without swelling or redness, that does not improve with rest or sleep. Associated with headaches, poor concentration and memory, sore throat, and tender lymph nodes in neck, armpits, and groin.

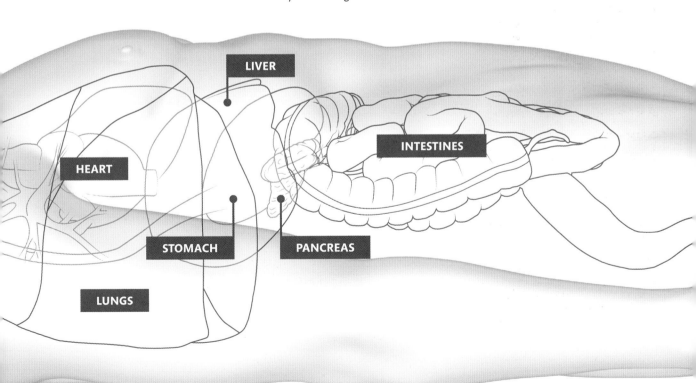

LIVER

HEART

INTESTINES

STOMACH

PANCREAS

LUNGS

FEVER

A fever is a body temperature over 38°C (100.4°F). Most commonly, fever is due to an infection, but it may also be caused by other conditions, such as heat exposure, or some cancers, such as lymphoma (p.188). Many of the well-known infectious diseases, such as chickenpox, rubella, and measles, typically produce a rash (pp.32–33) as well as fever.

Influenza *(p.232)* ⊕
High fever associated with generalized aches and pains, headache, dry cough, sore throat, and stuffy or runny nose. Also vomiting and diarrhoea. If symptoms are severe or in a child or older person, seek medical attention.

Pneumonia *(p.194)* ⊕ ⊕
High fever with abdominal pain (either side of body), cough (possibly coughing blood), and generally feeling unwell.

Kidney infection (pyelonephritis) *(p.208)* ⊕ ⊕
Vomiting with flu-like symptoms, blood in urine, and back pain. More common in women. Seek medical attention soon if symptoms severe.

Infectious mononucleosis (glandular fever) *(p.235)* ⊕ ⊕
Extreme tiredness with fever, sore throat, and enlarged lymph nodes in neck, armpit, and groin. Also puffiness around eyes and abdominal pain. If abdominal pain is severe, seek urgent medical attention.

Septicaemia *(p.234)* ⊕ ⊕ ⊕
Recent symptoms of infection such as fever, cough, or painful/frequent urination, and chills and violent shivering. Also with rapid heart beat, rapid, shallow breathing, and cold, pale hands and feet. Nausea and vomiting. Symptoms may progress to seizures, unconsciousness, and may be fatal. This is a medical emergency, dial 999.

Meningitis *(p.168)* ⊕ ⊕ ⊕
Fever and general neck stiffness, feeling very unwell, and light hurts eyes. May have a rash that doesn't fade after pressure is briefly applied. Seizures tend to occur in severe cases that do not receive prompt treatment. May rapidly be fatal. This is a medical emergency, dial 999.

Typhoid *(p.235)* ⊕ ⊕ ⊕
Fever associated with headache, tiredness, abdominal pain, and constipation. Diarrhoea may develop, along with rash on chest and abdomen.

Tuberculosis *(p.236)* ⊕ ⊕ ⊕
High fever and extreme tiredness with chest pain, night sweats, and weight loss. May be coughing up blood. Symptoms usually develop slowly, over several weeks.

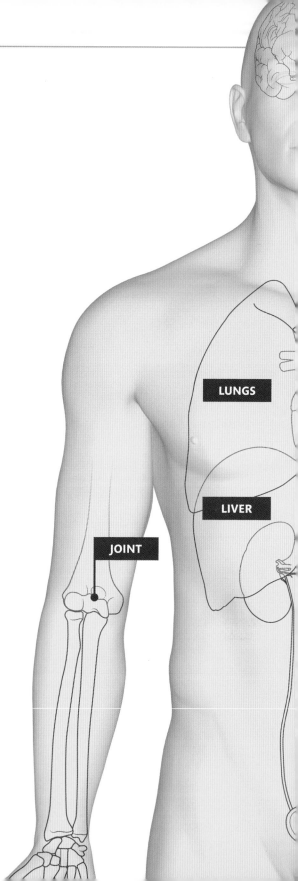

LUNGS

LIVER

JOINT

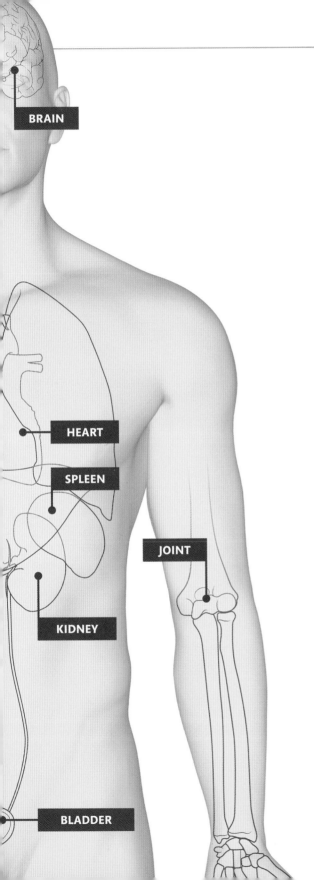

BRAIN

HEART

SPLEEN

JOINT

KIDNEY

BLADDER

⊕ SEEK URGENT MEDICAL ATTENTION IF:

FEVER IS HIGH – TEMPERATURE **OVER 38°C (100.4°F)**

YOU HAVE **STIFF NECK** WITH **RASH**

YOU HAVE **SHORTNESS** OF **BREATH**

A PERSON **LOSES CONSCIOUSNESS**

Infective endocarditis *(p.182)* ⊕⊕⊕
Fever, sweats, chills, and generally feeling unwell; loss of appetite/weight. May have chest pains when taking in a deep breath and swollen joints. Often occurs in those with heart valve problems or previous heart surgery.

Septic arthritis *(p.157)* ⊕⊕⊕
Fever and feeling unwell, associated with increasing pain, swelling, redness, and heat in a joint or joints. Pain worse with movement.

Tetanus *(p.235)* ⊕⊕⊕
High temperature, sweating, neck stiffness, and muscle spasms, which may cause difficulty with swallowing. There may be generalized rigidity of muscles, including the presence of lockjaw.

Lymphoma *(p.188)* ⊕⊕⊕
High fever with drenching night sweats, enlarged lymph nodes (typically in the neck or above the collarbone), and weight loss. May also have persistent cough, shortness of breath, and chest discomfort.

Heat exhaustion *(p.239)* ⊕
Profuse sweating, intense thirst, tiredness, muscle cramps, nausea and vomiting, faintness, unsteadiness, and headache. If heat exposure continues, heatstroke (see below) may develop.

Heatstroke *(p.239)* ⊕⊕⊕
Fever, confusion, disorientation, and fast, shallow breathing. May lead to seizures and loss of consciousness.

Malaria *(p.237)* ⊕⊕⊕
At first, flu-like symptoms, such as muscle and joint pains, headaches, shivering, fever, sweating, and loss of appetite. Additionally, there may be diarrhoea, vomiting, and cough.

WEIGHT GAIN

The most common cause of long-term weight gain is regularly eating or drinking too much, combined with lack of exercise. Many people tend to gain weight as they get older. This is usually because they are less active and the muscles get smaller so the body uses fewer calories. A health problem that may cause reduced mobility, fluid retention, or stress over-eating can lead to weight gain and medical advice should be sought.

DUE TO FLUID RETENTION

Heart failure (p.181) ➕➕
Weight gain with persistent breathlessness, worse on walking and lying flat. Associated with fatigue, swollen ankles, and a cough worse at night. Waking up to pass urine. Seek urgent medical attention if symptoms are severe or suddenly worsen.

Cirrhosis (p.201) ➕➕
Fluid build-up in feet, ankles, legs, and abdomen associated with pain in the abdomen and legs. Tiredness, poor appetite, and bruising and bleeding easily. Jaundice (yellowing of skin and eyes) and itch. Confusion.

FLUID RETENTION IN WOMEN

In women, fluid retention (oedema) may be linked to the menstrual cycle, and this may cause weight to fluctuate.

Premenstrual syndrome (p.212) ➕
Weight gain associated with bloating and fluid retention. May also include breast tenderness, irritability, and low mood. Symptoms occur up to two weeks before a period and disappear around the time the period finishes.

Idiopathic oedema ➕
Mild fluid retention without serious cause, often seen in women just before a period. Swelling is are usually worse at night and affects hands, feet, and abdomen.

Polycystic ovary syndrome (p.213) ➕➕
Weight gain with irregular or no menstrual periods. May also have excessive hair growth on the face, chin, back, or stomach, acne, and difficulty conceiving.

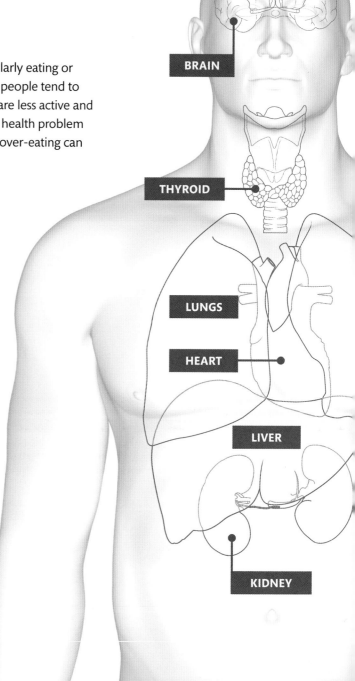

BRAIN

THYROID

LUNGS

HEART

LIVER

KIDNEY

Hypothyroidism *(p.220)* ✚✚

Weight gain and extreme tiredness in association with other symptoms of an underactive thyroid gland. This may include hair loss, dry skin, constipation, and a hoarse voice. Symptoms usually develop over months or years.

Restricted mobility ✚

Any condition that restricts movement, such as rheumatoid arthritis (p.157), can lead to weight gain if ability to exercise is significantly reduced.

Depression *(p.242)* ✚✚

Weight gain associated with persistent low mood; loss of enjoyment in leisure activities; feelings of guilt, worthlessness, and despair; difficulty in concentrating, remembering things, and making decisions.

Long-term stress/anxiety *(p.240)* ✚✚

Over-eating causing weight gain. May be problems sleeping, repetitive worrying thoughts, difficulty concentrating, irritability, headaches, and stomach cramps.

Cushing's syndrome *(p.221)* ✚✚

Weight gain, usually around the abdomen, with stretch marks. Associated with puffy, red face and thin skin that bruises easily, muscle weakness, mood swings, and depression. In women, irregular or no periods and growth of facial hair.

ARE YOU A HEALTHY WEIGHT?

You can check whether you are a healthy weight by using the height/weight graph below. Height and weight measurements can be used to calculate your body mass index (BMI), an indicator of body fat. Even if the graph indicates that you are a healthy weight, you are still at increased risk of cardiovascular disease if your waist measurement is greater than 89 cm (35 in) for women and 102 cm (40 in) for men.

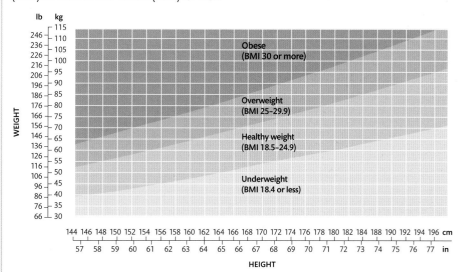

WEIGHT LOSS

Small fluctuations in weight due to temporary changes in your diet or the amount of exercise you take are normal. However, significant weight loss without an obvious cause, especially if there are also other symptoms, may indicate an underlying medical problem and you should see your doctor.

UNDERLYING DISORDERS

Diabetes *(p.219)* ✚ ✚
Weight loss associated with fatigue and muscle weakness. Excessive thirst and needing to pass urine more often than usual. Recurrent infections and slow healing of wounds.

Hyperthyroidism *(p.220)* ✚ ✚
Weight loss despite increased appetite, often with irritability, sweating, tremor of hands, palpitations (sensation of heart beating), diarrhoea, and feeling hot.

Inflammatory bowel disease *(p.203)* ✚ ✚
Abdominal pain, diarrhoea mixed with blood or mucus, weight loss, fever, feeling unwell, and sensation of fullness.

Malabsorption *(p.202)* ✚ ✚
Weight loss associated with prolonged diarrhoea with pale, foul-smelling, hard-to-flush stools. Fatigue and muscle weakness. In children, failure to grow at the expected rate.

Coeliac disease *(p.204)* ✚ ✚
Weight loss, abdominal pain, diarrhoea or constipation, bloating, and flatulence. Often there is a strong family history. In babies and infants, failure to put on weight.

Bowel cancer *(p.206)* ✚ ✚
Weight loss, diarrhoea (with or without blood), and sometimes constipation. May also have anaemia and abdominal pain.

Stomach cancer *(p.200)* ✚ ✚
Weight loss and poor appetite. Pain in upper abdomen. May have indigestion and nausea. Feeling unwell and anaemic (fatigue and pale skin); dark blood in the faeces.

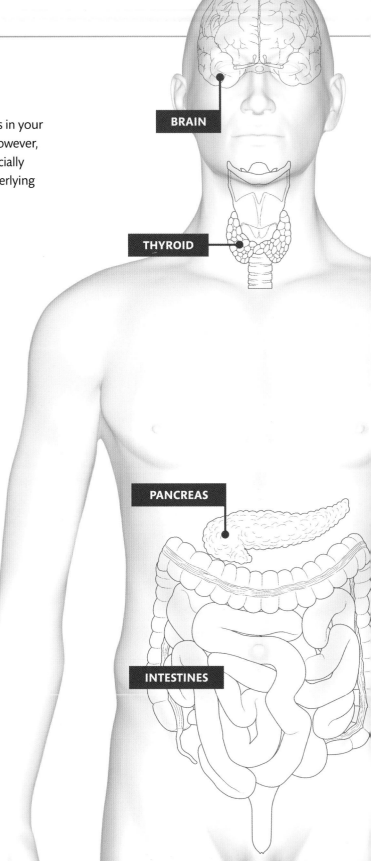

BRAIN

THYROID

PANCREAS

INTESTINES

WEIGHT LOSS AND CANCER

Cancer can cause unintentional weight loss in several ways: by speeding up the body's metabolism (so calories are used faster than normal), reducing appetite, and impairing absorption of nutrients from food. The amount of weight lost depends on the type of cancer and on how advanced it is. For example, many people with stomach cancer, pancreatic cancer, or oesophageal cancer have lost a large amount of weight by the time they are first diagnosed. In contrast, women with breast cancer or men with prostate cancer tend not to have lost a significant amount of weight at the time of diagnosis. Eventually, however, most types of cancer tend to cause weight loss, and when a cancer is at a very advanced stage, there may also be wasting away of the muscles and other body tissues.

Loss of appetite ⊕
A wide variety of conditions may cause loss of appetite and weight loss, including peptic ulcers, intestinal disorders, and conditions of the mouth and teeth, liver and kidney disease, and various cancers.

Medication effect ⊕
Many medications can cause weight loss. Some may cause loss of appetite, nausea, or vomiting, which may lead to weight loss. If severe or persistent, see your doctor.

Undernutrition (p.197) ⊕⊕
Weight loss, poor appetite, persistent tiredness, and weakness. Feeling cold, increased susceptibility to illness, and slow recovery time. In children, lower than expected growth.

Alcohol/drug misuse (p.243) ⊕
Loss of appetite due to feeling full; nausea; vomiting; and abdominal pain.

Stress or anxiety (p.240) ⊕
Loss of appetite and disinterest in food, resulting in weight loss.

Depression (p.242) ⊕⊕
Persistent low mood; loss of enjoyment in activities; feelings of guilt, worthlessness, and despair; difficulty in concentrating, remembering things, and making decisions.

Anorexia nervosa (p.243) ⊕⊕
Severe weight loss. Preoccupation with food, weight, and body image. Associated with constipation, fatigue, feeling cold, and fine, downy body hair. In girls and women, cessation of menstruation.

INFECTIONS AND INFESTATIONS

Tuberculosis (p.236) ⊕⊕
Weight loss, extreme fatigue with fever, night sweats, coughing up blood, and chest pains. Symptoms develop over several weeks.

HIV/AIDS (p.188) ⊕⊕
Fever, weight loss, night sweats, and persistent swollen lymph nodes. Also extensive genital warts, persistent diarrhoea, and infections of the mouth, gums, and skin.

Intestinal parasite (p.237) ⊕⊕
Weight loss with persistent diarrhoea due to infection, such as amoebiasis (p.237), hookworm infection (p.238), cryptosporidium (p.237), and giardiasis (p.237). Most common where access to clean water is limited.

Tapeworm infection (p.238)
Abdominal pain, nausea and vomiting, diarrhoea, loss or increase in appetite, jaundice (yellow skin or whites of eyes), and lack of energy. White, rice-like specks (tape worm eggs) seen in the faeces.

SKIN RASHES

Skin rashes may be diagnosed by the symptoms they produce, for example itch in allergy, by their colour, such as the purplish appearance of lichen planus, or by whether fever is present, suggesting infection as a cause.

RASHES WITH ITCH

Insect bites *(p.239)* ⊕
Raised bumps on skin, which may become intensely itchy. The bites may be in a group or a line. Causes include mosquitoes, fleas, and bedbugs.

Chickenpox *(p.233)* ⊕
A rash of red spots, which are initially flat and then become slightly raised. They then form a tiny blister and finally crust over. Crops of spots occur at different times over three to five days. May itch and there may also be a sore throat and fever.

Eczema *(p.222)* ⊕⊕
Itchy, dry skin that may become red. Intense scratching may cause the skin to break open. Skin thickens from prolonged scratching.

Seborrhoeic dermatitis *(p.222)* ⊕⊕
Scaly rash on the scalp which causes dandruff and redness of the skin. May be flaky skin in eyebrows and a red scaly rash at sides of nose.

Pityriasis rosea *(p.223)* ⊕
Presents usually with a "warning" (herald) patch. A few days later, smaller rose coloured patches appear on skin, which may have a fine scale on the border. Rash may cause a mild irritation.

Urticaria *(p.223)* ⊕
A blotchy red rash that can be very itchy. Rash comes and goes on different areas of the body. Rash may develop into raised areas, called wheals.

Contact dermatitis *(p.222)* ⊕⊕
Itchy, red skin that may resemble eczema. Develops as a result of an allergic reaction to something that has been in contact with skin, such as hair dye.

Scabies *(p.229)* ⊕⊕
Intense irritation, particularly at night. May be scratched spots and s-shaped lines (burrows) on sides of fingers and wrists particularly. Men may develop raised firm spots on the penis and scrotum.

Lichen planus *(p.222)* ⊕⊕
Small, raised, purplish, flat spots on inside of wrists, lower forearms, and legs. Extends to other parts of body including nails, mouth, and scalp. Usually affects the body symmetrically. May be some raised white lines on surface of spots. Can be very itchy.

RASHES WITH FEVER

Chickenpox (p.233)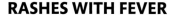
A rash of red spots, which are initially flat and then become slightly raised. They then form tiny blisters and finally crust over. Crops of spots occur at different times over three to five days. May itch and there may also be a sore throat and fever.

Cellulitis (p.228) ✚✚
Area of extending red skin that is painful. Most commonly affects lower leg on one side.

Parvovirus (p.234) ✚✚
Bright red rash on cheeks. After two to three days a fine non-itchy rash resembling a lace cloth spreads to rest of body. May be preceded by mild fever, feeling unwell, and headache.

Scarlet fever (p.235) ✚✚
A fine red rash made up of small flat spots all over body. May be an area of pale skin around the mouth. Associated with sore throat.

Measles (p.234) ✚✚
Rash made up flat spots, commencing on face and neck and spreading to trunk. Preceded by a fever, which may be high. Eyes may become red, along with runny nose and sore throat.

Rubella (p.233) ✚
In children, a red rash of flat spots that extends from behind the ears to the face, neck, and trunk. The rash may join up. In adults, also associated with fever, red eyes, and joint pains.

Lyme disease (p.236) ✚✚
May have spreading circular rash that appears like a target where tick bite has occurred. Associated with flu-like symptoms, fatigue, headache, fever, stiff neck, and muscle and joint pain.

Kawasaki disease (p.185) ✚✚✚
Fever, with redness of the hands and feet leading to skin peeling. A red blotchy rash then spreads to trunk. More common in children from Japan, Korea, and Taiwan.

RASHES WITHOUT ITCH

Acne vulgaris (p.223) ✚✚
Spots that may be found on the face, particularly the cheeks and forehead. May also occur on upper chest and back.

Psoriasis (p.222) ✚✚
Symmetrical rash with white scale (where the skin is dry). May affect back of elbows and front of knees. May also occur on scalp, lower back, genitals, belly button, and cause changes to the nails.

Rosacea (p.223) ✚✚
Redness, spots, and flushing of skin of cheeks. Spots may extend to chin and forehead. The skin of the nose may become thickened.

Lyme disease (p.236) ✚✚
May have spreading circular rash that appears like a target where tick bite has occurred. Associated with flu-like symptoms, fatigue, headache, fever, stiff neck, and muscle and joint pain.

SKIN MOLES AND DISCOLOURATION

Skin colour is determined by the type and quantity of melanin pigments in the skin's protective outer layer (epidermis). It is affected by external agents such as ultraviolet light, which after long-term, high exposure may cause skin cancer. It may also reflect internal conditions, such as infection.

ARMS AND LEGS

Eczema *(p.222)* ➕ ➕
Itchy, dry skin that may become red. Intense scratching may cause the skin to break open. Skin thickens from prolonged scratching.

Psoriasis *(p.222)* ➕ ➕
Symmetrical rash with white scale (where the skin is dry). May affect back of elbows and front of knees. May also occur on scalp, lower back, genitals, belly button, and cause changes to the nails.

Cellulitis *(p.228)* ➕ ➕
Area of extending red skin that is warm painful. Most commonly affects lower leg on one side.

Livedo reticularis *(p.224)* ➕
Mottled, faint, purple-coloured rash, usually affecting the legs. If it comes and goes, it is caused by sluggish circulation and is not a concern. If the rash persists, seek medical advice.

Lichen planus *(p.222)* ➕ ➕
Small raised, purplish, flat spots on inside of wrists, lower forearms, and legs. Extends to other parts of body including nails, mouth, and scalp. Usually affects the body symmetrically. Usually affects the body symmetrically. May be some raised white lines on surface of spots. Can be very itchy.

TRUNK

Seborrhoeic keratosis *(p.228)* ➕
Multiple raised yellow or brown skin lesions that may have a cracked surface and greasy texture, commonly found on trunk.

Psoriasis *(p.222)* ➕ ➕
Thick patches covered with white, scaly skin.

Cushing's syndrome *(p.221)* ➕ ➕
Reddish-purple stretch marks on body or limbs. Skin is thin and easily bruised. Acne may develop. Associated with weight gain, particularly on abdomen.

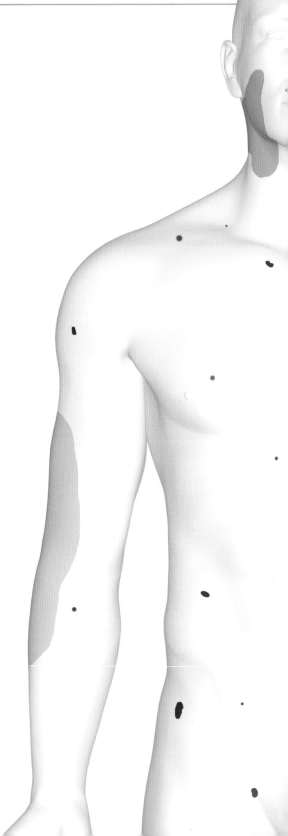

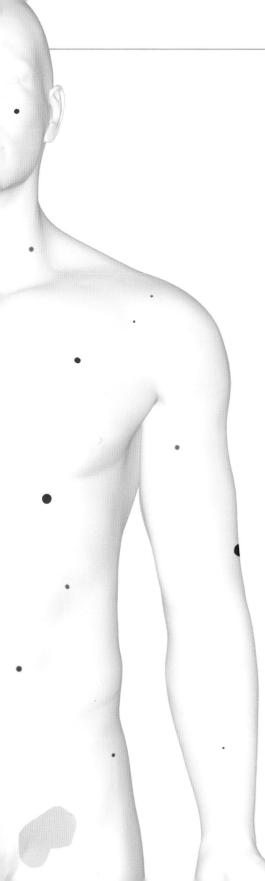

FACE AND NECK

Sunburn *(p.239)* ⊕
Redness of skin that may be painful after exposure to sunlight.

Eczema *(p.222)* ⊕ ⊕
Itchy, dry skin that may become red. Intense scratching may cause the skin to break open. Skin thickens from prolonged scratching.

Parvovirus *(p.234)* ⊕
Intense redness of the cheeks of a usually well child. More general fine, red rash occurs around two days later on rest of body.

Rosacea *(p.223)* ⊕ ⊕
Redness, spots, and flushing of skin of cheeks. Spots may extend to chin and forehead. The skin of the nose may become thickened.

Erysipelas *(p.228)* ⊕ ⊕ ⊕
Sudden development of one-sided redness of face. Associated with pain, fever, and skin blistering.

Photosensitivity *(see p.223)* ⊕ ⊕
Blistering in light-exposed areas. Redness and puffiness of skin after exposure to sunlight.

Chloasma *(p.224)* ⊕ ⊕
Increase in brown pigmentation on face that can occur in pregnancy and women taking the oral contraceptive.

GENERAL

Moles *(p.227)* ⊕
Brown pigmented lesions. Some may be present at birth and others develop up to the age of 30 years. They may be flat or sometimes a little raised.

Seborrhoeic keratosis *(p.228)* ⊕
Multiple raised yellow or brown skin lesions that may have a cracked surface and greasy texture, commonly found on trunk.

Vitiligo *(p.224)* ⊕ ⊕
Bright white patches in the skin with a clearly demarcated edge.

Jaundice *(p.201)* ⊕ ⊕
Yellowing of skin and whites of eyes, usually associated with liver problems.

Melanoma *(p.226)* ⊕ ⊕ ⊕
Usually dark skin patch that may newly develop in the skin or come from an existing mole. May develop variation in pigmentation (colour) or become intensely black. May have non-symmetrical shape, irregular border, and enlarge with a diameter of more than 7 mm (¼ in). May also itch and bleed. Some may melanomas become raised from the skin.

SKIN LUMPS AND BUMPS

Growths may develop on the skin surface and range from noncancerous, such as a skin tag, to cancerous, such as a melanoma. Swellings may also originate from under the skin and develop from structures such as tendons.

Moles *(p.227)*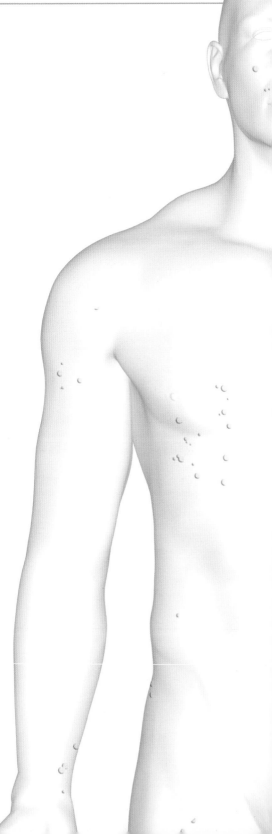
Brown pigmented lesions. Some may be present at birth and others develop up to the age of 30 years. They may be flat or sometimes a little raised.

Skin tag *(p.226)*
Piece of skin hanging from the skin surface. They may vary in size. May be multiple, particularly on the neck and in the armpits.

Haemangioma *(p.224)*
Raised red swelling caused by a dilated (widened) blood vessel. Turns whiter when pressure is applied.

Sebaceous cyst *(p.225)*
Firm swelling, just under the skin, that has a rounded shape. Some may have a black dot on the surface. Occasionally may become infected.

Lipoma *(p.226)*
Soft swelling that lies just below the skin surface. A small lipoma may be more easy to feel than see. There may be multiple lipomas on the body.

Boil *(p.227)*
Painful spot with yellow pus surrounded by a red border that develops at base of a hair follicle. May occasionally become multi-headed (a carbuncle).

Lymphadenopathy *(p.187)*
Enlargement of lymph nodes that are found in neck (back and front), groin, and armpits.

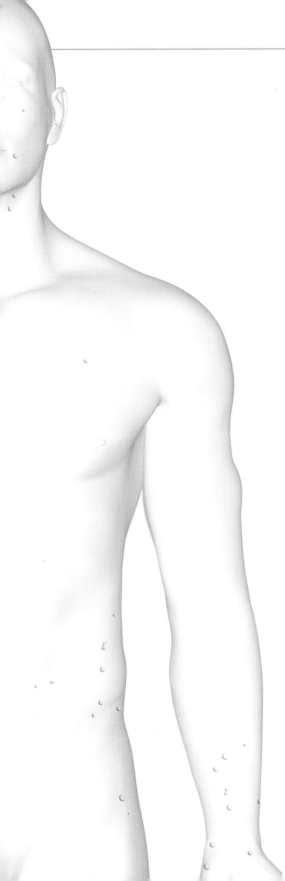

Seborrhoeic keratosis (p.228)
Raised lesion on the skin that is soft and a little greasy on its surface. May be skin-coloured, but may develop a yellow-brown colour. Surface may have cracked appearance.

Viral warts (p.229)
May appear as small, slightly raised skin lesions with a light brown colour (such as plane warts on the face), raised lesions with black dots (hands and feet), or lesions with finger-like projections (filiform warts).

Solar keratosis (p.226)
May range from small patches of rough skin on sun-exposed areas to raised crusty growths.

Basal cell carcinoma (p.226)
May develop as a flat patch with possibly some scale and a slightly raised edge. May also develop as a raised round or irregular growth. May show some prominent blood vessels on surface. Some may develop a non-healing ulcer (crater). Firm to touch.

Xanthelasma (p.179)
Yellow patches that may develop above and below the eyelids. May be associated with raised cholesterol.

Molluscum contagiosum (p.228)
Small, raised round lesions on skin with a dip at centre.

Squamous cell carcinoma (p.226)
Raised skin growth in sun-exposed skin that fails to heal. The surface may become crusty and hard; ultimately, an ulcer that does not heal may develop on the surface.

Melanoma (p.226)
Usually dark skin patch that may newly develop in the skin or come from an existing mole. May develop variation in pigmentation (colour) or become intensely black. May have non-symmetrical shape, irregular border, and enlarge with a diameter of more than 7 mm (¼ in). May also itch and bleed. Some may melanomas become raised from the skin.

MOOD CHANGES

Most people have minor ups and downs in mood, but they often have an identifiable cause – such as a stressful event – and tend to resolve by themselves. However, persistent or repeated feelings of depression or mood swings, particularly if they are severe enough to interfere with everyday life, may indicate an underlying health problem and medical advice should be sought.

DRUGS, ALCOHOL, AND MOOD

Certain medications (such as some drugs used to treat high blood pressure and oral contraceptives), complementary remedies, and recreational drugs can cause depression or other disturbances of mood. Regularly drinking too much alcohol (p.243) can have a similar effect. Abrupt withdrawal of some medications, recreational drugs, or alcohol in those who have become dependent on them may also cause psychological disturbances.

PHYSICAL ILLNESS AND MOOD

Changes in mental state are a common response to physical illness, and a serious illness may cause anxiety or depression. Such reactions usually disappear when the illness is successfully treated or the person adjusts to their physical condition. However, an illness that is long-term or involves persistent disability may cause persistent mood problems.

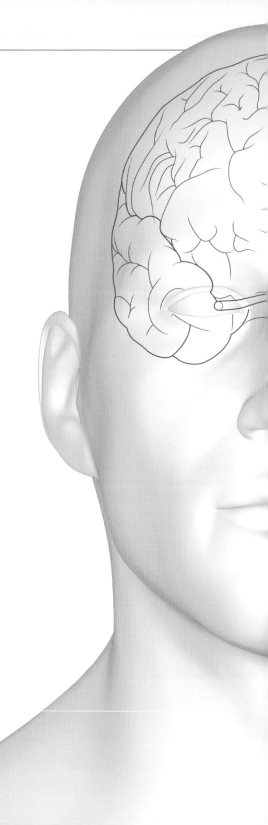

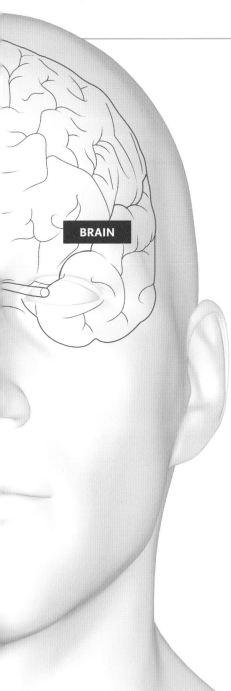

BRAIN

⊕ SEEK URGENT MEDICAL ATTENTION IF:
YOU ARE HAVING **SUICIDAL THOUGHTS**

A **NEW MOTHER** DEVELOPS THOUGHTS OF **HARMING HER BABY** OR **HERSELF**

Depression *(p.242)* ⊕ ⊕
Persistent low mood with loss of enjoyment in leisure activities, and feelings of guilt, despair, and worthlessness. Difficulty in concentrating, remembering things, and making decisions.

Generalized anxiety disorder *(p.240)* ⊕ ⊕
Constantly feeling worried and unable to relax. Sense of foreboding with no apparent cause. Sleeping difficulty, irritability, panic attacks, and rapid heartbeat (palpitations).

Bipolar disorder *(p.241)* ⊕ ⊕
Extreme mood swings over the course of months, alternating between profound highs (mania or hypomania) and lows (depression). During highs, elation, confidence, decreased need for sleep, and loss of inhibitions. During lows, symptoms of depression. Get urgent help if thoughts of self harm or suicide.

Cyclothymia *(p.241)* ⊕
A mild, less extreme form of bipolar disorder. See a doctor if mood swings occur persistently and are severe enough to disrupt everyday life.

Seasonal affective disorder *(p.242)* ⊕ ⊕
Same symptoms as depression, but symptoms usually start in autumn or winter and improve in spring.

IN WOMEN ONLY

Postnatal depression *(p.242)* ⊕ ⊕
Symptoms of depression (see above). Feeling overwhelmed by responsibilities of looking after a new baby and frightening thoughts about hurting the baby. Get urgent medical help if having thoughts of harming self or the baby or if actual harm has occurred.

Premenstrual syndrome *(p.212)* ⊕
Mood swings and irritability associated with bloating, nausea, breast tenderness, and joint and muscle pain. Symptoms occur up to two weeks before a period and disappear around the time a period has finished.

BEHAVIOUR PROBLEMS

Everybody has their own characteristic range of behaviour that enables them to function normally in their work, social, and emotional life. Sometimes, however, a person's behaviour falls outside socially accepted norms or causes persistent difficulties with everyday life, relationships, or activities. In such cases, there may be a mental health or psychological problem and expert advice should be sought.

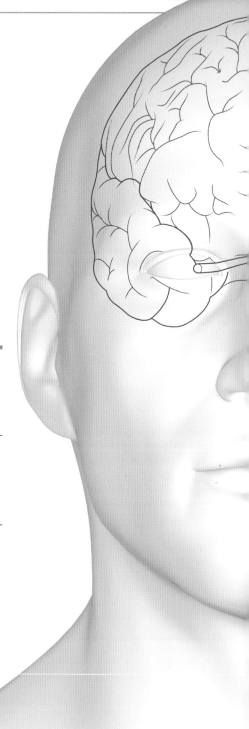

ANXIETY-RELATED PROBLEMS

Generalized anxiety disorder
(p.240) ➕➕
Constantly feeling worried and unable to relax. Sense of foreboding with no apparent cause, sleeping difficulty, irritability, panic attacks, and rapid heartbeat (palpitations).

Obsessive–compulsive disorder
(p.242) ➕➕
Unwanted intrusive thoughts or images that cause anxiety (obsessions). Repetitive behaviours or thoughts carried out to resist the obsession and relieve the anxiety it causes (compulsions).

Addictions *(p.243)* ➕➕
Compulsively and excessively using a substance or activity (alcohol, drugs, gambling) to the extent that it causes harm to the person and/or their family. May be associated with secretive behaviour.

Panic disorder *(p.240)* ➕➕
Repeated panic attacks with symptoms such as sweating, rapid heartbeat, breathlessness, and dizziness or faintness. May also be chest pain, pins-and-needles; and a feeling of dread.

Phobias *(p.240)* ➕➕
Overwhelming fear of objects or situations that are usually regarded as harmless, resulting in anxiety attacks (rapid heartbeat, sweating, breathlessness). Altered behaviour or activities to avoid the feared thing.

Post-traumatic stress disorder
(p.240) ➕➕
After a stressful event: flashbacks and nightmares; avoiding reminders of the event; numbing of emotions; feeling anxious; depression; and drug or alcohol misuse.

Hypochondria (health anxiety)
(p.240) ➕➕
Constant anxiety about health, which disrupts relationships, work, and everyday activities; interpreting even trivial symptoms as signs of serious illness; frequent visits to the doctor.

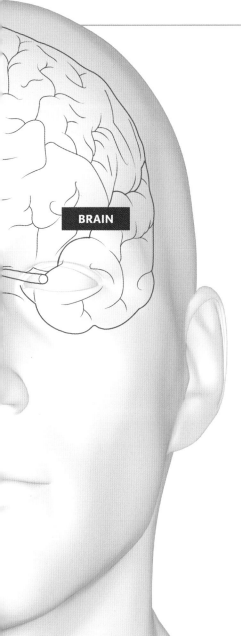

BRAIN

Schizophrenia *(p.241)* ➕➕
Hallucinations and irrational beliefs not based on reality (delusions). Also confused thoughts, incoherent speech, lack of insight into one's condition, agitation, and social withdrawal.

Personality disorders *(p.242)* ➕➕
Difficulty maintaining social relationships and regulating mood. Feeling emotionally disconnected and often unpredictable behaviour. Overwhelmed by negative feelings.

Eating disorders *(p.243)* ➕➕
Obsession with weight and body image. May involve avoiding meals, excessive exercising, deliberately vomiting after eating. Associated with weight loss (anorexia nervosa), weight gain (binge eating disorder), or no major change in weight (bulimia).

Attention deficit hyperactivity disorder (ADHD) *(p.242)* ➕➕
Short attention span with inability to follow instructions and finish tasks. Constant fidgeting, talking excessively, interrupting others, and difficulty in taking turns. Usually diagnosed in childhood.

Tourette's syndrome *(p.243)* ➕➕
Repetitive, involuntary physical and vocal tics including head jerks, grunting, coughing, or swearing. Usually starts in childhood and continues to a less severe extent into adulthood.

MEMORY AND CONFUSION

People may become confused either as part of a long-term condition (such as dementia) or more suddenly, often with physical symptoms such as fever (delerium). They may not be able to answer simple questions such as their age, name, or the date. A degree of forgetfulness can be normal with older age.

✚ SEEK URGENT MEDICAL ATTENTION IF:

A PERSON SUDDENLY BECOMES **SEVERELY CONFUSED, AGITATED, DISORIENTATED,** OR HAS **HALLUCINATIONS**

A PERSON HAS **FACIAL DROOPING, ARM WEAKNESS, OR TROUBLE SPEAKING**

WITH PHYSICAL SYMPTOMS

Stroke *(p.169)* ✚✚✚
Confusion associated with drooping of one side of face, weakness down one side of body, and difficulty speaking. Other symptoms can include dizziness, numbness, headache, and loss of balance and coordination. This is a medical emergency, dial 999.

Transient ischaemic attack (TIA) *(p.169)* ✚✚✚
Symptoms of a stroke (see above) but short-lived, clearing up completely within 24 hours. This is a medical emergency, dial 999.

High fever ✚✚
Confusion associated with temperature over 38°C (100.4°F), chills, headache, weakness, poor concentration, sleepiness in the day, and nausea and vomiting.

Hypoglycaemia *(p.219)* ✚✚✚
Confusion and slurred speech may follow lightheadedness, sweating, nausea, shaking, and feeling of hunger. Without treatment may lead to unconsciousness and seizures. Usually associated with diabetes. This is a medical emergency, dial 999.

Head injury *(p.167)* ✚✚✚
Confusion preceded by lump, bruise, or bleeding at the injury site, headache, nausea and vomiting. There may be loss of recollection of the event, clear fluid or blood leaking from ears, drowsiness, seizures, and unconsciousness. Symptoms may develop hours or days after the event. Seek urgent medical attention.

Parkinson's disease *(p.171)* ✚✚
Involuntary tremors that occur at rest (often in one hand); slow movements; muscle stiffness; shuffling walk; stooped posture; expressionless face; insomnia; depression.

Brain tumour *(p.168)* ✚✚✚
Memory problems with associated headache that is worsened by bending or coughing, more severe in the morning, and with increase in frequency and severity. Other signs include nausea and vomiting, personality change, and stroke symptoms, such as slurred speech and weakness on one side of body.

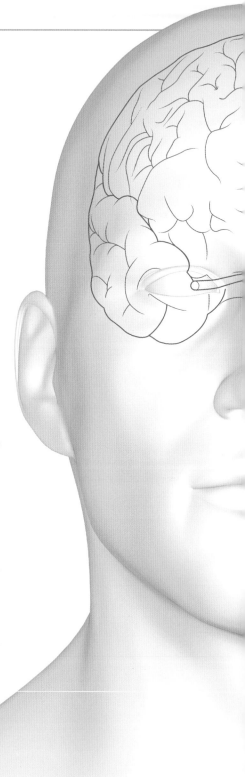

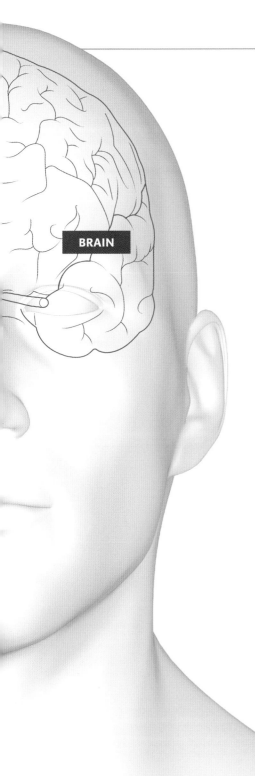

BRAIN

MEDICATION AND MEMORY

Some prescription and over-the-counter medications and recreational drugs can affect normal mental functioning, causing confusion, memory problems, or mental slowness. Sedative and sleeping drugs are well-known examples, but other drugs, such as anti-epileptic medications, can also affect memory and mental functioning. Abrupt withdrawal from some drugs may also cause confusion.

WITHOUT PHYSICAL SYMPTOMS

Dementia (p.170) ⊕⊕
Increasing forgetfulness. Difficulties understanding written and spoken language, poor concentration, and difficulty with simple tasks. Also wandering and getting lost, mood swings, and personality changes. Uncommon under 65.

Depression (p.242) ⊕⊕
Confusion and forgetfulness alongside persistent low mood with loss of enjoyment in leisure activities, and feelings of guilt, despair, and worthlessness. Difficulty in concentrating, remembering things, and making decisions.

Anxiety disorders (p.240) ⊕⊕
Constantly feeling on edge, a sense of foreboding with no obvious cause, sweating, rapid heartbeat, breathlessness and dizziness, and insomnia.

Persistent sleep deprivation/persistent insomnia (p.241) ⊕⊕
Tiredness, yawning, difficulty concentrating, forgetfulness, irritability, difficulty making decisions, anxiety, and depression.

Alcohol misuse (p.243) ⊕⊕
Symptoms of intoxication. Maybe violent behaviour, confusion, memory loss (such as being unable to recall what happened the night before), and hangover.

Schizophrenia (p.241) ⊕⊕
Confused thoughts, with hallucinations and irrational beliefs not based on reality (delusions). Also incoherent speech, lack of insight into one's condition, agitation, and social withdrawal.

SLEEPING PROBLEMS

Some conditions directly affect the ability to fall asleep or remain asleep, such as asthma, sleep apnoea, and restless legs. Other medical conditions that may disturb sleep include an enlarged prostate (causing frequent urination), an overactive thyroid, and conditions that cause long-term pain. Sleep problems are also a significant symptom in illnesses such as depression and anxiety.

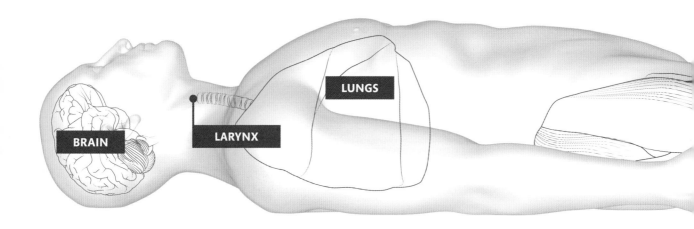

LUNGS

LARYNX

BRAIN

WITH BREATHING PROBLEMS

Sleep apnoea *(p.191)*
Episodes of temporary pauses in breathing for around 10 seconds whilst sleeping. At the end of the pause the person may gasp and wake briefly. There may also be daytime sleepiness, snoring, frequent waking to urinate and irritability.

Asthma *(p.193)*
Wheezing, difficulty breathing, tightness in the chest, and a dry, persistent cough. Symptoms often worse at night.

SNORING

Noisy breathing during sleep is due to the narrowing of the airways causing the soft tissues at the back of the mouth, nose, or throat to vibrate. Snoring may be due to various factors, including drinking alcohol, taking sedatives, smoking, or having a large amount of fat around the neck. It may also be a symptom of sleep apnoea *(p.191)*, an infection of the airways, such as the common cold, hay fever *(p.190)*, enlarged adenoids, or, rarely, a structural abnormality, such as a deviated nasal septum *(p.190)*.

Depression *(p.242)* ⊕ ⊕
Insomnia and unrefreshing sleep associated with persistent low mood, loss of enjoyment in leisure activities, and feelings of guilt, worthlessness, and despair. Difficulty in concentrating, remembering things, and making decisions.

Anxiety disorders *(p.240)* ⊕ ⊕
Sleep disturbances include insomnia, early morning waking, or nightmares. Other symptoms may include constantly being on edge, a sense of foreboding with no obvious cause, sweating, rapid heart beat, breathlessness, and dizziness.

Nightmares and night terrors *(p.241)* ⊕
Woken by vivid, unpleasant dreams that occur late at night. Typically with strong feelings of fear, distress, and anxiety.

Alzheimer's disease *(p.170)* ⊕ ⊕
Disturbed sleep is one of the many possible symptoms of Alzheimer's disease. Others include memory problems, poor judgement, mood changes, anxiety, agitation, confusion, delusions, and behavioural changes.

Parkinson's disease *(p.171)* ⊕ ⊕
The main symptoms of Parkinson's disease are involuntary tremors that occur at rest (usually in one hand), slow movements, and muscle stiffness, but insomnia is also a common problem.

Narcolepsy *(p.167)* ⊕
Repeated daytime sleep attacks during which the person falls asleep suddenly and without warning. Also daytime tiredness, temporary paralysis when waking up and falling asleep, and temporary loss of muscle control when awake (cataplexy).

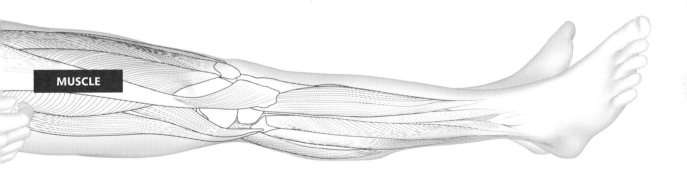

MUSCLE

Restless leg syndrome *(p.162)* ⊕ ⊕
An unpleasant crawling, burning, prickling, or aching sensation in legs, typically accompanied by an overwhelming urge to move the legs. May also be involuntary jerking of legs and arms while asleep. Symptoms usually come on at night and can severely disrupt sleep, causing insomnia.

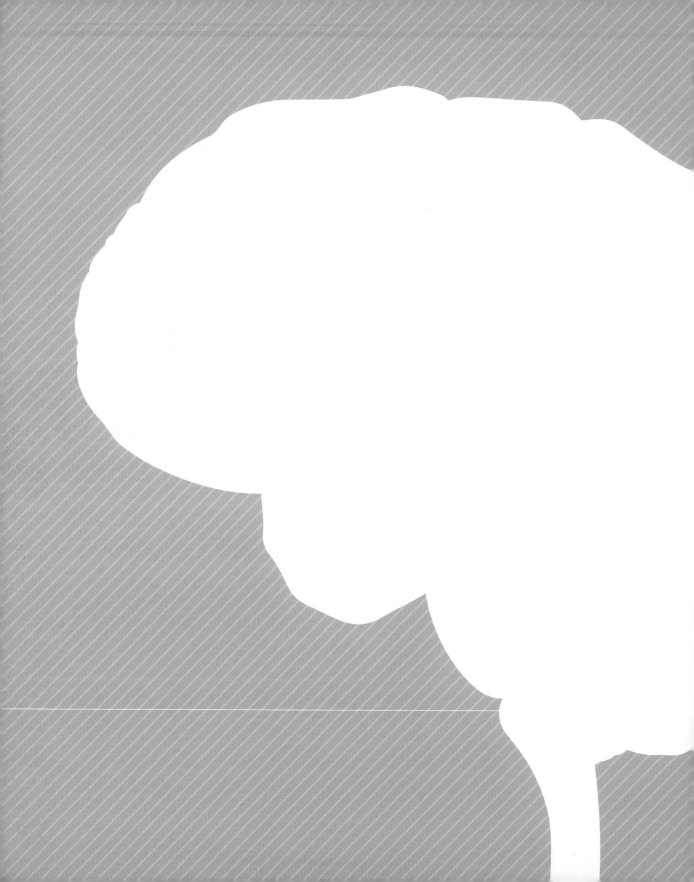

PART 2
HEAD-TO-TOE SYMPTOM GUIDE

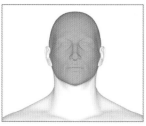

SEE ALSO Head side *pp.50–51*
Hair and scalp *pp.52–53* **Nose**
pp.64–65

HEAD
FRONT

The head houses many important structures, including the brain. Headaches, including tension-type and migraines, can be debilitating. Injuries may need urgent attention. Unless otherwise indicated, symptoms can occur on one or both sides.

Tension-type headache *(p.166)* ⊕
Ache or pressure in temple area and eyes, possibly extending all around head and feeling like a headband. Associated with stress.

Medication-overuse headache *(p.166)* ⊕⊕
Headaches, such as tension-type or migraine, that do not improve, or get worse, despite taking regular painkillers.

Cluster headache *(p.166)* ⊕⊕
One-sided, extremely sharp pain in head, usually around eye. May occur many times a day; associated with eye redness and watering. Face may become red, flushed, and sweaty.

LIGHTHEADEDNESS AND FAINTING

Feeling lightheaded or faint can be a result of a number of disorders. Repeated episodes of fainting may indicate an underlying medical problem (see pp.14–15).

Vasovagal syncope (fainting) ⊕
Fainting episode that follows nausea, cold sweat, lightheadedness, and blurred vision. Usually occurs as a result of emotional stress.

Hypoglycaemia (low blood glucose) *(p.219)* ⊕⊕⊕
Lightheadedness, sweating, nausea, shaking, and feeling of hunger. May progress to slurred speech, confusion, unconsciousness, and seizures. Usually associated with diabetes. This is a medical emergency, call 999.

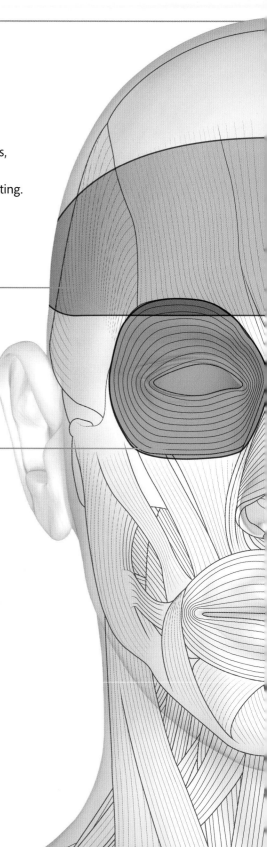

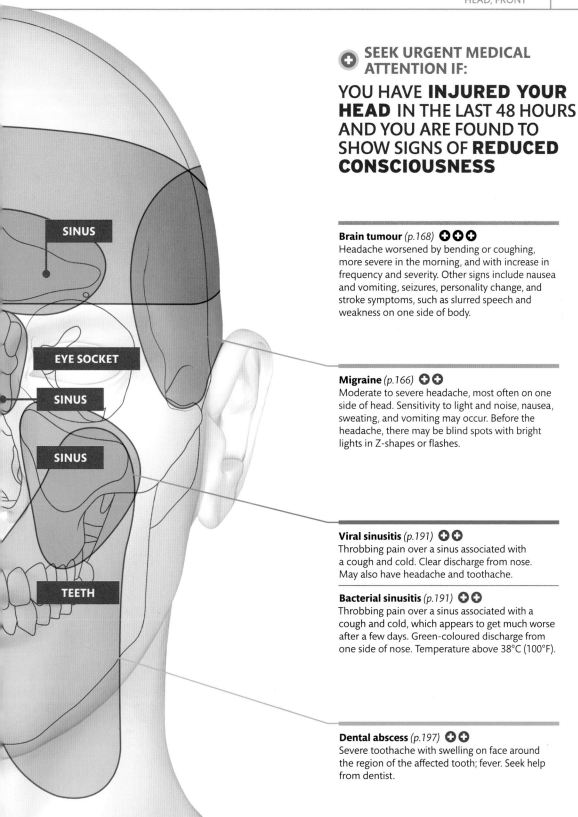

SINUS

EYE SOCKET

SINUS

SINUS

TEETH

➕ **SEEK URGENT MEDICAL ATTENTION IF:**

YOU HAVE **INJURED YOUR HEAD** IN THE LAST 48 HOURS AND YOU ARE FOUND TO SHOW SIGNS OF **REDUCED CONSCIOUSNESS**

Brain tumour *(p.168)* ➕➕➕
Headache worsened by bending or coughing, more severe in the morning, and with increase in frequency and severity. Other signs include nausea and vomiting, seizures, personality change, and stroke symptoms, such as slurred speech and weakness on one side of body.

Migraine *(p.166)* ➕➕
Moderate to severe headache, most often on one side of head. Sensitivity to light and noise, nausea, sweating, and vomiting may occur. Before the headache, there may be blind spots with bright lights in Z-shapes or flashes.

Viral sinusitis *(p.191)* ➕➕
Throbbing pain over a sinus associated with a cough and cold. Clear discharge from nose. May also have headache and toothache.

Bacterial sinusitis *(p.191)* ➕➕
Throbbing pain over a sinus associated with a cough and cold, which appears to get much worse after a few days. Green-coloured discharge from one side of nose. Temperature above 38°C (100°F).

Dental abscess *(p.197)* ➕➕
Severe toothache with swelling on face around the region of the affected tooth; fever. Seek help from dentist.

HEAD
SIDE

Jaw problems and ear and sinus pain may be felt or seen here. Symptoms may arise from injury or through an underlying disorder, such as an infection, stroke, or blood clot.

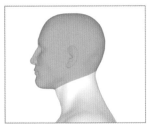

SEE ALSO Head, front *pp.48–49*, Nose *pp.64–65*, Neck *pp.72–73*

Giant cell arteritis *(p.183)* ✚✚✚
Burning pain in temple region affecting one or both sides of head. Sore scalp and pain in face that comes on after chewing. Fever and tiredness. May be vision loss. May also be stiffness and pain in the shoulders.

Parotid (salivary gland) stone *(p.198)* ✚✚
Painful swelling at angle of jaw in front, just below ear. May have increased discomfort and swelling when eating.

Parotitis *(p.198)* ✚✚
Swelling of the parotid gland (one of the salivary glands). Pain, with redness of the overlying skin.

Mumps *(p.233)* ✚✚
Headache, fever, feeling unwell. Visible lump in front and below ears on one or both sides of face. Occasionally, may have lower abdominal pain and, in men, tenderness of testicles.

Parotid (salivary gland) tumour *(p.198)* ✚✚
Gradual swelling of part of cheek. Noncancerous tumours have a rubbery feel and grow slowly. Cancerous growths feel hard, may cause pain, grow quickly, and may cause that side of the face to droop.

Temporo-mandibular joint dysfunction *(p.159)* ✚✚
Pain in ear, headache, and pain around jawline. Clicking of jaw when opening and closing mouth.

Trigeminal neuralgia *(p.172)* ✚✚
Recurrent electric shock-like pain affecting the cheek, gum, teeth, or jaw on one side of face. Usually, attacks last a few seconds but can go on for days.

Atypical facial pain *(p.172)* ✚✚
Severe aching, burning pain on one side of face, which has an unknown cause.

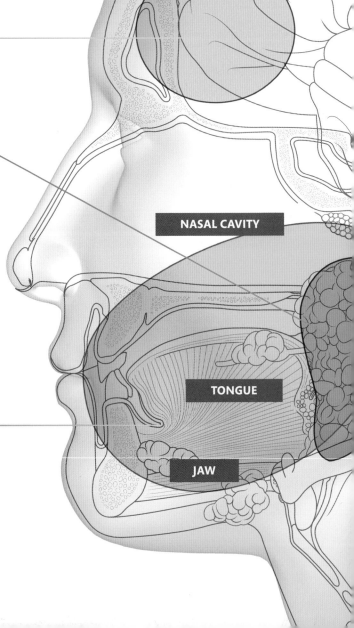

NASAL CAVITY

TONGUE

JAW

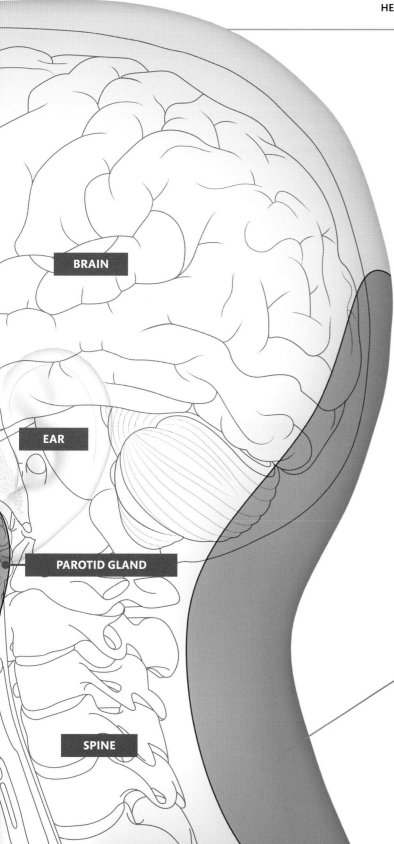

BRAIN

EAR

PAROTID GLAND

SPINE

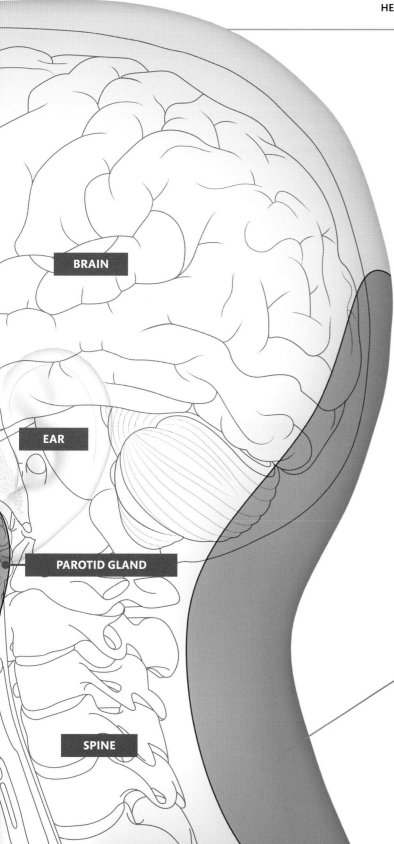 SEEK URGENT MEDICAL ATTENTION IF:

YOU HAVE **INJURED YOUR HEAD** IN THE LAST 48 HOURS AND YOU ARE FOUND TO SHOW SIGNS OF **REDUCED CONSCIOUSNESS**

Migraine *(p.166)*
Moderate to severe headache, most often on one side of head. Nausea, sweating, and vomiting may occur. Before the headache, there may be blind spots with bright lights in Z-shapes or flashes.

Stroke *(p.169)*
Sudden start of symptoms include: drooping of face on one side, loss of power down one side of body, slurred speech, difficulty with swallowing, double vision, and loss of coordination. This is a medical emergency, dial 999.

Transient ischaemic attack *(p.169)*
Symptoms of a stroke (see above) that resolves within 24 hours. This is a medical emergency, dial 999.

Subdural haematoma *(p.170)*
Loss of consciousness after a head injury. Symptoms may also develop slowly over days or weeks, with headache, nausea, vomiting, and stroke symptoms, such as slurred speech and weakness on one side of the body. This is a medical emergency, dial 999.

Extradural haematoma *(p.170)*
Loss of consciousness after a head injury, followed by appearing normal then loss of consciousness again. Sometimes nausea, headache, vomiting, and stroke symtoms (see above) may occur with no loss of consciousness. This is a medical emergency, dial 999.

Cervical spondylosis *(p.158)*
Mild to moderate pain extending from the neck to back and side of head.

Subarachnoid haemorrhage *(p.170)*
Severe sudden pain at back of head. May be associated with neck stiffness, vomiting, aversion to light, and stroke symptoms, such as slurred speech, weakness on one side of body, and unconsciousness. This is a medical emergency, dial 999.

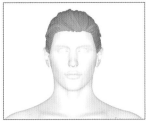

SEE ALSO Face pp.54–55

HAIR AND SCALP

Problems with the hair and scalp can be distressing as they may cause itching, irritation, or hair loss. Stress such as caused by crash diets and major illness may result in abnormal hair loss. It may also happen in the months after childbirth.

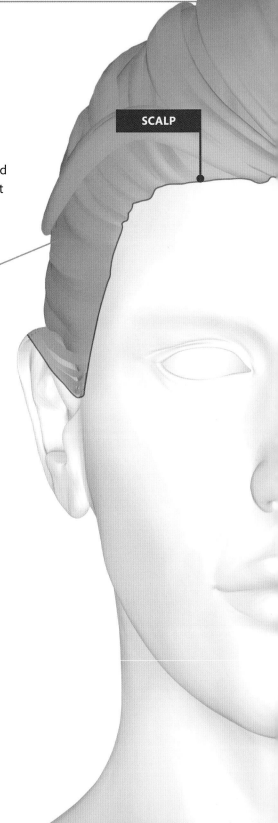

SCALP

HAIR LOSS

Telogen effluvium *(p.230)* ✚✚
Dramatic general hair loss. No visible changes to remaining hair, and scalp appears normal.

Diffuse alopecia *(p.230)* ✚✚
General hair thinning of the scalp. Hairs may look finer.

Alopecia areata *(p.230)* ✚✚
Circular patch of complete hair loss, with short stubs ("exclamation mark" hairs) on border of the patch.

Tinea capitis (ringworm) *(p.230)* ✚✚
Patchy hair loss, with possibly red scalp and flaky skin. Occasionally, the infection develops as a soft, spongy swelling. More common in children.

Traction alopecia *(p.230)* ✚✚
Hair loss in temple region following hair being repeatedly straightened, plaited, or pulled.

Discoid lupus erythematosus (DLE) *(p.189)* ✚✚
Patches of complete hair loss, with skin looking shiny and scarred. Skin may be red or flaky.

Lichen planus (scarring alopecia) *(p.222)* ✚✚
Patches of complete hair loss, with skin looking shiny and scarred. Skin may look scaly and have a purplish colour.

Trichotillomania *(p.230)* ✚✚
Patch of hair thinning with long hairs missing, but short hairs present. Due to impulsive compulsion to pull out hair.

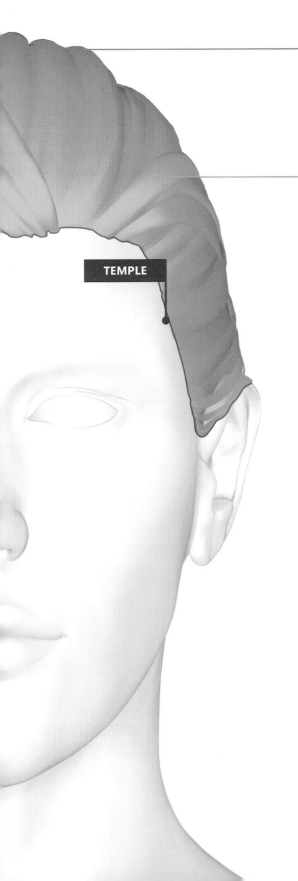

TEMPLE

Head lice *(p.231)*
Itching; beige coloured nit cases around 2.5cm
(1 in) from scalp; black and red "dots" on skin of
scalp; moving head lice may be seen. Seek help
from pharmacist.

SCALP SKIN CHANGES

Dandruff *(p.230)*
Fine white flakes, without redness of scalp.
Seek help from pharmacist.

Solar keratosis *(p.226)*
Areas of skin change ranging from rough skin
to raised hard crusts, resulting from sun damage,
usually where there is hair loss or thinning.

Seborrhoeic dermatitis *(p.230)*
Large amount of fine white flakes on scalp
(dandruff), redness, and itching of skin. May be
associated with red rash and flakes in eyebrows
and at sides of nose.

Psoriasis *(p.222)*
Thick patches covered with white scaly skin affecting
any part of scalp. There may be similar white scaly
patches affecting other parts of the body.

Epidermoid cyst *(p.225)*
Raised, firm, painless swelling in the skin of the scalp.
Pain and redness may suggest infection.

FACE

The face is controlled by nerves, and when these malfunction, weakness of the muscles may cause it to droop. Skin disease may be a major cause of embarrassment or social anxiety, so it is important to get medical advice on how to improve the condition.

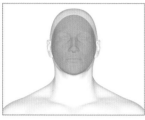

SEE ALSO Head, front *pp.48–49,*
Eye, physical *pp.56–57,*
Nose *pp.64–65*

FOREHEAD

EYELID

Syringoma *(p.226)* ➕ ➕
Small, raised swellings above and below the eyes.

Erysipelas *(p.228)* ➕ ➕ ➕
Sudden development of one-sided redness of the face. Pain, fever, and skin blistering.

FACIAL WEAKNESS

Facial nerve palsy *(p.173)* ➕ ➕ ➕
Sudden onset of one-sided weakness of the face with inability to fully close eye, reduced wrinkling of forehead, and loss of ability to smile or put lips in a whistling position.

Transient ischaemic attack *(p.169)* ➕ ➕ ➕
Symptoms of a stroke (see below) that resolves within 24 hours. This is a medical emergency, dial 999.

Stroke *(p.169)* ➕ ➕ ➕
Sudden onset of facial weakness, associated with possible loss of speech and paralysis of one side of body. This is a medical emergency, dial 999.

Myasthenia gravis *(p.163)* ➕ ➕
Weakening in the use of muscles in face and throat, such as difficulty opening eyes or swallowing. Develops as the day goes on.

Dental abscess *(p.197)* ➕ ➕
Sudden development of swelling around the upper and/or lower jaw; may be associated with toothache. Seek urgent dental care.

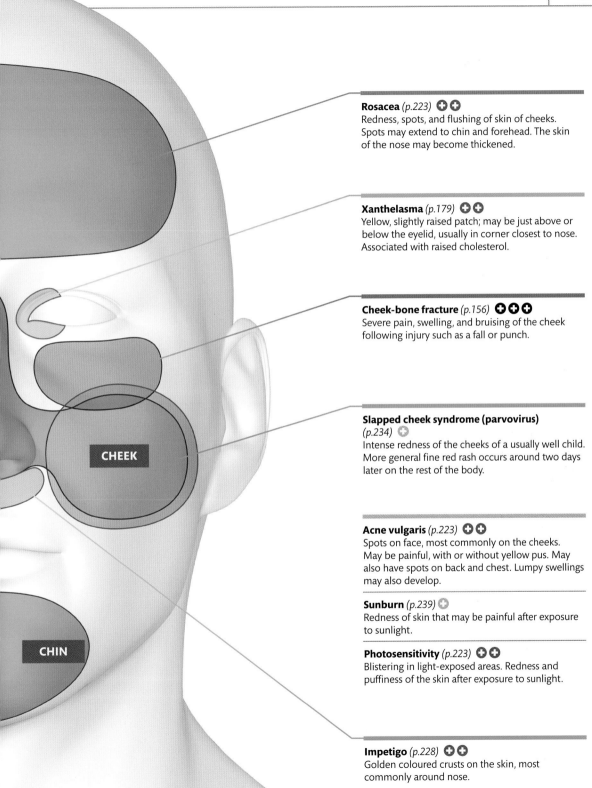

CHEEK

CHIN

Rosacea *(p.223)* ✚ ✚
Redness, spots, and flushing of skin of cheeks.
Spots may extend to chin and forehead. The skin
of the nose may become thickened.

Xanthelasma *(p.179)* ✚ ✚
Yellow, slightly raised patch; may be just above or
below the eyelid, usually in corner closest to nose.
Associated with raised cholesterol.

Cheek-bone fracture *(p.156)* ✚ ✚ ✚
Severe pain, swelling, and bruising of the cheek
following injury such as a fall or punch.

Slapped cheek syndrome (parvovirus)
(p.234) ✚
Intense redness of the cheeks of a usually well child.
More general fine red rash occurs around two days
later on the rest of the body.

Acne vulgaris *(p.223)* ✚ ✚
Spots on face, most commonly on the cheeks.
May be painful, with or without yellow pus. May
also have spots on back and chest. Lumpy swellings
may also develop.

Sunburn *(p.239)* ✚
Redness of skin that may be painful after exposure
to sunlight.

Photosensitivity *(p.223)* ✚ ✚
Blistering in light-exposed areas. Redness and
puffiness of the skin after exposure to sunlight.

Impetigo *(p.228)* ✚ ✚
Golden coloured crusts on the skin, most
commonly around nose.

EYE
PHYSICAL

Being exposed to the environment, the eye is at risk of infection and allergy. Inflammation that occurs in conditions such as shingles may cause eye pain requires medical attention.

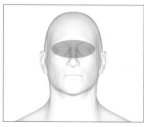

SEE ALSO Eye vision pp.58–59

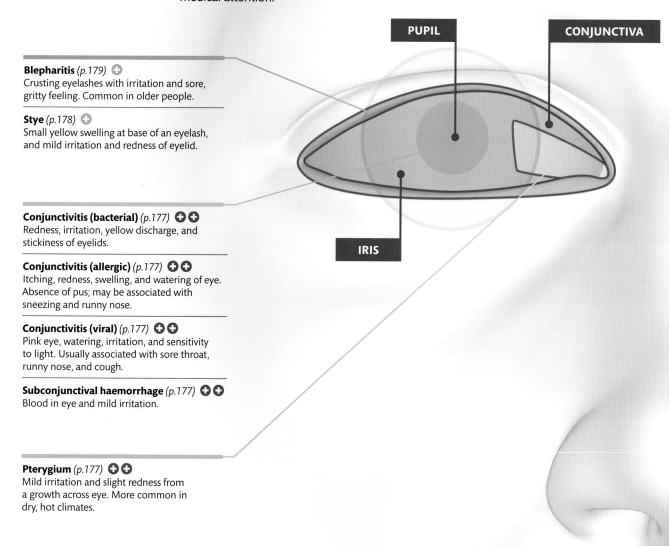

PUPIL

CONJUNCTIVA

IRIS

Blepharitis *(p.179)* ⊕
Crusting eyelashes with irritation and sore, gritty feeling. Common in older people.

Stye *(p.178)* ⊕
Small yellow swelling at base of an eyelash, and mild irritation and redness of eyelid.

Conjunctivitis (bacterial) *(p.177)* ⊕⊕
Redness, irritation, yellow discharge, and stickiness of eyelids.

Conjunctivitis (allergic) *(p.177)* ⊕⊕
Itching, redness, swelling, and watering of eye. Absence of pus; may be associated with sneezing and runny nose.

Conjunctivitis (viral) *(p.177)* ⊕⊕
Pink eye, watering, irritation, and sensitivity to light. Usually associated with sore throat, runny nose, and cough.

Subconjunctival haemorrhage *(p.177)* ⊕⊕
Blood in eye and mild irritation.

Pterygium *(p.177)* ⊕⊕
Mild irritation and slight redness from a growth across eye. More common in dry, hot climates.

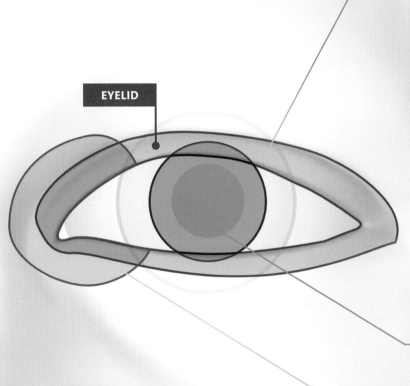

EYELID

Stye *(p.178)*
Mild irritation and redness of eyelid with small yellow swelling at base of an eyelash.

Entropion *(p.179)*
Eyelid turned in, irritation, watering, and mild redness.

Ectropion *(p.179)*
Eyelid turned out, sore, watering, and redness. Generallly affects only the lower lid.

Ptosis *(p.179)*
Upper eyelid droops over the eye. The eyelid may droop a little or enough to cover the pupil.

Eczema *(p.222)*
Itchy, dry, cracked, and flaky skin.

Chalazion *(p.178)*
Swollen lump (cyst) on eyelid with mild discomfort. Cyst may also be red. More common on upper lid.

Cellulitis *(p.228)*
Painful redness, swelling, and warmth of eyelid and possibly eyebrow and cheek. Seek medical advice soon.

Trachoma *(p.177)*
Discharge from eyes; pain, swollen eyelids, irritation, and sensitivity to light. Common in tropical countries.

Acute uveitis *(p.177)*
Redness, sensitivity to light, and moderate pain. Blurring of vision.

Xanthelasma *(p.179)*
Yellow, slightly raised patch; may be just above or below the eyelid, usually in corner closest to nose. Associated with raised cholesterol.

Shingles *(p.233)*
Red eye with moderate to severe pain. Bubbly rash on skin affecting one side of face.

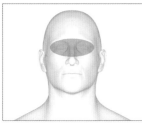

SEE ALSO Eye, physical *pp.56–57*

EYE
VISION

Gradual change in vision can occur throughout life and may be remedied by the use of glasses provided by an optician. Sudden loss of vision is an emergency and you should seek urgent medical help.

LOSS OF VISION

Diabetic retinopathy *(p.220)* ✚✚✚
Blurred vision or gradual loss of central vision. Sudden loss of vision may also occur. Diabetic retinopathy only occurs in people with diabetes.

Chronic glaucoma *(p.178)* ✚✚
Gradual loss of vision, starting with side vision. Common in old age. Seek advice from an optician.

Retinal vein thrombosis *(p.178)* ✚✚✚
Sudden loss of vision in one eye, which may be painless or painful.

Retinal artery thrombosis *(p.178)* ✚✚✚
Sudden, painless loss of vision in one eye.

Acute glaucoma *(p.178)* ✚✚✚
Acute, severe pain in the eye, with a reduction in vision, redness, seeing haloes, watering, light sensitivity, and vomiting.

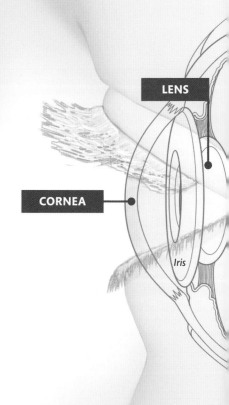

LENS

CORNEA

Iris

BLURRED VISION

Cataract *(p.177)* ✚✚
Blurred or misty vision, bright lights sparkle, altered colours to yellow/brown. Seek advice from an optician.

Diabetic retinopathy *(p.220)* ✚✚✚
Blurred vision or gradual loss of central vision. Sudden loss of vision may also occur. Diabetic retinopathy only occurs in people with diabetes.

Squint *(p.178)* ✚✚
Blurred or double vision. Both eyes are not straight (in parallel), and the eyes do not look in the same direction. Often develops in childhood. Seek advice from an optician.

Acute uveitis *(p.177)* ✚✚✚
Redness, sensitivity to light, and moderate pain. Blurring of vision.

SPOTS AND FLASHES IN VISION

Migraine *(p.166)* ✚✚
Severe headache that may be associated with bright lights in Z-shapes or flashes.

Vitreous detachment *(p.178)* ✚✚✚
Flashes of light and floating black spots ("floaters").

Retinal detachment *(p.178)* ✚✚✚
Flashes of light, with large numbers of floating black spots, and the development of a black "curtain" coming into the field of vision.

DIFFICULTY SEEING OBJECTS

Shortsightedness *(p.179)* ✚✚
Difficulty seeing objects in the distance. Seek advice from an optician.

Longsightedness *(p.179)* ✚✚
Difficulty seeing objects that are close. Seek advice from an optician.

Macular degeneration *(p.178)* ✚✚
Difficulty with fine detail: recognizing faces, reading, watching TV. Straight lines seem wavy.

Astigmatism *(p.179)* ✚✚
Difficulty seeing objects both close-up and in the distance. Seek advice from an optician.

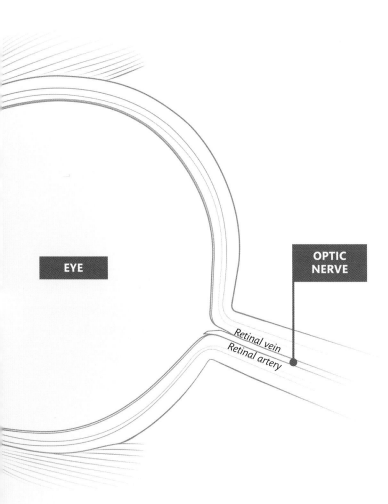

EYE

OPTIC NERVE

Retinal vein
Retinal artery

EAR
PHYSICAL

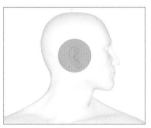

SEE ALSO Head, side *pp.50–51*, Ear, hearing *pp.62–63*

Pain in the ear may result from a middle ear infection, which occurs most commonly in young children. Changes to the ear itself may result from procedures such as piercing or from trauma in sports such as rugby.

Gouty tophus *(p.159)* ➕ ➕
Small white growth, usually on the outer curve of the ear. May be painful.

Keloid scar *(p.227)* ➕ ➕
A lump at site on ear where it has been pierced.

Auricular chondritis *(p.174)* ➕ ➕
Redness of the ear with pain; associated with outer ear infection or previous ear piercing through the hard part of the ear.

Auricular haematoma *(p.174)* ➕ ➕
Swelling and pain following injury to ear with bleeding.

OUTER EAR

Otitis externa *(p.174)* ➕ ➕
Itching or pain inside the ear that worsens when pulling on it.

Contact dermatitis *(p.222)* ➕ ➕
Red, itchy rash after wearing jewellery or applying creams or drops.

Shingles *(p.233)* ➕ ➕
Painful bubbly rash, which may appear on ear and face, mouth, and tongue. May be associated with drooping of one side of face along with deafness, tinnitus (ringing in ear), and vertigo (dizziness).

AURICLE (PINNA)

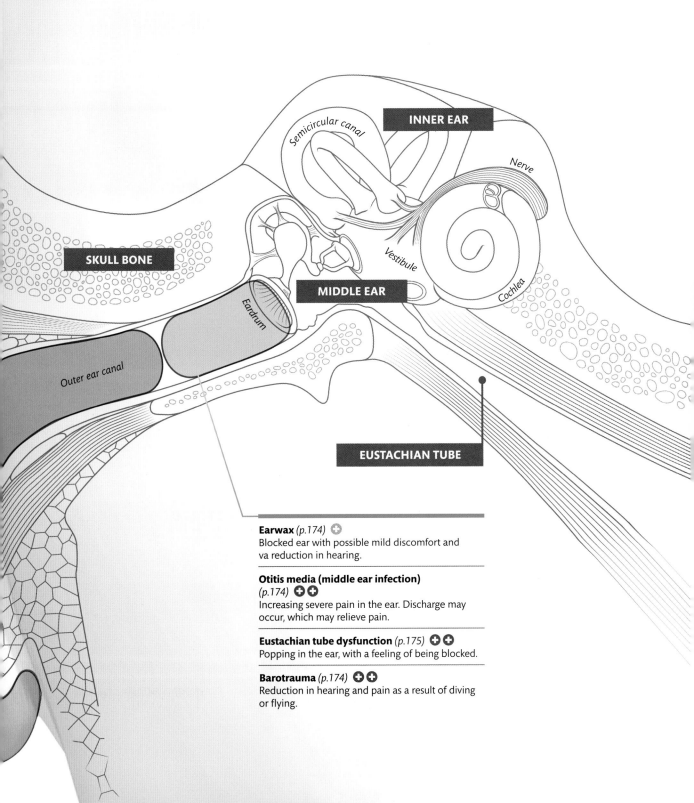

INNER EAR

Semicircular canal

Nerve

SKULL BONE

Vestibule

Cochlea

MIDDLE EAR

Eardrum

Outer ear canal

EUSTACHIAN TUBE

Earwax *(p.174)* ⊕
Blocked ear with possible mild discomfort and
va reduction in hearing.

Otitis media (middle ear infection)
(p.174) ⊕⊕
Increasing severe pain in the ear. Discharge may
occur, which may relieve pain.

Eustachian tube dysfunction *(p.175)* ⊕⊕
Popping in the ear, with a feeling of being blocked.

Barotrauma *(p.174)* ⊕⊕
Reduction in hearing and pain as a result of diving
or flying.

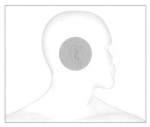

SEE ALSO Ear, hearing pp.60–61

EAR
HEARING

Loss of hearing may gradually occur with age. In younger people, hearing loss may result from problems such as a build-up of wax or having had an infection of the middle ear. Hearing loss affecting one side will require medical investigation.

HEARING LOSS

Presbycusis *(pp.174)* ⊕
Gradually increasing hearing loss affecting both ears. Develops with advancing age. Higher notes affected initially, then lower notes. Background noise makes it harder to hear conversation. Seek medical advice if hearing aid required.

Otitis media (glue ear) *(p.174)* ⊕⊕
Reduced hearing (such as needing the volume high on the television); speech that is quieter than normal. May have had a recent cold. More common in children.

Labyrinthitis *(p.176)* ⊕⊕
Vertigo (dizziness), worsened by change of head position; tinnitus (noises in ears); hearing loss. Fever, and feeling of fullness or pressure in the ear may also be present.

Ménière's disease *(p.176)* ⊕⊕
Attacks of dizziness, hearing loss, and tinnitus (noises in ears). Lasts between a few minutes and several days.

Earwax *(p.174)* ⊕
Blocked ear with possible mild discomfort and a reduction in hearing.

Otosclerosis *(p.174)* ⊕⊕
Increasing level of hearing loss affecting both ears; may be unequal. Hearing may be improved when there is a noisy background. Tinnitus (noises in ears) and vertigo (dizziness) may be present. More common in women.

Acoustic neuroma *(p.176)* ⊕⊕⊕
One-sided, slowly developing hearing loss with tinnitus (noises in ears). Loss of balance may develop along with headaches and numbness or weakness of the face on the affected side.

Sensorineural hearing loss *(p.174)* ⊕⊕
Sudden hearing loss, usually on one side only. See doctor soon.

Ruptured eardrum *(p.175)* ⊕⊕
Slight hearing loss following brief, intense pain. There may be slight bleeding or discharge from ear.

WITH DIZZINESS

Labyrinthitis *(p.176)* ⊕⊕
Vertigo (dizziness), worsened by change of head position; tinnitus (noises in ears); hearing loss. Fever, and feeling of fullness or pressure in the ear may also be present.

Ménière's disease *(p.176)* ⊕⊕
Attacks of dizziness, hearing loss, and tinnitus (noises in ears). Lasts between a few minutes and several days.

Vestibular neuritis *(p.176)* ⊕⊕
Sudden onset of dizziness with nausea and vomiting. Associated with feeling of being unsteady.

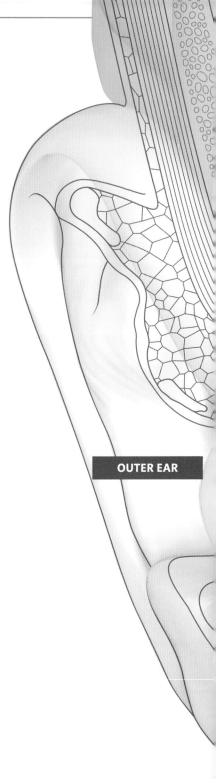

OUTER EAR

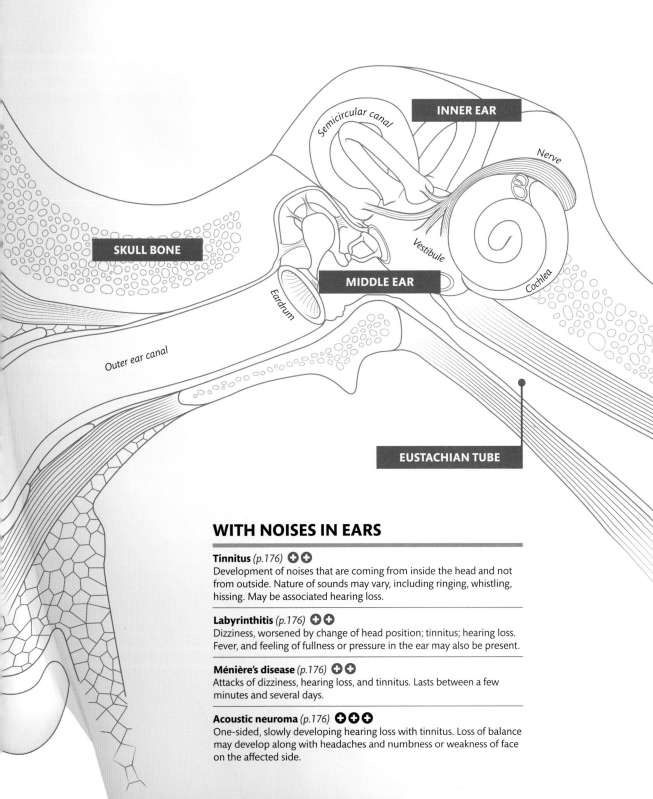

INNER EAR

Semicircular canal

Nerve

SKULL BONE

Vestibule

Cochlea

MIDDLE EAR

Eardrum

Outer ear canal

EUSTACHIAN TUBE

WITH NOISES IN EARS

Tinnitus *(p.176)* ➕➕
Development of noises that are coming from inside the head and not from outside. Nature of sounds may vary, including ringing, whistling, hissing. May be associated hearing loss.

Labyrinthitis *(p.176)* ➕➕
Dizziness, worsened by change of head position; tinnitus; hearing loss. Fever, and feeling of fullness or pressure in the ear may also be present.

Ménière's disease *(p.176)* ➕➕
Attacks of dizziness, hearing loss, and tinnitus. Lasts between a few minutes and several days.

Acoustic neuroma *(p.176)* ➕➕➕
One-sided, slowly developing hearing loss with tinnitus. Loss of balance may develop along with headaches and numbness or weakness of face on the affected side.

NOSE

A stuffy nose may be the result of structural damage to the inside or viral conditions such as the common cold. Changes in the skin of the nose may be a sign of an inflammatory condition, so you should see a doctor.

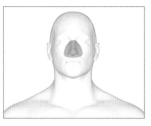

SEE ALSO Face *pp.54–55*

Sinusitis *(p.191)* ⊕
Pain in face, feeling unwell, clear runny nose, and cough. Seek medical advice if discharge from nose turns green.

Allergic rhinitis *(p.190)* ⊕
Sneezing and runny nose. May be associated with itchiness and a feeling of a stuffy nose while feeling well. Itchy eyes and throat may be present.

Deviated nasal septum *(p.190)* ⊕ ⊕
Feeling blocked on one side of nose. Outside of nose may not look straight. Seek urgent medical advice if newly developed from an injury or similar.

Nasal polyps *(p.190)* ⊕ ⊕
Stuffy nose with purplish coloured growths inside. Associated with sneezing, runny nose, catarrh at back of throat, and reduced ability to smell.

SINUS

SINUS

SINUS

JAW

⊕ SEEK URGENT MEDICAL ATTENTION IF:

A NOSEBLEED FAILS TO STOP AFTER **20 MINUTES**

SKIN CHANGES

Impetigo *(p.228)* ⊕ ⊕
Golden coloured crusts on the skin, extending from nose onto face.

Rhinophyma *(p.223)* ⊕ ⊕
Thickening of soft tissues on outside of nose, causing it to enlarge. May have pus-filled spots. May also have spots on face and intermittent flushing.

Lupus pernio *(p.224)* ⊕ ⊕
Bluish-red discolouration of nose, which may be lumpy.

Systemic lupus erythematosus (SLE) *(p.189)* ⊕ ⊕
Red rash affecting nose and cheeks. May be painful or itchy and worsened by exposure to sunlight.

Nosebleed *(p.190)* ⊕
Sudden, continuous blood loss from nose. Seek urgent medical attention if it fails to stop after 20 minutes despite home treatment.

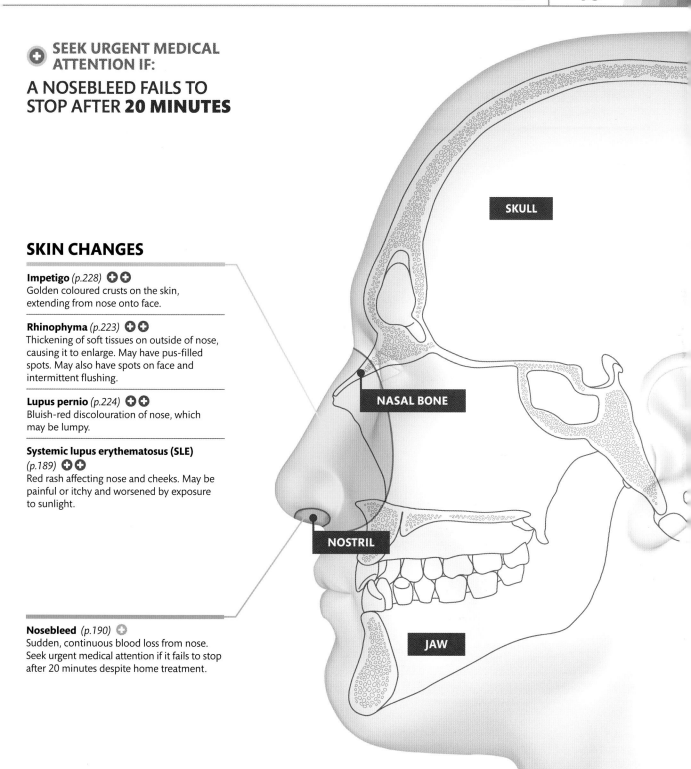

SKULL

NASAL BONE

NOSTRIL

JAW

MOUTH

The mouth can be affected by painful ulceration. If recurrent, a check with your doctor is recommended. Any mouth ulcer that fails to heal should be checked by a dentist or doctor.

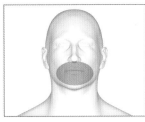

SEE ALSO Throat *pp.68–69*

Herpes simplex (cold sore) *(p.229)* ⊕
Acutely painful bubbly rash that may occur recurrently in the same place on lip. May also occur inside mouth, causing pain when eating.

Hand, foot, and mouth disease *(p.229)* ⊕ ⊕
Small spots turning to ulcers on lips and in mouth. Associated with fever, sore throat, and small blisters on hands and feet. Spots may also appear elsewhere on body.

Dental abscess *(p.197)* ⊕ ⊕
Swelling, pain, and redness of the gum in region of a possibly painful tooth. Consult a dentist.

Oral thrush *(p.238)* ⊕ ⊕
White coating to tongue with soreness and alteration in taste. May also be some red patches.

Geographic tongue *(p.199)* ⊕ ⊕
Tongue surface looks like a map with raw red patches and white borders. The tongue may feel sore or develop a burning sensation when eating certain foods.

Oral lichen planus *(p.222)* ⊕ ⊕
Lines of white inside cheeks, on tongue and gums, with a pattern like lace cloth. May also appear as flat white patches and be associated with a rash on certain areas of the body. May be soreness or burning worsened by eating acidic or spicy foods.

Fibroepithelial polyp ⊕ ⊕
Small, soft, pinkish-red swelling usually growing on side of tongue or inside of cheek. Consult a dentist.

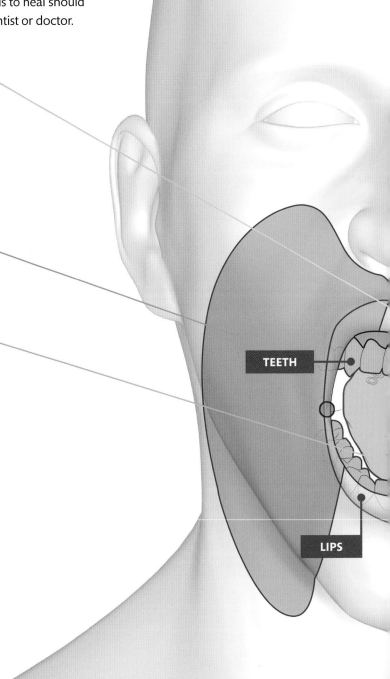

TEETH

LIPS

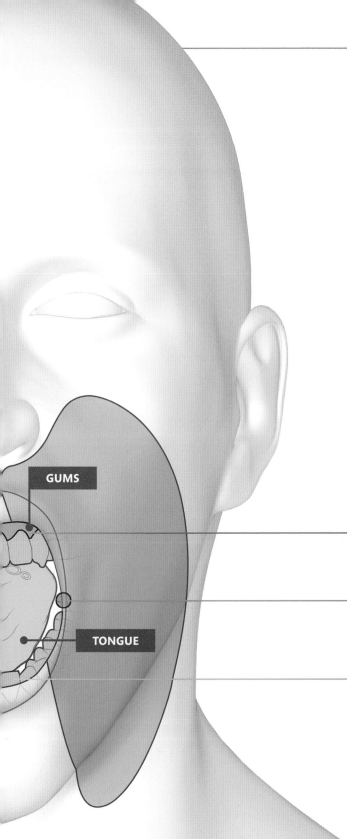

GUMS

TONGUE

INSIDE MOUTH

Mouth ulcer *(p.198)* ✚
Single or multiple shallow ulcers inside mouth. Painful. Seek medical advice if recurrent or fail to heal after three weeks.

Hand, foot, and mouth disease *(p.229)* ✚ ✚
Small spots turning to ulcers on lips and in mouth. Associated with fever, sore throat, and small blisters on hands and feet. Spots may also appear elsewhere on body.

Fibroepithelial polyp ✚ ✚
Small, soft, pinkish-red swelling usually growing on side of tongue or inside of cheek. Consult a dentist.

Oral lichen planus *(p.222)* ✚ ✚
Lines of white inside cheeks, tongue, and gums with a pattern like lace cloth. May also appear as flat white patches. May be soreness or burning worsened by eating acidic or spicy foods. Can be associated with a rash on certain areas of body.

Leukoplakia *(p.198)* ✚ ✚
White or red patch anywhere in mouth that does not disappear.

Oral (mouth) cancer *(p.198)* ✚ ✚ ✚
Firm, solitary ulcer anywhere in mouth that fails to heal after three weeks. New hard lumps may be a developing cancer.

Gingivitis *(p.198)* ✚ ✚
Painful, red gums with swelling. Consult a dentist.

Angular stomatitis *(pp228)* ✚
Cracking of the skin at the corners of the mouth, redness, and mild discomfort.

Tooth decay *(p.197)* ✚ ✚
Black or brown spots on tooth, pain in tooth on eating, bad breath. Consult a dentist.

THROAT

The back of the throat contains lymphatic tissues, such as the tonsils, that are positioned to defend against infection entering the body. Sore throat may develop as a result of infections with viruses, which get better on their own or due to bacteria as in tonsillitis, which requires antibiotic treatment.

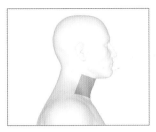

SEE ALSO Throat, voice *pp.70–71*, Neck *pp.72–73*

Viral sore throat (pharyngitis) *(p.192)* ✚
Mild fever with redness at back of throat. May occur with or without runny nose and cough.

Bacterial tonsillitis *(p.192)* ✚✚
Very painful sore throat, high fever, enlarged lymph nodes by angle of jaw; white spots on tonsils at back of throat. May be red rash on body and redness on cheeks with pale skin around the lips and a "strawberry" appearance to tongue. Common in children and young adults.

Herpangina *(p.192)* ✚✚
High fever, sore throat, ulcers at back of throat that have a white base and red border. Lumps in front of neck (enlarged lymph nodes). More common in children.

Tonsil stone *(p.191)* ✚✚
White-coloured material lying in one of the dips in the tonsil. No sore throat but may be associated with bad breath.

Acute epiglottitis *(p.191)* ✚✚✚
High fever, severe sore throat, difficulty swallowing, and altered voice. Inability to swallow own saliva or a loud noise on breathing in are very serious signs. Hospital treatment is urgently required, dial 999. (Now rare in UK).

Croup *(p.192)* ✚✚
Fever, runny nose, hoarse voice, noise on breathing in, harsh barking cough that sounds like a seal or a dog. Rarely, breathing may become a problem. In this situation seek urgent medical help. Usually only affects children.

Glandular fever *(p.235)* ✚✚
Slowly developing sore throat, enlarged lumps (lymph nodes) particularly at front and back of neck and possibly in armpits and groin. Tonsils covered in an off-white membrane. Skin around eyes may become puffy; may be a red rash on roof of mouth. Mostly affects children and young adults.

Herpangina *(p.192)* ✚✚
High fever, sore throat, ulcers at back of throat that have a white base and red border. Enlarged lymph nodes at front of neck.

Acute epiglottitis *(p.191)* ✚✚✚
High fever, severe sore throat, difficulty swallowing, and altered voice. Inability to swallow saliva, or a loud noise on breathing in, are very serious signs. Hospital treatment is urgently required, dial 999.

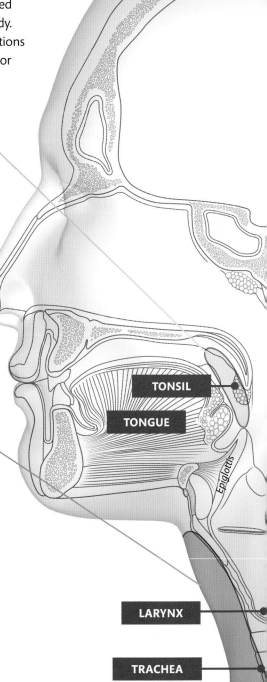

TONSIL

TONGUE

Epiglottis

LARYNX

TRACHEA

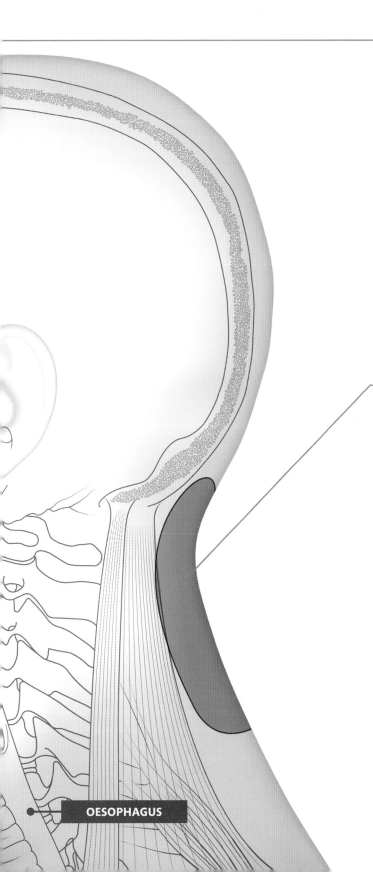

OESOPHAGUS

⊕ **SEEK URGENT MEDICAL ATTENTION IF:**

A PERSON IS **UNABLE TO SWALLOW** OR **BREATHING IS IMPAIRED**

Snoring ⊕
Loud noise that may be associated with stuffy nose. In children, there may be enlarged adenoids and tonsils.

Obstructive sleep apnoea *(p.191)* ⊕⊕
Snoring associated with intermittent stopping of breathing. Restarting of breathing is signalled by a "snort". Most common in middle-aged men, but may also occur in small children who have enlarged tonsils and adenoids.

Glandular fever *(p.235)* ⊕⊕
Slowly developing sore throat, enlarged lumps (lymph nodes) particularly at front and back of neck. Tonsils covered in an off-white membrane. Skin around eyes may become puffy; may be a red rash on roof of mouth. Mostly affects children and young adults.

SWOLLEN LYMPH NODES

Several disorders cause enlarged lymph nodes ("glands"). These can be felt under the jawline and on the neck. Examples are bacterial tonsillitis *(p.192)*, glandular fever *(p.235)*, and herpangina *(p.192)*. Lymphoma *(p.188)* and leukaemia *(p.187)* are rare causes of swollen lymph nodes.

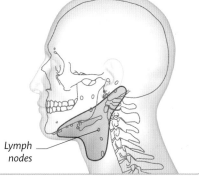

Lymph nodes

THROAT
VOICE

A sudden change in one's voice is usually caused by a viral infection, and it will get better with simple remedies. However, if hoarseness lasts longer than three weeks, you should seek medical advice.

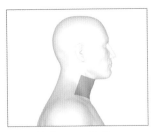

SEE ALSO Throat *pp.68–69*

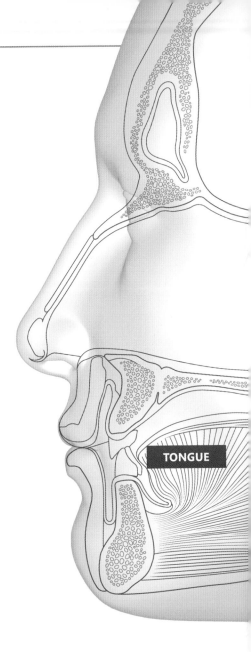

TONGUE

Voice overuse *(p.192)* ✚✚
Hoarseness from longterm overuse, such as shouting.

Functional dysphonia *(p.192)* ✚✚
Hoarse voice in the absence of any abnormality of the vocal cords – possibly resulting from stress (p.240).

Hypothyroidism *(p.220)* ✚✚
Hoarse voice in association with other symptoms of an underactive thyroid gland, such as hair loss, dry skin, constipation, and tiredness.

Vocal cord polyp *(p.192)* ✚✚
Loss or alteration of the voice as a result of long-standing overuse. Most common in singers.

Laryngeal cancer *(p.193)* ✚✚
Hoarseness lasting more than three weeks, usually in someone who is a long-term smoker.

HOARSENESS WITH COUGH

Gastro-oesophageal reflux disease (acid reflux) *(p.199)* ✚✚
Sensation of something in the throat, cough, and hoarseness. Associated with heartburn (burning sensation in the chest).

Croup *(p.192)* ✚✚
Fever, harsh barking cough, and voice change. Any difficulty in breathing should result in an urgent medical assessment. Affects children.

Lung cancer *(p.195)* ✚✚✚
Hoarseness and prolonged cough, which may be associated with bringing up blood, chest pain, shortness of breath, loss of weight, and reduced appetite; usually in someone who is a long-term smoker.

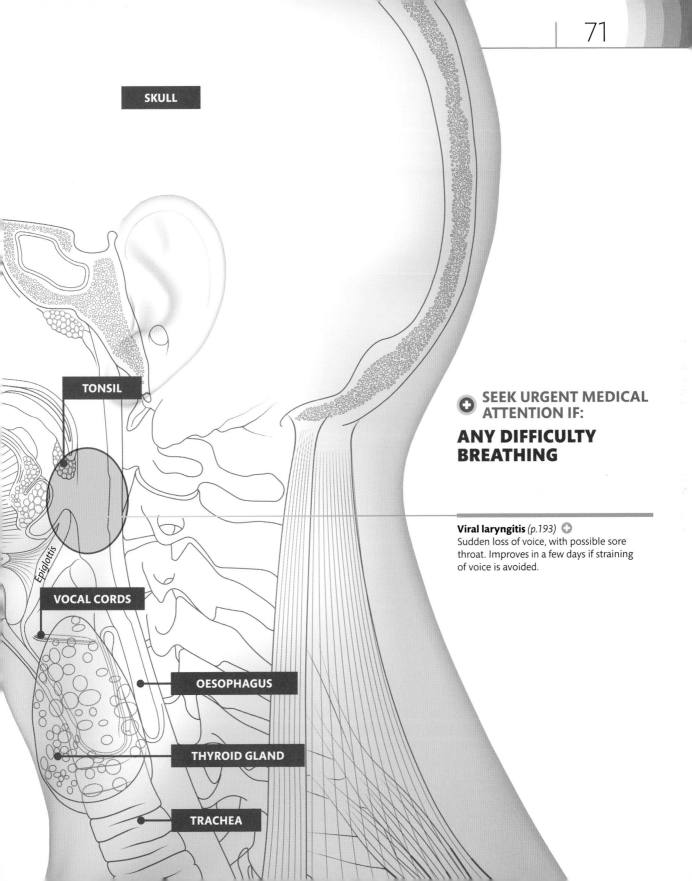

SKULL

TONSIL

Epiglottis

VOCAL CORDS

OESOPHAGUS

THYROID GLAND

TRACHEA

SEEK URGENT MEDICAL
ATTENTION IF:

ANY DIFFICULTY
BREATHING

Viral laryngitis *(p.193)*
Sudden loss of voice, with possible sore
throat. Improves in a few days if straining
of voice is avoided.

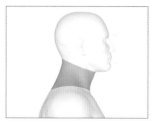

SEE ALSO Head, front *pp.48–49*, Throat *pp.68–69*, **Throat, voice** *pp.70–71*

NECK

Problems in the surrounding muscles and in the spine may cause pain and neck stiffness. Most neck pain gets better on its own. However, when combined with other symptoms it may be a sign of a more serious condition, such as meningitis (p.168).

Swollen lymph nodes *(p.187)* ⊕
Tender moveable lump(s) under the skin. Usually there is a localized infection or viral illness that settles within two to three weeks. If it persists, seek medical advice.

Whiplash *(p.161)* ⊕ ⊕
Tender; restricted movement and headache, localized pain. Get urgent help if numbness in hands, arms, shoulders, or chest.

Stiff neck ⊕
Pain and restricted movement. Result of sleeping awkwardly and/or poor posture. Settles in one to three days. Painkillers and heat applied to the area may help.

Muscle tension/stress ⊕
Tender muscles, headache, and pain in a specific area reulting from stress and poor posture. Try exercises to improve flexibility and strengthen core muscles. Keep hydrated.

Cervical spondylosis *(p.158)* ⊕ ⊕
Stiffness and dull pain in neck, which sometimes extends to shoulder and upper arm. Grinding noise when turning head. Common with increasing age.

TRAPEZIUS

SHOULDER BLADE

Meningitis *(p.168)* ✚✚✚
General neck stiffness, fever, feeling very unwell, and light hurts eyes. May have a rash that doesn't fade after pressure is briefly applied. May rapidly be fatal. This is a medical emergency, dial 999.

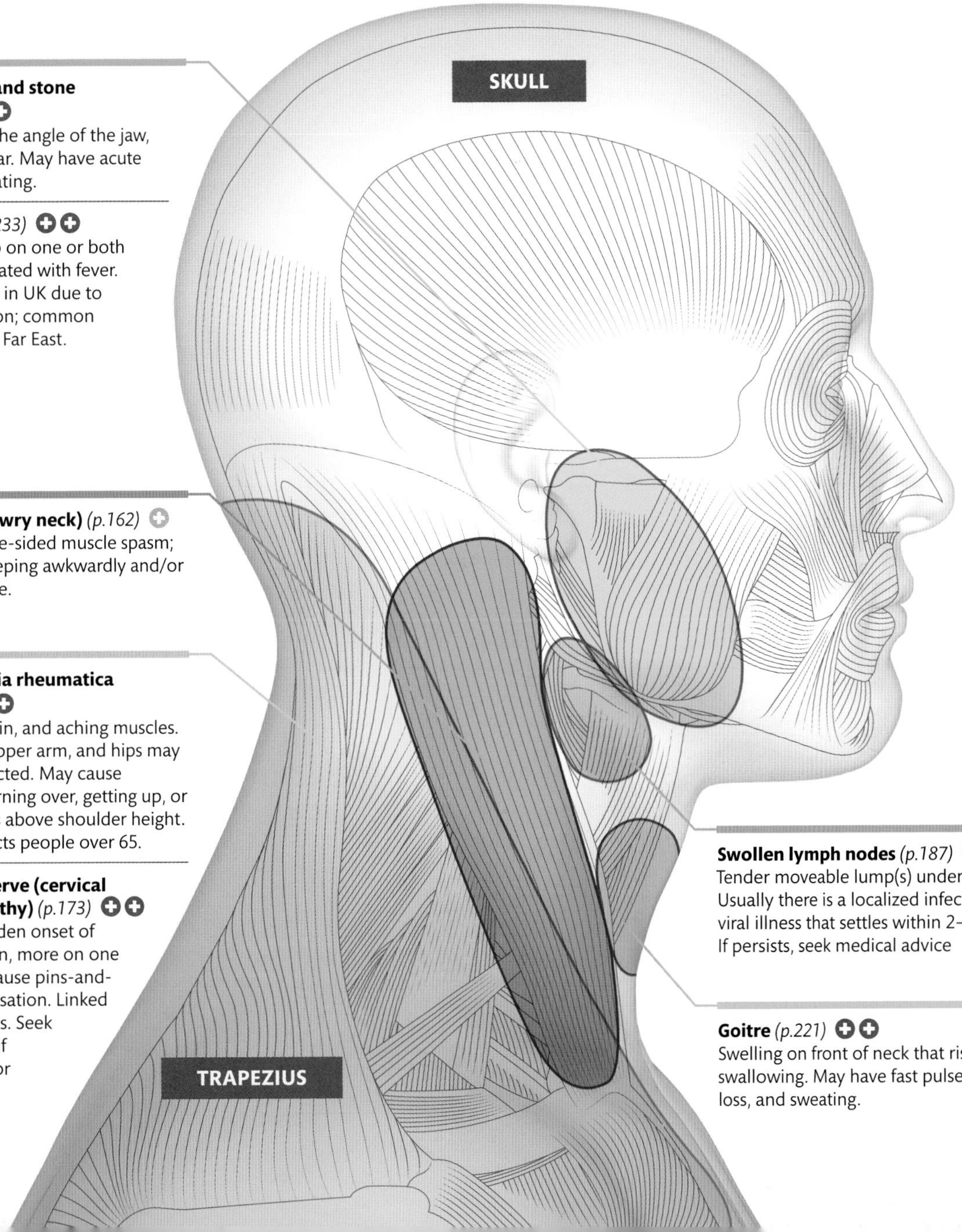

Salivary gland stone *(p.198)* ✚✚
Swelling at the angle of the jaw, in front of ear. May have acute pain after eating.

Mumps *(p.233)* ✚✚
Visible lump on one or both sides; associated with fever. Uncommon in UK due to immunization; common in India and Far East.

Torticollis (wry neck) *(p.162)* ✚
Pain and one-sided muscle spasm; result of sleeping awkwardly and/or poor posture.

Polymyalgia rheumatica *(p.189)* ✚✚
Stiffness, pain, and aching muscles. Shoulder, upper arm, and hips may also be affected. May cause difficulty turning over, getting up, or raising arms above shoulder height. Mainly affects people over 65.

Trapped nerve (cervical radiculopathy) *(p.173)* ✚✚
Usually sudden onset of burning pain, more on one side. May cause pins-and-needles sensation. Linked with arthritis. Seek ugent help if numbness or weakness.

✚ **SEEK URGENT MEDICAL ATTENTION IF:**

YOU HAVE A **STIFF NECK** WITH **FEVER**, **RASH**, AND **AVERSION TO BRIGHT LIGHT**

SKULL

TRAPEZIUS

Swollen lymph nodes *(p.187)* ✚
Tender moveable lump(s) under the skin. Usually there is a localized infection or viral illness that settles within 2–3 weeks. If persists, seek medical advice

Goitre *(p.221)* ✚✚
Swelling on front of neck that rises with swallowing. May have fast pulse, weight loss, and sweating.

SHOULDER
FRONT

Shoulder disorders are common. The shoulder
is the joint with the greatest range of movement
and the least stability, so it is prone to strains,
repetitive injuries, and wear. Unless otherwise
stated, symptoms can affect both sides.

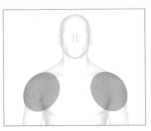

SEE ALSO Neck *pp.72–73*, **Shoulder,
back** *pp.76–77*, **Upper arm** *pp.78–79*

Collarbone fracture *(p.156)* ✚✚✚
Sudden severe pain and swelling and
deformity, resulting from injury. Sharp
pain with any arm movement.

Humerus fracture *(p.156)* ✚✚✚
Sudden severe pain and swelling, and
possible deformity, resulting from injury.
Pain with any attempt to move arm.

REFERRED PAIN

Various diseases that originte in the
chest or abdomen may cause shoulder
pain. This is usually gnawing in nature,
but it can be sharp. Such conditions
include heart attack *(p.180)*, angina
(p.181), and lung problems, including
lung cancer *(p.195)*, pneumonia
(p.194), and pleurisy *(p.194)*. The pain
is deep and not made worse with
movement, and the area does not
feel tender when touched.

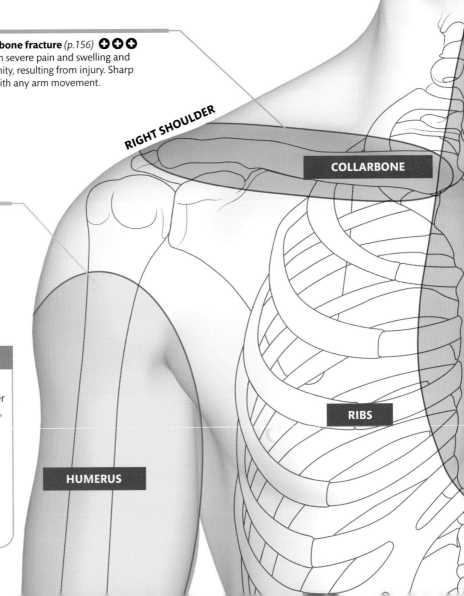

RIGHT SHOULDER

COLLARBONE

RIBS

HUMERUS

Angina *(p.181)*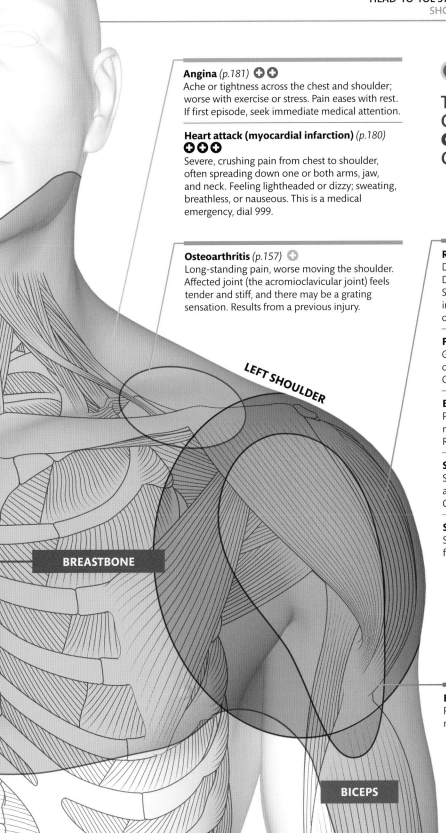
Ache or tightness across the chest and shoulder; worse with exercise or stress. Pain eases with rest. If first episode, seek immediate medical attention.

Heart attack (myocardial infarction) *(p.180)*
Severe, crushing pain from chest to shoulder, often spreading down one or both arms, jaw, and neck. Feeling lightheaded or dizzy; sweating, breathless, or nauseous. This is a medical emergency, dial 999.

Osteoarthritis *(p.157)*
Long-standing pain, worse moving the shoulder. Affected joint (the acromioclavicular joint) feels tender and stiff, and there may be a grating sensation. Results from a previous injury.

SEEK URGENT MEDICAL ATTENTION IF:

THERE ARE SIGNS OF **REDUCED CONSCIOUSNESS** OR **PAIN IS SEVERE**

Rotator cuff disorders *(p.163)*
Deep, dull ache, worse lying on affected side. Difficulty doing hair or reaching behind back. Some arm weakness. More likely with increasing age and in people playing sports or working above head level.

Frozen shoulder *(p.159)*
Gradually increasing pain and restriction of movement over days or weeks. Common in people over 50.

Bursitis *(p.159)*
Pain and stiffness with certain arm movements. Worse when reaching up. Results from injury of repetitive motion.

Shoulder dislocation *(p.161)*
Sudden, severe pain and inability to move arm. Usually lump at front of shoulder. Often a result of injury.

Shoulder instability *(p.160)*
Shoulder feels unstable and weak. Results from a previous shoulder dislocation.

LEFT SHOULDER

BREASTBONE

Biceps tendinitis *(p.164)*
Pain and stiffness with certain arm movements, particularly overhead.

BICEPS

SHOULDER
BACK

From the rear, most of the shoulder is made up of large muscles and the shoulder blade. Pain can be caused by minor injury, bad posture, or an underlying disorder. Range of movement reduces with age and may produce painless grinding or clicking noises. Unless otherwise stated, conditions can affect both shoulders.

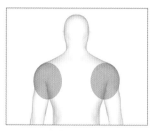

SEE ALSO Neck *pp.72–73*, **Shoulder, front** *pp.74–75*, **Upper back** *pp.96–97*

Muscle tension *(p.163)* ⊕
Localized muscle tenderness and pain over shoulder blade, usually on one side only. Results from poor posture or sleeping awkwardly.

Polymyalgia rheumatica *(p.161)* ⊕ ⊕
Stiffness, pain, aching muscles. May cause difficulty turning over, getting up, or raising arms above shoulder height. Worst first thing in the morning. Mainly affects people over 65; more common in women.

REFERRED PAIN

Pain in the back of the shoulder that is not made worse by movement, and where there is no specific tenderness, may be caused by problems in the chest or abdomen. This is referred pain and results from pain signals from the original source impinging on nerves in the shoulder. Conditions include heart attack *(p.180)*, angina *(p.181)*, and lung problems such as lung cancer *(p.195)*, pneumonia *(p.194)*, and pleurisy *(p.194)*.

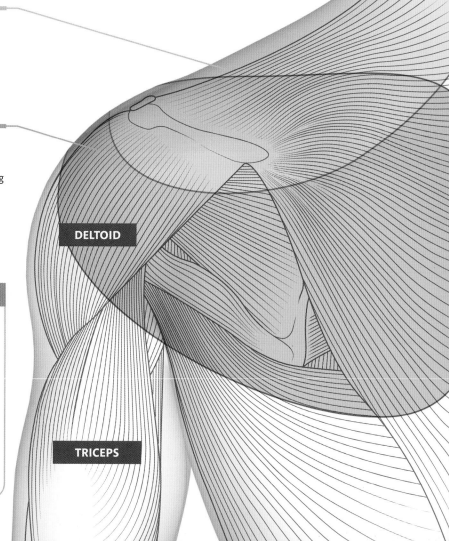

DELTOID

TRICEPS

Rotator cuff disorders *(p.163)*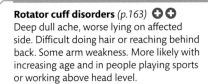
Deep dull ache, worse lying on affected side. Difficult doing hair or reaching behind back. Some arm weakness. More likely with increasing age and in people playing sports or working above head level.

Frozen shoulder *(p.159)*
Gradually increasing pain and restriction of movement over days or weeks. Common especially in people over 50.

Cholecystitis *(p.202)*
Right shoulder tip pain (referred pain, see opposite) and tenderness below shoulder blade. Associated with severe, constant stomach pain; nausea and vomiting; tenderness below ribs. Affects women over 40 more than men.

Bursitis *(p.159)*
Pain and stiffness with certain arm movements; worse if reaching up. Results from injury or repetitive motion.

Shoulder instability *(p.160)*
Joint feels unstable and weak. Results from a previous shoulder dislocation.

Osteoarthritis *(p.157)*
Long-standing pain and stiffness, worse with moving arm. Some weakness.

VERTEBRA

COLLARBONE

SHOULDER
BLADE

RIB

HUMERUS

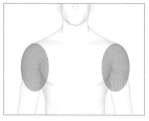

SEE ALSO Shoulder, front *pp.74–75*, Shoulder, back *pp.76–77*, Chest, upper *pp.88–89*

UPPER ARM

This major "lever" is prone to injury through overuse. Problems affecting the neck and shoulder can spread down the arms. Some serious conditions can be felt here: pain down the left arm is a potential sign of angina or heart attack. Unless otherwise stated, symptoms can affect one or both arms.

RIGHT SHOULDER

SHOULDER

BICEPS

Trapped nerve (cervical radiculopathy) *(p.173)* ✚✚
Usually, pain that starts suddenly on one side. A pins-and-needles sensation may be felt down arm to fingers. Associated with arthritis of neck. Seek urgent medical advice if any numbness or weakness.

Polymyalgia rheumatica *(p.161)* ✚✚
Stiffness, pain, aching muscles. Neck and hips may also be affected. Difficulty turning over, getting up, or raising arms above shoulder height. Worst first thing in the morning. Mainly affects people over 65. More common in women.

Biceps tendinitis *(p.164)* ✚
Gradual onset of pain in front or side of shoulder and upper arm. Worse at night and when sleeping on affected side. Pain when moving, especially raising arm above the head or reaching behind. Shoulder weakness and stiffness. Results from overuse or strain.

Biceps rupture *(p.165)* ✚✚✚
Sudden pain after lifting heavy weight, in elbow initially. Bruising around elbow and forearm developing over two to three days, changed shape (higher bulge in biceps muscle), weakness when turning palm up.

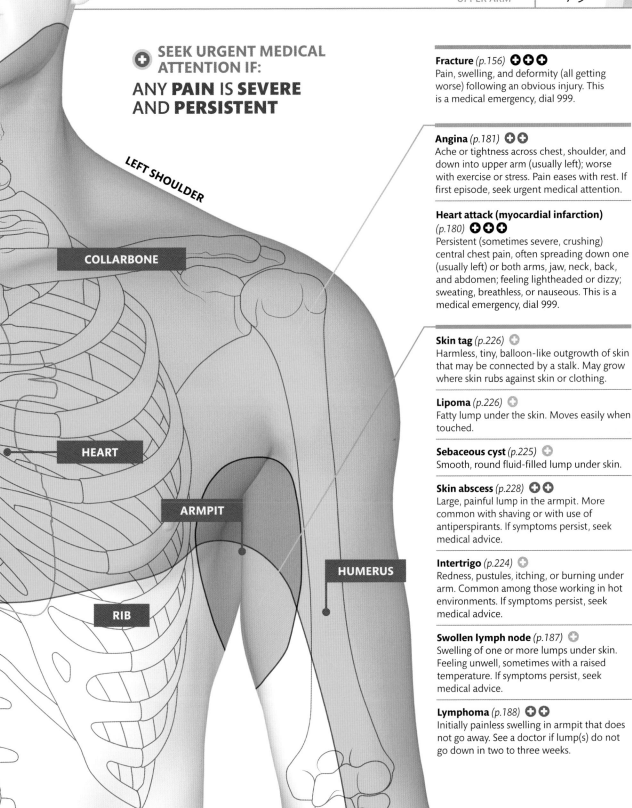

⊕ **SEEK URGENT MEDICAL ATTENTION IF:**
ANY **PAIN** IS **SEVERE** AND **PERSISTENT**

LEFT SHOULDER

COLLARBONE

HEART

ARMPIT

HUMERUS

RIB

Fracture *(p.156)* ⊕⊕⊕
Pain, swelling, and deformity (all getting worse) following an obvious injury. This is a medical emergency, dial 999.

Angina *(p.181)* ⊕⊕
Ache or tightness across chest, shoulder, and down into upper arm (usually left); worse with exercise or stress. Pain eases with rest. If first episode, seek urgent medical attention.

Heart attack (myocardial infarction) *(p.180)* ⊕⊕⊕
Persistent (sometimes severe, crushing) central chest pain, often spreading down one (usually left) or both arms, jaw, neck, back, and abdomen; feeling lightheaded or dizzy; sweating, breathless, or nauseous. This is a medical emergency, dial 999.

Skin tag *(p.226)* ⊕
Harmless, tiny, balloon-like outgrowth of skin that may be connected by a stalk. May grow where skin rubs against skin or clothing.

Lipoma *(p.226)* ⊕
Fatty lump under the skin. Moves easily when touched.

Sebaceous cyst *(p.225)* ⊕
Smooth, round fluid-filled lump under skin.

Skin abscess *(p.228)* ⊕⊕
Large, painful lump in the armpit. More common with shaving or with use of antiperspirants. If symptoms persist, seek medical advice.

Intertrigo *(p.224)* ⊕
Redness, pustules, itching, or burning under arm. Common among those working in hot environments. If symptoms persist, seek medical advice.

Swollen lymph node *(p.187)* ⊕
Swelling of one or more lumps under skin. Feeling unwell, sometimes with a raised temperature. If symptoms persist, seek medical advice.

Lymphoma *(p.188)* ⊕⊕
Initially painless swelling in armpit that does not go away. See a doctor if lump(s) do not go down in two to three weeks.

ELBOW

The elbow is a hinge joint where the upper arm meets the two bones of the forearm. Elbow pain is usually due to overuse or injury. Many sports, hobbies, and jobs require repetitive hand, wrist, or arm movements that contribute to this.

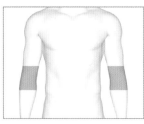

SEE ALSO Upper arm *pp.78–79*, Forearm and wrist *pp.82–83*

SWELLING

Rheumatoid arthritis *(p.157)* ➕➕
Painful swelling with possible joint deformity in later stages. Other joints, such as knees and hips, also usually affected. May be associated with tiredness and weight loss.

Gout *(p.159)* ➕➕
Painful swelling around elbow. Skin over joint may be shiny and red.

Biceps rupture *(p.165)* ➕➕➕
Sudden pain (in elbow initially) after lifting excessive weight. Bruising around elbow or forearm. Characteristic changed shape (higher bulge in biceps muscle) and weakness when turning palm up. More common in men over 30.

Olecranon bursitis (student's elbow) *(p.159)* ➕➕
Warm, swollen, tender cyst. Restricted movement. May result from trauma, such as falling on the elbow, or from prolonged overuse, such as with leaning elbow on desk whilst studying.

Familial hypercholesterolaemia *(p.221)* ➕➕
Fatty lumps underneath the skin, especially on knees and elbows and around eyelids.

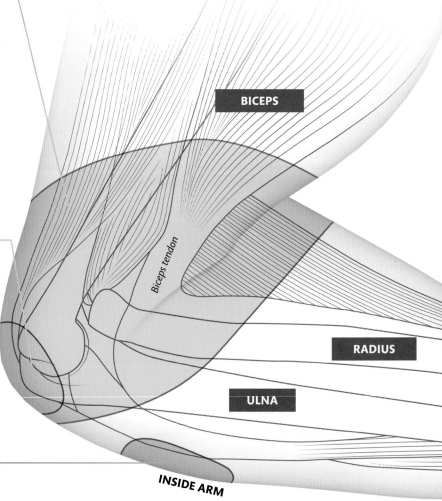

BICEPS

Biceps tendon

RADIUS

ULNA

INSIDE ARM

Biceps tendinitis *(p.164)*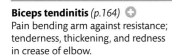
Pain bending arm against resistance;
tenderness, thickening, and redness
in crease of elbow.

Sprain *(p.162)* ◯
Aching and some stiffness. Improves in a few
days. Rest helps.

Osteoarthritis *(p.157)* ◯
Aching pain and stiffness that is worse
with movement.

Rheumatoid arthritis *(p.157)* ◯◯
Painful swelling with possible joint deformity
in later stages. Other joints, such as knees
and hips, also commonly affected. May be
associated with tiredness and weight loss.

Gout *(p.159)* ◯◯
Painful swelling around elbow. Skin over joint
may be shiny and red.

Fibromyalgia *(p.162)* ◯
Deep, burning, aching pain that may move
around body. Worse with activity, stress, and
weather changes. Muscle stiffness, tingling,
and tiredness. See doctor if persists.

Tennis elbow *(p.165)* ◯
Constant soreness and pain, worse when
twisting forearm. Common, especially
in 40- to 60-year-olds.

Golfer's elbow *(p.165)* ◯
Constant soreness and pain on inside
of elbow. Worse with repeated flexing
and gripping from wrist.

Fracture *(p.156)* ◯◯◯
Pain, swelling, and deformity (all getting
worse) following an obvious injury.

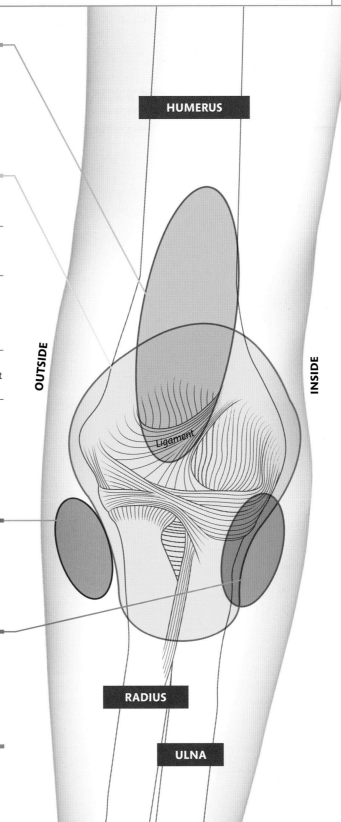

HUMERUS

OUTSIDE

INSIDE

Ligament

RADIUS

ULNA

FOREARM AND WRIST

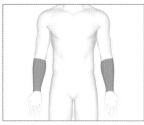

SEE ALSO Elbow *pp.80–81*, **Hand, back** *pp.84–85*, **Hand, palm** *pp.86–87*

The two bones of the forearm – the radius and ulna – meet the eight bones that make up the wrist. Wrist injuries can be debilitating because they may limit hand movement. Symptoms can affect one or both sides of the body unless otherwise stated.

Osteoarthritis *(p.157)* ⊕
Stiff, painful, swollen joints; difficulty with tasks such as writing, opening jars, or turning keys; bumps may develop around affected joints. More common with increasing age.

Tendinitis *(p.164)* ⊕
Aching and stiffness that improves with rest. May happen during sports or activities that involve sudden, sharp movements, such as throwing, or with repetitive daily work.

FRONT

ELBOW

WRIST

PALM OF HAND

Rheumatoid arthritis *(p.157)* ⊕ ⊕
Long-term condition with pain, swelling, and stiffness in several joints, usually on both sides of body. May be associated with tiredness and weight loss.

Ganglion (cyst) *(p.160)*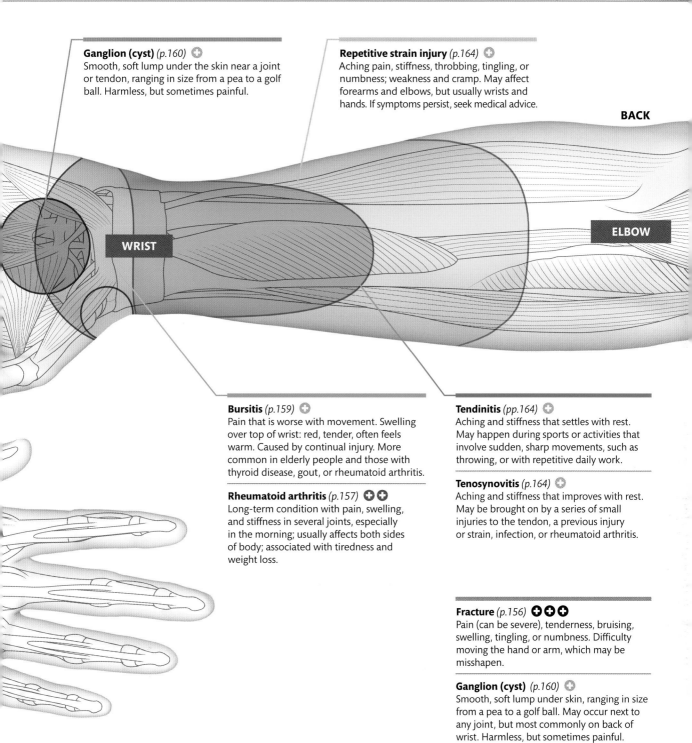
Smooth, soft lump under the skin near a joint or tendon, ranging in size from a pea to a golf ball. Harmless, but sometimes painful.

Repetitive strain injury *(p.164)*
Aching pain, stiffness, throbbing, tingling, or numbness; weakness and cramp. May affect forearms and elbows, but usually wrists and hands. If symptoms persist, seek medical advice.

BACK

WRIST

ELBOW

Bursitis *(p.159)*
Pain that is worse with movement. Swelling over top of wrist: red, tender, often feels warm. Caused by continual injury. More common in elderly people and those with thyroid disease, gout, or rheumatoid arthritis.

Rheumatoid arthritis *(p.157)*
Long-term condition with pain, swelling, and stiffness in several joints, especially in the morning; usually affects both sides of body; associated with tiredness and weight loss.

Tendinitis *(pp.164)*
Aching and stiffness that settles with rest. May happen during sports or activities that involve sudden, sharp movements, such as throwing, or with repetitive daily work.

Tenosynovitis *(p.164)*
Aching and stiffness that improves with rest. May be brought on by a series of small injuries to the tendon, a previous injury or strain, infection, or rheumatoid arthritis.

Fracture *(p.156)*
Pain (can be severe), tenderness, bruising, swelling, tingling, or numbness. Difficulty moving the hand or arm, which may be misshapen.

Ganglion (cyst) *(p.160)*
Smooth, soft lump under skin, ranging in size from a pea to a golf ball. May occur next to any joint, but most commonly on back of wrist. Harmless, but sometimes painful.

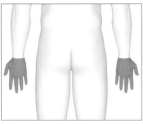

SEE ALSO Forearm and wrist
pp.82–83, **Hand, palm** *pp.86–87*

HAND
BACK

The hands have many joints, small muscles, and nerves needed for grip and touch. They are in constant use, so overuse and injuries are common. The fingernails are subject to potential damage and infection.

Fracture *(p.156)* ✚✚✚
Pain (can be severe), tenderness, bruising, swelling, deformity, tingling, or numbness. Difficulty moving affected finger or hand. Occurs after injury.

Gouty tophi *(p.159)* ✚✚
Usually painless chalk-like lumps under skin, especially of fingers, toes, knees, and ears. May become inflamed and produce a toothpaste-like discharge. More common in men.

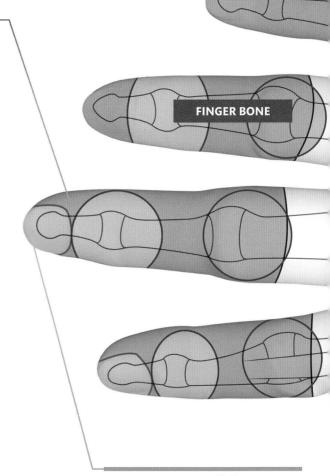

FINGER BONE

Raynaud's disease *(p.185)* ✚✚
Fingers go white, numb, and cool. Bright red when warmed, causing tingling, throbbing, and pain. Sometimes other extremities (toes, ears, and nose) are affected. More common in women, people with a family history, and smokers.

Hand-arm vibration syndrome *(p.185)* ✚✚
Numbness, tingling, and pain. Cold, white fingers. Impaired dexterity and grip. Results from working with vibrating tools or machinery.

NAIL SYMPTOMS

Healthy nails are normally smooth and consistent in colour. Abnormalities may be caused by skin disease and infections, but can also indicate more general medical illnesses. Some nail changes are common with older age.

Paronychia (whitlow) *(p.231)* Infection of nail skin fold. Area is sore, tender, swollen, and warm, eventually with visible pustule.

Horizontal ridges More common in elderly people and those with rheumatoid arthritis *(p.157)*, lichen planus *(p.222)*, or eczema *(p.222)*.

Pitting May be associated with psoriasis *(p.222)* and eczema *(p.222)*.

Onycholysis Separation of nail from the nailbed. It may occur with psoriasis *(p.222)*, lichen planus *(p.222)*, and thyroid diseases *(p.220)*.

Yellowing May be from tobacco use or medical conditions such as fungal infection (onychomycosis, *p.231*), or liver and lung disorders.

Spoon-shaped nails May be a sign of iron deficiency.

Clubbed nails Curving down around fingertips with bulging nailbeds. May be a sign of lung, heart, or liver disease.

Finger clubbing *(p.231)* ✚✚
Painless increase in the soft tissue around ends of fingers (and sometimes toes). Nail base curves down and extends halfway up nail.

Rheumatoid arthritis *(p.157)*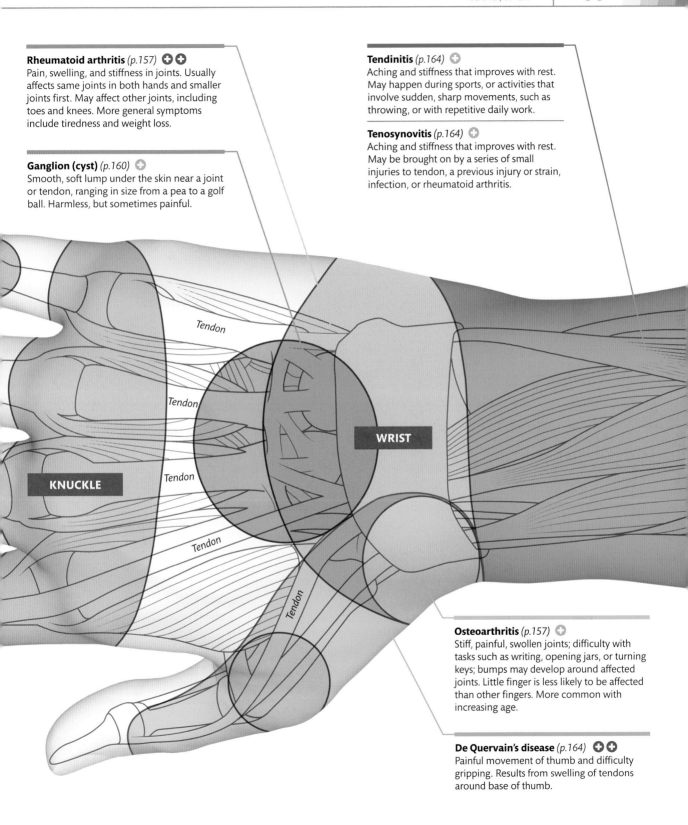
Pain, swelling, and stiffness in joints. Usually affects same joints in both hands and smaller joints first. May affect other joints, including toes and knees. More general symptoms include tiredness and weight loss.

Ganglion (cyst) *(p.160)*
Smooth, soft lump under the skin near a joint or tendon, ranging in size from a pea to a golf ball. Harmless, but sometimes painful.

Tendinitis *(p.164)*
Aching and stiffness that improves with rest. May happen during sports, or activities that involve sudden, sharp movements, such as throwing, or with repetitive daily work.

Tenosynovitis *(p.164)*
Aching and stiffness that improves with rest. May be brought on by a series of small injuries to tendon, a previous injury or strain, infection, or rheumatoid arthritis.

Tendon

Tendon

WRIST

Tendon

KNUCKLE

Tendon

Tendon

Osteoarthritis *(p.157)*
Stiff, painful, swollen joints; difficulty with tasks such as writing, opening jars, or turning keys; bumps may develop around affected joints. Little finger is less likely to be affected than other fingers. More common with increasing age.

De Quervain's disease *(p.164)*
Painful movement of thumb and difficulty gripping. Results from swelling of tendons around base of thumb.

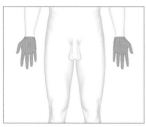

SEE ALSO Forearm and wrist
pp.82–83, **Hand, back** *pp.84–85*

HAND
PALM

The palm (front) of the hand is prone to many of the same conditions that affect the back of the hand. Some joint disorders produce pain and deformities.

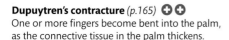

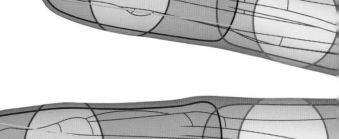

Trigger finger or thumb *(p.164)* ⊕
Finger (or thumb) clicks or locks when bent towards palm. Pain, stiffness, and a small lump in palm at base of affected digit. More common in women, people older than 40, and people with diabetes or rheumatoid arthritis.

Dupuytren's contracture *(p.165)* ⊕⊕
One or more fingers become bent into the palm, as the connective tissue in the palm thickens.

Raynaud's disease *(p.185)* ⊕⊕
Fingers turn white, numb, and cool. Bright red when warmed, causing tingling, throbbing, and pain. Sometimes other extremities (toes, ears, and nose) are affected. More common in women, people with a family history of Raynaud's disease, and smokers.

SKIN CONDITIONS

Pompholyx (dyshidrotic eczema) *(p.222)* ⊕⊕
Tiny blisters across fingers and palms of hands, and sometimes soles of feet. Can affect people of any age, but most often adults under 40.

Hand, foot, and mouth disease *(p.229)* ⊕
Small painful blisters on the fingers and palms, and mouth ulcers. Mainly affects young children. If symptoms persist more than a few days, or mouth ulcers prevent drinking fluids, seek medical advice.

Warts *(p.229)* ⊕
Small, rough lumps caused by a virus. Can be contagious. If symptoms persist, seek medical advice.

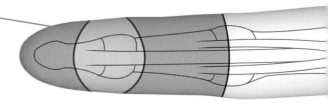

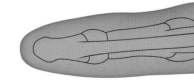

Fracture *(p.156)* ⊕⊕⊕
Pain (can be severe), tenderness, bruising, swelling, deformity, tingling, or numbness. Difficulty moving the affected finger or hand.

Hand-arm vibration syndrome *(p.185)* ⊕⊕
Numbness, tingling, and pain. Cold, white fingers. Impaired dexterity and grip.

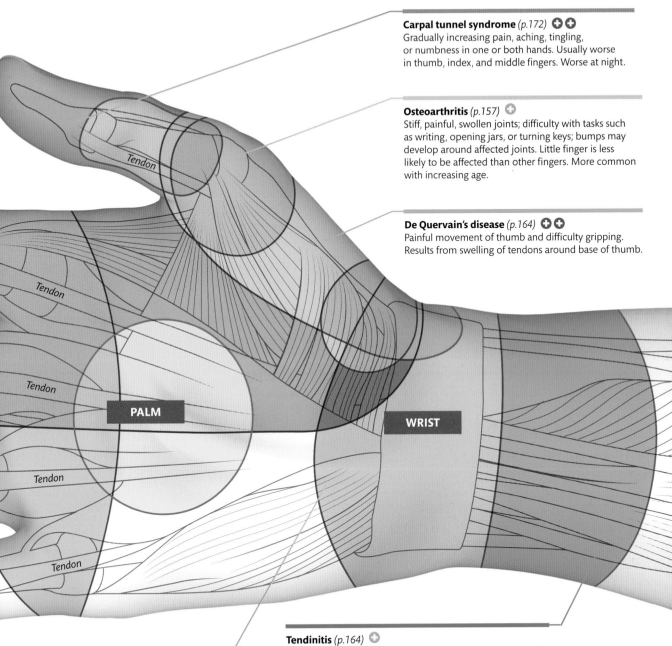

Carpal tunnel syndrome *(p.172)* ➕➕
Gradually increasing pain, aching, tingling, or numbness in one or both hands. Usually worse in thumb, index, and middle fingers. Worse at night.

Osteoarthritis *(p.157)* ➕
Stiff, painful, swollen joints; difficulty with tasks such as writing, opening jars, or turning keys; bumps may develop around affected joints. Little finger is less likely to be affected than other fingers. More common with increasing age.

De Quervain's disease *(p.164)* ➕➕
Painful movement of thumb and difficulty gripping. Results from swelling of tendons around base of thumb.

Tendon

Tendon

Tendon

PALM

WRIST

Tendon

Tendon

Rheumatoid arthritis *(p.157)* ➕➕
Pain, swelling, and stiffness in joints. Usually affects same joints in both hands and smaller joints first. May affect other joints, including toes and knees. More general symptoms include tiredness and weight loss.

Tendinitis *(p.164)* ➕
Aching and stiffness that settles with rest. May happen during sports, or activities that involve sudden, sharp movements, such as throwing, or with repetitive daily work.

Tenosynovitis *(p.164)* ➕
Aching and stiffness that settles with rest. May be brought on by a series of small injuries to the tendon, a previous injury or strain, infection, or rheumatoid arthritis. If persists, seek medical advice.

CHEST
UPPER

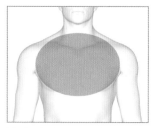

SEE ALSO Chest, central *pp.90–91*, Chest, side *pp.92–93*

Most problems in the upper chest originate from the heart and lungs, or from the stomach and gastrointestinal tract (the food gullet). Trauma can lead to a fractured bone, causing severe pain. Breathlessness is a symptom of several disorders.

Collarbone fracture *(p.156)* ✚✚
Swelling or tenderness around the injured area, bruising to the skin; numbness or pins-and-needles sensation if nerves in arm are injured.

Bronchitis *(p.193)* ✚✚
Fever, cough, headache, flu-like symptoms; green/yellow sputum.

Lung cancer *(p.195)* ✚✚✚
Pain combined with weight loss, persistent cough, and coughing up blood.

Tuberculosis *(p.236)* ✚✚✚
Chest pain with night sweats, weight loss, and coughing up blood.

Rib fracture *(p.156)* ✚
Pain that worsens with any movement of the affected area; can also cause shortness of breath as it is too painful to breath in deeply.

OESOPHAGUS

COLLARBONE

AIRWAYS

RIB

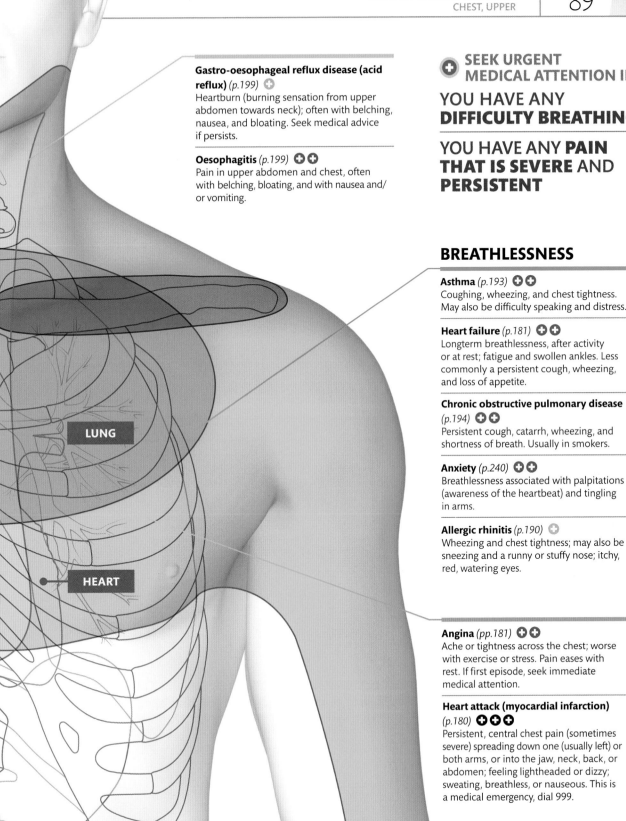

Gastro-oesophageal reflux disease (acid reflux) *(p.199)* ⊕
Heartburn (burning sensation from upper abdomen towards neck); often with belching, nausea, and bloating. Seek medical advice if persists.

Oesophagitis *(p.199)* ⊕⊕
Pain in upper abdomen and chest, often with belching, bloating, and with nausea and/or vomiting.

⊕ **SEEK URGENT MEDICAL ATTENTION IF:**

YOU HAVE ANY DIFFICULTY BREATHING

YOU HAVE ANY PAIN THAT IS SEVERE AND PERSISTENT

BREATHLESSNESS

Asthma *(p.193)* ⊕⊕
Coughing, wheezing, and chest tightness. May also be difficulty speaking and distress.

Heart failure *(p.181)* ⊕⊕
Longterm breathlessness, after activity or at rest; fatigue and swollen ankles. Less commonly a persistent cough, wheezing, and loss of appetite.

Chronic obstructive pulmonary disease *(p.194)* ⊕⊕
Persistent cough, catarrh, wheezing, and shortness of breath. Usually in smokers.

Anxiety *(p.240)* ⊕⊕
Breathlessness associated with palpitations (awareness of the heartbeat) and tingling in arms.

Allergic rhinitis *(p.190)* ⊕
Wheezing and chest tightness; may also be sneezing and a runny or stuffy nose; itchy, red, watering eyes.

Angina *(pp.181)* ⊕⊕
Ache or tightness across the chest; worse with exercise or stress. Pain eases with rest. If first episode, seek immediate medical attention.

Heart attack (myocardial infarction) *(p.180)* ⊕⊕⊕
Persistent, central chest pain (sometimes severe) spreading down one (usually left) or both arms, or into the jaw, neck, back, or abdomen; feeling lightheaded or dizzy; sweating, breathless, or nauseous. This is a medical emergency, dial 999.

LUNG

HEART

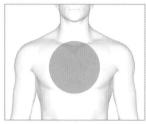

SEE ALSO Chest, side *pp.92–93*, Chest, upper *pp.88–89*, **Upper abdomen** *pp.100–01*

CHEST
CENTRAL

Pain that feels localized in the central chest area can originate from the heart, airways, or from the stomach and oesophagus (food gullet). The oesophagus passes behind the heart and any irritation of this tube can produce "heartburn".

⊕ **SEEK URGENT MEDICAL ATTENTION IF:**

YOU HAVE **SEVERE CHEST PAIN** THAT DOESN'T GET BETTER WITH REST

COUGHING UP BLOOD

Costochondritis *(p.158)* ⊕ ⊕
Sharp and stabbing pain. Painful area is tender when pressed. Worse with deep breathing or when coughing.

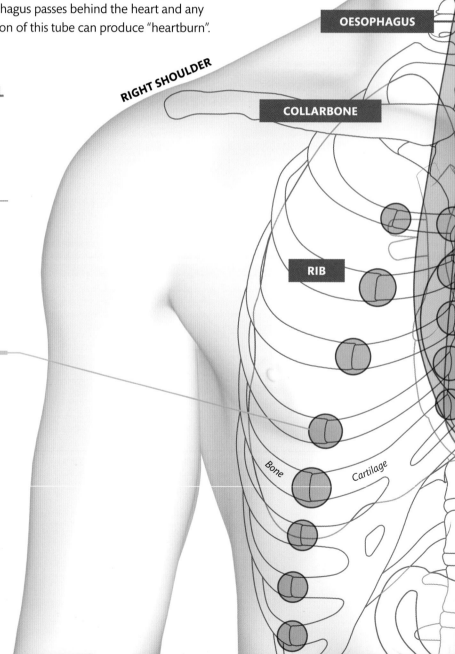

OESOPHAGUS

RIGHT SHOULDER

COLLARBONE

RIB

Bone

Cartilage

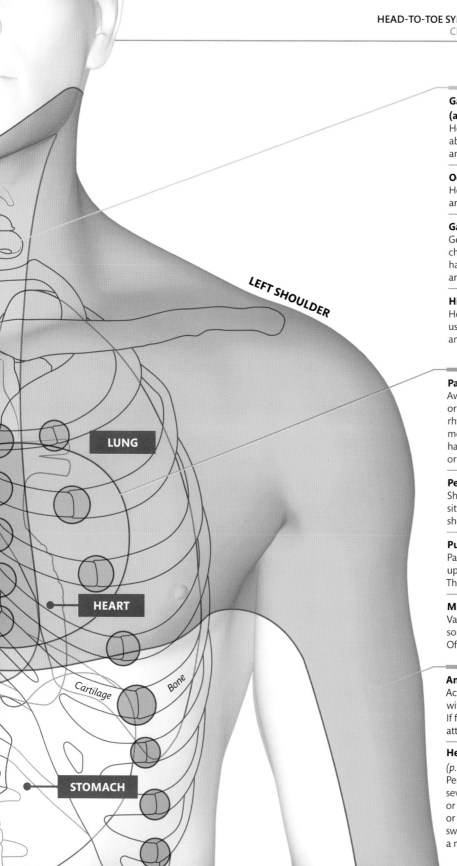

LEFT SHOULDER

LUNG

HEART

Cartilage

Bone

STOMACH

Gastro-oesophageal reflux disease (acid reflux) *(p.199)* ➕➕
Heartburn (burning sensation from upper abdomen towards neck); belching, nausea, and bloating.

Oesophagitis *(p.199)* ➕➕
Heartburn; belching, nausea and/or vomiting, and bloating.

Gastritis *(p.199)* ➕➕
Generally mild burning or pain in central chest area and left upper abdomen. May also have bloating, burping, and feel nauseous and full after a meal.

Hiatus hernia *(p.204)* ➕➕
Heartburn; pain in upper abdomen; usually with belching, bloating, and nausea and vomiting.

Palpitations *(p.181)* ➕
Awareness of heart beating fast or slow or with "skipping" beats. May indicate heart rhythm disorder (p.181). Seek immediate medical advice if pulse is irregular or if you have any shortness of breath, chest pain, or dizziness, or if sensation persists.

Pericarditis *(p.182)* ➕➕➕
Sharp central chest pain that is better when sitting or leaning forwards. May also cause shortness of breath.

Pulmonary embolism *(p.183)* ➕➕➕
Pain with breathlessness, and coughing up blood. Pain may also affect sides of chest. This is a medical emergency, dial 999.

Mitral valve prolapse *(p.182)* ➕➕
Vague, mild central chest pain and sometimes sensation of "skipping" beats. Often with exercise.

Angina *(p.181)* ➕➕
Ache or tightness across the chest; worse with exercise or stress. Pain eases with rest. If first episode, seek immediate medical attention.

Heart attack (myocardial infarction) *(p.180)* ➕➕➕
Persistent, central chest pain (sometimes severe) spreading down one (usually left) or both arms, or into the jaw, neck, back, or abdomen; feeling lightheaded or dizzy; sweating, breathless, or nauseous. This is a medical emergency, dial 999.

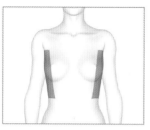

SEE ALSO Chest, upper *pp.88–89*, Chest, central *pp.90–91*

CHEST
SIDE

Injuries affecting the ribs and muscles may be felt at the side of the chest. Disorders that affect the lower part of the lung and the kidneys can also produce symptoms here. Unless otherwise stated, symptoms can occur on one or both sides.

Osteoarthritis of spine *(p.157)* ✚✚
Pain from back of chest around to front, due to pressure on nerve where it leaves the spine.

Kidney stones *(p.208)* ✚✚
Sudden, severe pain that comes and goes in waves. Pain often starts in lower back and moves to front. Fever, excessive shivering and shaking, and pain when passing urine. Blood in urine and possible vomiting. Seek medical attention soon if symptoms severe.

Kidney infection (pyelonephritis) *(p.208)* ✚✚
Fever, vomiting, blood in urine, lower back pain or pain between ribs and hips. Seek medical attention soon if symptoms severe.

KIDNEYS

SPINE

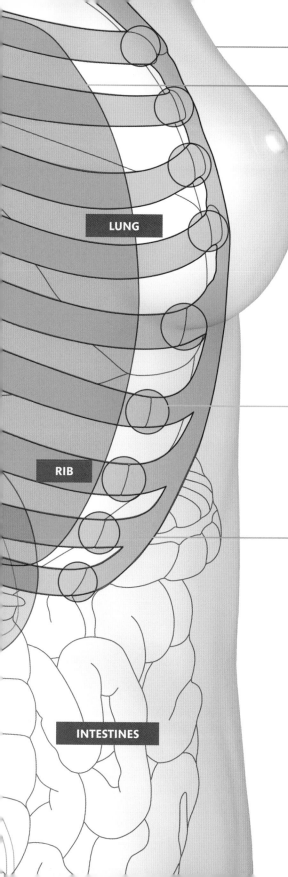

LUNG

RIB

INTESTINES

Strained muscles *(p.163)* ⊕
Pain can develop after heavy lifting or prolonged coughing. Worse when moving and breathing in deeply.

Pleurisy *(p.194)* ⊕⊕⊕
Sharp stabbing pain anywhere in chest. Fever and aching body; lethargy. Pain worse when breathing in or coughing.

Pulmonary embolism *(p.183)* ⊕⊕⊕
Pain with breathlessness; coughing with or without blood. Medical emergency, dial 999.

Pneumothorax *(p.195)* ⊕⊕⊕
Sudden, sharp stabbing pain on one side of chest with breathlessness. Pain worse with breathing in. Most common in young men.

Shingles *(p.233)* ⊕⊕
Severe pain that follows course of a nerve in the chest wall. Affects one side of chest, usually with a rash. Can cause long-term pain.

Costochondritis *(p.158)* ⊕⊕
Sharp and stabbing pain. Painful area is tender when pressed. Worse with deep breathing or when coughing.

Rib fracture *(p.156)* ⊕⊕⊕
Pain that worsens with any movement of affected area; can also cause shortness of breath because it is too painful to breathe in deeply.

Bone cancer *(p.155)* ⊕⊕⊕
Persistent and often very severe pain, usually accompanied by other symptoms, such as weight loss.

Lung cancer *(p.195)* ⊕⊕⊕
Pain (felt anywhere in chest) with shortness of breath, weight loss, persistent cough, and coughing up blood. Pain if the cancer starts to involve ribs or outer parts of lungs.

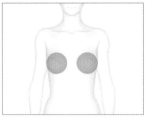

SEE ALSO Chest, central *pp.90–91*
Chest, side *pp.92–93*

BREAST

In women, the breast can change in shape, size, and appearance during puberty, pregnancy, and lactation, and over the course of the menstrual cycle and even menopause. Most breast problems occur in women and are harmless.

Eczema *(p.222)* ⊕
Scaly, itchy rash. Can be on one or both nipples.

Cracked nipples *(p.216)* ⊕⊕
Common when breastfeeding. Seek advice from a midwife, pharmacist, or health visitor.

Nipple discharge *(p.216)* ⊕⊕
May be normal for pregnant or breastfeeding woman. In menstruating woman, if does not resolve within one month, medical seek advice. If blood-stained or in a postmenopausal woman or a man, seek medical advice sooner.

Nipple inversion *(p.216)* ⊕⊕
Nipple retracts into breast. Can be present at birth, but when a normal nipple becomes inverted, seek medical advice soon.

Breast cancer *(p.216)* ⊕⊕⊕
Dimpling of skin or changes in skin around nipple, or blood-stained discharge. Usually with a hard, firm, irregular lump in the breast that does not move. Rare before mid-30s.

Intertrigo *(p.224)* ⊕⊕
Redness, burning, and itching in the skin folds under the breast. Also occurs in the armpits, and (most commonly) in the groin.

BREAST PROBLEMS IN MEN

Men have breast tissue just like women, though it is less developed. It can become enlarged due to excess weight, hormone issues, or other disorders, but these changes are generally harmless (see Gynaecomastia, p.212). Men can get breast cancer, but it is much less common than in women. Older men who find a hard lump in the breast tissue should seek urgent medical attention.

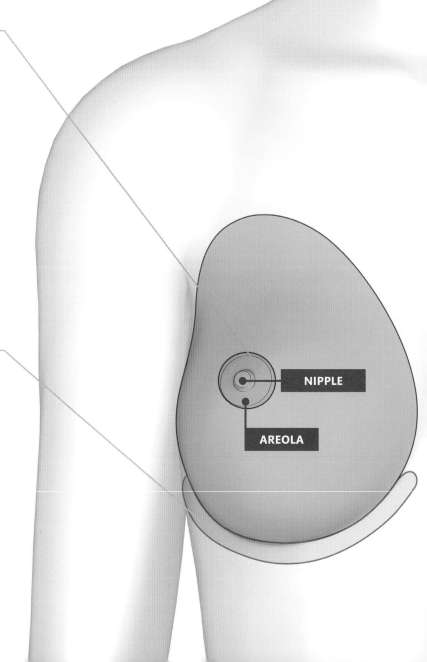

NIPPLE

AREOLA

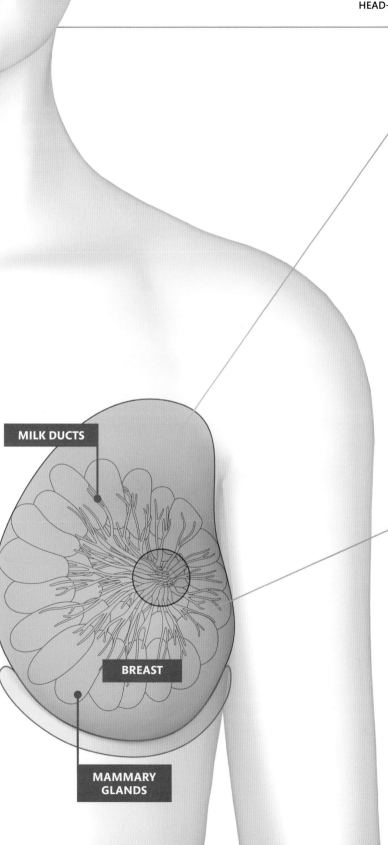

MILK DUCTS

BREAST

MAMMARY GLANDS

LUMPS

Fibrocystic breast disease *(p.217)* ⊕
Lumpy and sometimes painful breasts; usually multiple lumps that change in size with the menstrual cycle.

Fibroadenoma *(p.217)* ⊕⊕
Smooth, solid lump that moves easily when touched. Most common in women aged 20–25.

Cyst *(p.217)* ⊕⊕
Smooth lump that moves easily when touched. Often develops quite suddenly, and can be painful. Most common in women aged 30–50.

Breast cancer *(p.216)* ⊕⊕⊕
Hard, firm, irregular lump that does not move. Can have dimpling of the skin or changes in the skin around the nipple. Not usually painful. Rare before mid-30s.

Lipoma *(p.226)* ⊕⊕
Doughy lump just under the skin. Moves easily when touched. Medical advice needed to confirm diagnosis.

Fat necrosis *(p.216)* ⊕⊕
Painful lump due to injury. Medical advice needed to confirm diagnosis.

PAIN

Cyclical breast pain *(p.216)* ⊕
Monthly pain, soreness, or tenderness in one or both breasts caused by the menstrual cycle.

Breast pain *(p.216)* ⊕
Not related to menstrual cycle. May be a result of an infection or from the muscles of the chest wall. If any skin redness or warmth, seek medical advice.

Mastitis *(p.216)* ⊕⊕
Fever, redness, and pain. Usually occurs when breastfeeding.

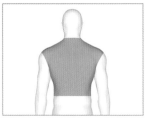

SEE ALSO Shoulder, back *pp.76–77*, Lower, back *pp.102–03*

UPPER BACK

Most of the problems in the upper back come from the muscles in the back or the bones of the spine, with muscle pain often made worse by moving. Problems in the front of the chest or upper abdomen can also lead to upper back pain.

Muscular pain *(pp.163)* ⊕
Pain related to poor posture and strain such as from carrying bags and using computers. Worse in certain positions.

Lung cancer *(p.195)* ⊕⊕⊕
Severe and persistent upper back pain. Persistent cough, coughing up blood, and weight loss. Most common in smokers.

Stomach ulcer *(p.200)* ⊕⊕
Gnawing pain that penetrates through to back. Usually associated with heartburn and feeling unwell after eating, with nausea and vomiting.

Pancreatitis *(p.202)* ⊕⊕⊕
Deep, penetrating back pain that is often severe and relentless. May have nausea, vomiting, and loss of appetite. Usually associated with jaundice (yellowing of skin and eyes) and weight loss.

Cancer of pancreas *(p.202)* ⊕⊕⊕
Deep, penetrating back pain that is often severe and relentless. May have nausea, vomiting, and loss of appetite. Usually associated with jaundice and weight loss.

Ruptured abdominal aortic aneurysm *(p.184)* ⊕⊕⊕
Pain in abdomen, back, or chest. Often associated with older age (men over 60), especially those with high blood pressure. This is a medical emergency, dial 999.

Kidney infection (pyelonephritis) *(p.208)* ⊕⊕
Pain usually in one side, often with fever, shaking, shivering, and blood in urine.

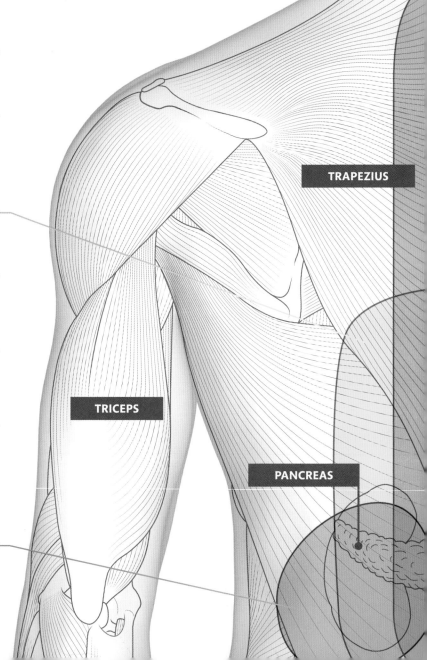

TRAPEZIUS

TRICEPS

PANCREAS

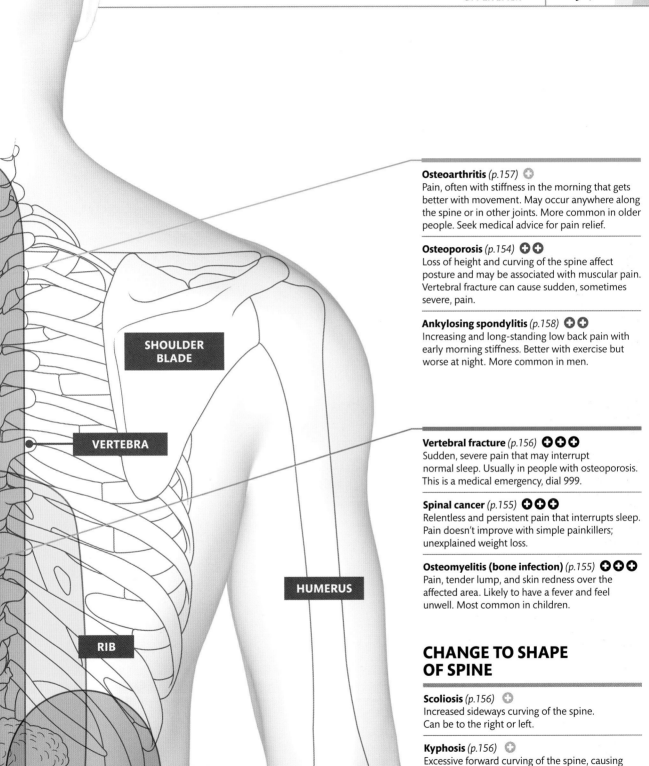

SHOULDER BLADE

VERTEBRA

HUMERUS

RIB

KIDNEY

Osteoarthritis *(p.157)* ✚
Pain, often with stiffness in the morning that gets better with movement. May occur anywhere along the spine or in other joints. More common in older people. Seek medical advice for pain relief.

Osteoporosis *(p.154)* ✚ ✚
Loss of height and curving of the spine affect posture and may be associated with muscular pain. Vertebral fracture can cause sudden, sometimes severe, pain.

Ankylosing spondylitis *(p.158)* ✚ ✚
Increasing and long-standing low back pain with early morning stiffness. Better with exercise but worse at night. More common in men.

Vertebral fracture *(p.156)* ✚ ✚ ✚
Sudden, severe pain that may interrupt normal sleep. Usually in people with osteoporosis. This is a medical emergency, dial 999.

Spinal cancer *(p.155)* ✚ ✚ ✚
Relentless and persistent pain that interrupts sleep. Pain doesn't improve with simple painkillers; unexplained weight loss.

Osteomyelitis (bone infection) *(p.155)* ✚ ✚ ✚
Pain, tender lump, and skin redness over the affected area. Likely to have a fever and feel unwell. Most common in children.

CHANGE TO SHAPE OF SPINE

Scoliosis *(p.156)* ✚
Increased sideways curving of the spine. Can be to the right or left.

Kyphosis *(p.156)* ✚
Excessive forward curving of the spine, causing a hump. Often develops gradually. Seek medical advice if painful or breathing is difficult.

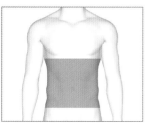

ABDOMEN
GENERAL

Abdominal pain is sometimes difficult
to pinpoint. Generalized pain can have several
causes: some of them may be associated with
vomiting, diarrhoea, or constipation. In children,
abdominal pain can be a sign of a problem
elsewhere in the body.

⊕ SEEK URGENT MEDICAL ATTENTION IF:

YOU HAVE **SUDDEN, SEVERE STOMACH PAIN**

YOU ARE **VOMITING BLOOD**

YOU HAVE **BLOODY** OR **BLACK, STICKY STOOLS**

Appendicitis *(p.205)* ⊕⊕⊕
Pain felt generally or in centre of abdomen. Within hours,
pain travels to lower right-hand side and becomes
constant and severe.

Peritonitis *(p.205)* ⊕⊕⊕
Severe abdominal pain that usually begins suddenly but
can start more gradually. Tense and hard belly. Feeling very
unwell; fever; pale and sweaty. Medical emergency, dial 999.

Parasitic infection *(p.237)* ⊕⊕
Parasites such as *Giardia* (p.237) may cause abdominal
pain or cramping; wind and bloating; weight loss.

Sickle cell crises *(p.186)* ⊕⊕⊕
Severe crippling pain that can affect many parts
of body, including the abdomen. More common
in people of African, Caribbean, Middle Eastern,
Eastern Mediterranean, and South Asian origin.

Cirrhosis *(p.201)* ⊕⊕
Pain and swelling of abdomen and legs. Tiredness, poor
appetite, and easy bruising and bleeding. Jaundice
(yellowing of skin and eyes) and itching. Confusion.

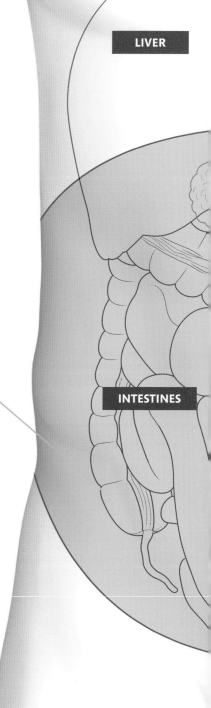

LIVER

INTESTINES

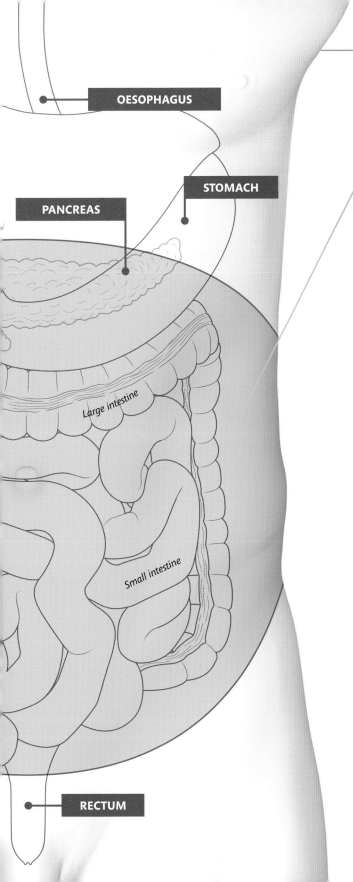

OESOPHAGUS

STOMACH

PANCREAS

Large intestine

Small intestine

RECTUM

WITH DIARRHOEA OR CONSTIPATION

Gastroenteritis *(p.196)*
Upper abdominal pain or tenderness, but can be all over abdomen. Nausea and/or vomiting and diarrhoea. Seek medical advice if vomiting frequently, if symptoms are persistent, and in children.

Food poisoning *(p.197)*
Generalized pain, but can be felt in any part of abdomen; nausea and/or vomiting and diarrhoea. Seek medical advice if vomiting frequently, if symptoms are persistent, and in children.

Irritable bowel syndrome *(p.203)*
Episodes of pain anywhere in abdomen with diarrhoea and/or constipation. Can have mucus in the stools. Bloating and excessive wind.

Lactose intolerance
Wind, abdomen pain, bloating, and diarrhoea.

Diverticulitis *(p.205)*
Pain all over abdomen or on lower left side; change in bowel habits (such as diarrhoea or constipation), and fever.

Diverticular disease *(p.205)*
Often lower abdominal discomfort and tenderness, but can be all over abdomen. Bleeding and passing mucus with stools; diarrhoea and/or constipation.

Coeliac disease *(p.204)*
Abdominal pain associated with diarrhoea or constipation; tiredness and itching. May have smelly stools and anaemia.

Crohn's disease *(p.203)*
Pain anywhere in abdomen. May cause diarrhoea mixed with blood or mucus. Often with cracks around anus. Weight loss, anaemia, fever, and feeling unwell. Symptoms come and go.

STOMACH PAIN IN CHILDREN

In children under 8 years, the source of pain is not necessarily the same as where it is felt. Abdominal pain may actually be a sign of ear infection, sore throat *(p.192)*, emotional distress, constipation *(p.196)*, or urinary tract infection *(p.209)*. Usually, other symptoms are present too, such as vomiting, diarrhoea, blood in stools, or constipation.

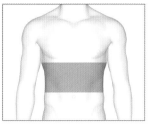

SEE ALSO Chest, central *pp.90–91,* Abdomen, general *pp.98–99*

UPPER ABDOMEN

This contains the stomach, spleen, liver, gallbladder, pancreas, and duodenum. Pain is the most common symptom experienced here. Others include bloating, vomiting, poor appetite, weight loss, jaundice, and heartburn. If you vomit blood you should seek urgent medical advice.

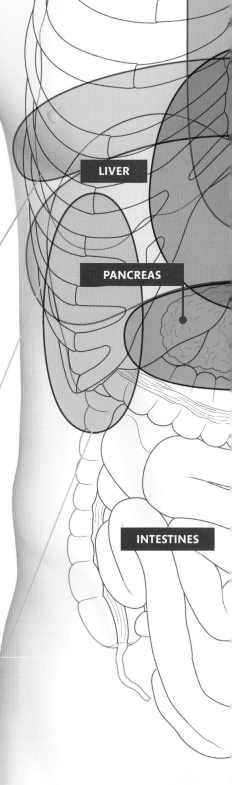

LIVER

PANCREAS

INTESTINES

Costochondritis *(p.158)* ✚ ✚
Sharp and stabbing pain. Painful area is tender when pressed. Worse with deep breaths or when coughing.

Pneumonia *(p.194)* ✚ ✚
Abdominal pain (either side of body), with cough, fever, coughing blood, and generally feeling unwell.

Pleurisy *(p.194)* ✚ ✚ ✚
Pain breathing in, may be felt in side of chest and abdomen (either side); coughing blood.

Hepatitis *(p.200)* ✚ ✚
Jaundice (yellowing of skin and eyes) and itchy skin. Feeling generally unwell, tiredness, and right-sided abdominal discomfort.

Cirrhosis *(p.201)* ✚ ✚
Pain and swelling of abdomen and legs. Tiredness, poor appetite, and bruising and bleeding easily. Jaundice and itch. May also be confusion.

Liver cancer *(p.201)* ✚ ✚ ✚
Upper right abdominal pain, jaundice, swollen abdomen, and general itching.

Leptospirosis *(p.236)* ✚ ✚
Jaundice, itchy skin. Feeling generally unwell, tiredness, and right-sided discomfort.

Liver flukes *(p.238)* ✚ ✚
Jaundice, flu-like symptoms, tiredness, and right-sided discomfort.

Amoebiasis *(p.237)* ✚ ✚
General lower abdominal pain with bloody diarrhoea. More common in countries with limited access to good sanitation and clean water and in people travelling from these areas.

Hydatid cyst *(p.238)* ✚ ✚
Abdominal pain, with jaundice, flu-like symptoms, tiredness, and right-sided abdominal discomfort. It develops over a period of years. Usually in travellers to and immigrants from Africa, Asia, the Middle East, and Central and South America.

Gallstones *(p.202)* ✚ ✚
Intermittent episodes of spasmodic pain; with nausea and vomiting. Can be associated with jaundice (yellowing of skin and eyes).

Cholangitis *(p.201)* ✚ ✚ ✚
Constant pain in right side, just below ribcage; fever and chills; jaundice.

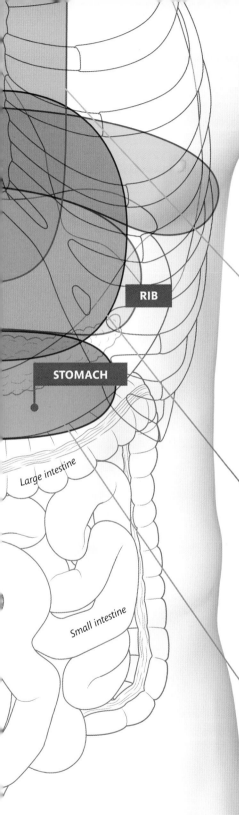

RIB

STOMACH

Large intestine

Small intestine

⊕ SEEK URGENT MEDICAL ATTENTION IF:
YOU HAVE **PERSISTENT ABDOMINAL PAIN**
OR YOU **VOMIT BLOOD**

Gastro-oesophageal reflux disease (dyspepsia/acid reflux) *(p.199)* ⊕
Pain in upper abdomen and/or upper central chest. Belching, nausea, and bloating. Seek medical advice if continues.

Gastritis *(p.199)* ⊕
Generally mild central chest and left upper abdominal burning or pain. May also cause bloating, burping, and feelings of nausea and fullness after a meal.

Angina *(p.181)* ⊕⊕
Ache or tightness across the chest; worse with exercise or stress. Pain eases with rest. If first episode, seek immediate medical attention.

Heart attack *(p.180)* ⊕⊕⊕
Persistent, central chest pain (sometimes severe) spreading down one (usually left) or both arms, or into the jaw, neck, back, or abdomen; feeling lightheaded or dizzy; sweating, breathless, or nauseous. This is a medical emergency, dial 999.

Gastroenteritis *(p.196)* ⊕
Pain with nausea/vomiting and diarrhoea. Seek medical advice in children or if persistent or very frequent vomiting.

Stomach ulcer *(p.200)* ⊕⊕
Intermittent central and/or left or right-sided gnawing, burning pain. May have loss of appetite, feel bloated, and burp or belch. May feel sick and full after a meal.

Stomach cancer *(p.200)* ⊕⊕⊕
Pain in upper abdomen. Weight loss and poor appetite. May have indigestion and nausea. Feeling unwell and anaemic (fatigue and pale skin); dark blood in the stools.

Perforated ulcer *(p.200)* ⊕⊕⊕
Severe pain in central upper abdomen; smelly black stools or obvious blood in stools; may vomit blood. May collapse. This is a medical emergency, dial 999.

Pancreatic cancer *(p.202)* ⊕⊕⊕
Severe upper abdominal pain that may spread to back. Associated with weight loss, nausea and vomiting, and jaundice (yellowing of skin and eyes).

Acute pancreatitis *(p.202)* ⊕⊕⊕
Severe pain in centre of abdomen that develops over a few days. Associated with vomiting, diarrhoea, fever, and feeling generally unwell.

Chronic pancreatitis *(p.202)* ⊕⊕
Repeated episodes of abdominal pain that may be severe. May spread to back. Stools (faeces) are pale and smelly. More common in men over 40.

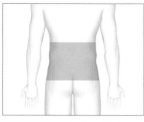

SEE ALSO Upper back *pp.96–97*, Buttocks and anus *pp.120–21*, Hip, back *pp.130–31*

LOWER BACK

The lower back is a frame that allows us to walk upright. Most problems here come from muscles in the lower back or bones of the spine (vertebrae). Pain is the most common symptom.

PANCREAS

KIDNEY

GLUTEUS MAXIMUS

⊕ SEEK URGENT MEDICAL ATTENTION IF:

YOU HAVE **SEVERE PAIN**

ARE **UNABLE TO PASS URINE** OR **CONTROL BOWEL MOVEMENTS**

HAVE **WEAKNESS IN ONE** OR **BOTH LEGS**

Kidney infection (pyelonephritis) *(p.208)* ⊕ ⊕
Pain, usually on just one side; often with fever, shaking, shivering, and blood in urine. More common in women. Seek medical attention soon if symptoms severe.

Kidney stones *(p.208)* ⊕ ⊕ ⊕
Pain that comes and goes, beginning in lower back and moving to abdomen. May need to pass urine more often; possibly with blood in urine.

Ruptured abdominal aortic aneurysm *(p.184)* ⊕ ⊕ ⊕
Pain in the abdomen, back, or chest. Often associated with older age (men over 60), especially with high blood pressure. This is a medical emergency, dial 999.

Muscle strain *(p.163)* ⊕
Short-term pain, but can come and go. Responds to heat and simple painkillers.

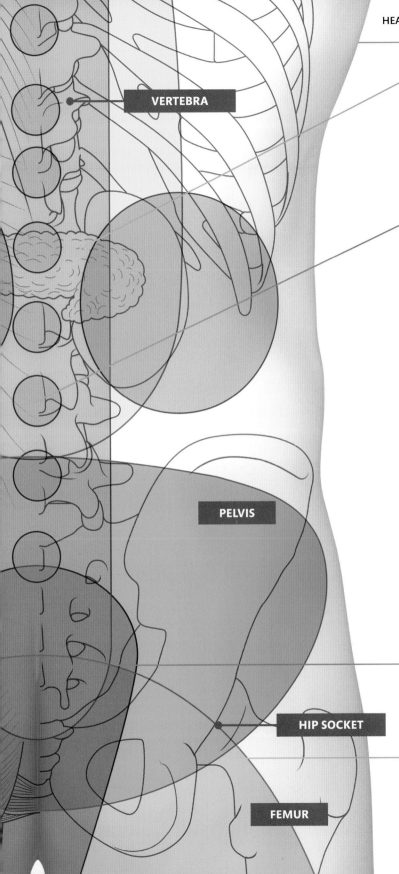

VERTEBRA

PELVIS

HIP SOCKET

FEMUR

Osteoarthritis *(p.157)* ⊕
Back pain often with stiffness in morning that gets better with movement. May be associated with pain in other joints. Seek medical advice for pain relief.

Osteoporosis *(p.154)* ⊕ ⊕
Loss of height and curving of the spine affect posture and may be associated with muscular pain. Vertebral fracture can cause sudden, sometimes severe, pain.

Vertebral fracture *(p.156)* ⊕ ⊕ ⊕
Sudden, severe pain, most common in middle or lower spine. Worse when standing or moving. This is a medical emergency, dial 999.

Rheumatoid arthritis *(p.157)* ⊕ ⊕
Pain and stiffness. May affect several other joints, including toes and wrists. More general symptoms include mild fever, aches, tiredness, and weight loss.

Bone cancer *(p.155)* ⊕ ⊕ ⊕
Often pain is relentless and worse at night. Not affected by position. Fails to respond to painkillers.

Spondylolisthesis *(p.158)* ⊕ ⊕
Pain and stiffness, usually worse when leaning backwards. Most common in physically active adolescents and young people.

Spondylolysis *(p.154)* ⊕ ⊕
Pain from a stress fracture in lower back. Often causes pain in a specific area when playing sports. Most common in adolescents.

Ankylosing spondylitis *(p.158)* ⊕ ⊕
Increasing and long-standing low back pain with early morning stiffness. Better with exercise but worse at night. More common in men.

Slipped disc *(p.158)* ⊕ ⊕
Severe low back pain accompanied by sciatica (p.173). Can have tingling, weakness, and/or numbness. Worse with moving, coughing, or sneezing.

Cauda equina syndrome *(p.171)* ⊕ ⊕ ⊕
Low back pain and numbness around sacrum. Bladder and bowel disturbance; usually inability to pass urine or to control bowel movements. Weakness in one or both legs. This is a medical emergency, dial 999.

Sciatica *(p.173)* ⊕
Low back pain associated with pain down leg to calf or big toe. May lead to a pins-and-needles sensation and numbness or weakness in buttock, leg, or foot. If symptoms persist, seek medical advice.

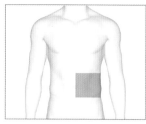

SEE ALSO Abdomen, general
pp.98–99, **Lower abdomen, right**
pp.106–07

LOWER ABDOMEN
LEFT

This contains part of the large intestine and is where the solid matter from the digestive processes is stored and expelled periodically. If you have bleeding from the rectum, either bright red or mixed in with the stools, then you should seek medical advice. If you have discharge from your rectum or a change in your bowel habits, you should also see your doctor.

LIVER

Gastroenteritis *(p.196)* ✚
General lower abdominal pain or pain felt specifically anywhere in abdomen. Associated with nausea and/or vomiting and diarrhoea. Seek medical advice in children or in those with persistent or very frequent vomiting.

Food poisoning *(p.197)* ✚
General lower abdominal pain or pain felt specifically anywhere in abdomen after eating contaminated food. Associated with nausea and/or vomiting and diarrhoea.

Irritable bowel syndrome *(p.203)* ✚✚
Episodes of pain anywhere in abdomen with diarrhoea and/or constipation. Can have mucus in the stools. Bloating and excessive wind.

Dysentery *(p.237)* ✚✚
Bloody diarrhoea often with mucus. Abdominal cramps and fever. Can cause dehydration, especially in children and elderly people who should seek urgent medical advice.

Amoebiasis *(p.237)* ✚✚
General lower abdominal pain with bloody diarrhoea. More common in countries with limited access to good sanitation and clean water and in people travelling from these areas.

Crohn's disease *(p.203)* ✚✚
Pain anywhere in abdomen and feeling of fullness. Can cause diarrhoea mixed with blood or mucus. Weight loss, anaemia, and feeling unwell. Episodic. Often with anal fissures. More common in young adults.

Cholera *(p.235)* ✚✚✚
Profuse watery diarrhoea that can quickly lead to severe dehydration and death. Often occurs following natural disasters, as it is transmitted by contaminated water.

Bowel obstruction *(p.204)* ✚✚✚
Pain in lower abdomen and vomiting; not passing wind nor having bowels move. Abdomen is tense (hard) and often bloated.

Volvulus *(p.204)* ✚✚✚
Pain and symptoms of bowel obstruction (see above). Abdomen is tense (hard) and often bloated. More common in elderly people.

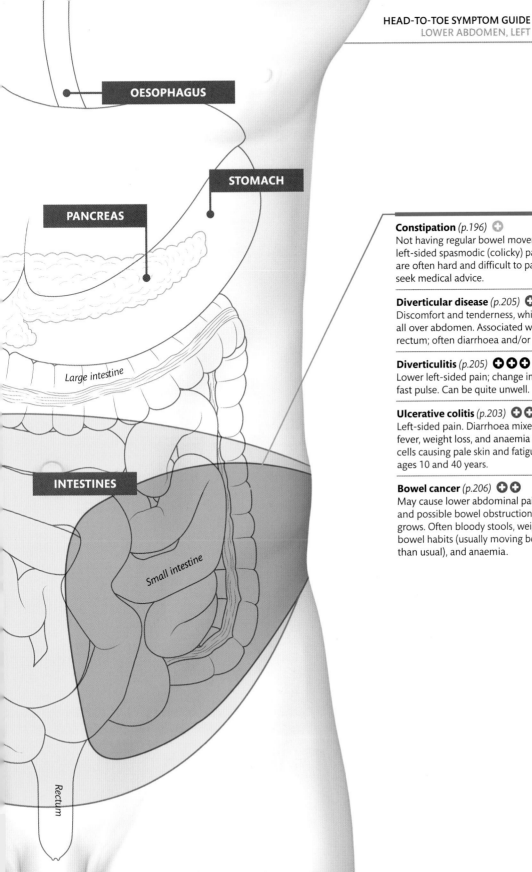

OESOPHAGUS

STOMACH

PANCREAS

Large intestine

INTESTINES

Small intestine

Rectum

Constipation *(p.196)*
Not having regular bowel movements can cause lower left-sided spasmodic (colicky) pain and discomfort. Stools are often hard and difficult to pass. If symptoms persist, seek medical advice.

Diverticular disease *(p.205)*
Discomfort and tenderness, which can be left-sided or all over abdomen. Associated with blood and mucus from rectum; often diarrhoea and/or constipation.

Diverticulitis *(p.205)*
Lower left-sided pain; change in bowel habits, fever, and fast pulse. Can be quite unwell.

Ulcerative colitis *(p.203)*
Left-sided pain. Diarrhoea mixed with blood. Unwell with fever, weight loss, and anaemia (low number of red blood cells causing pale skin and fatigue). Usually starts between ages 10 and 40 years.

Bowel cancer *(p.206)*
May cause lower abdominal pain (usually left-sided) and possible bowel obstruction (see opposite) as cancer grows. Often bloody stools, weight loss, change in bowel habits (usually moving bowels more often than usual), and anaemia.

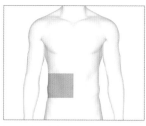

SEE ALSO Abdomen, general
pp.98–99, **Lower abdomen, left**
pp.104–05, **Female lower abdomen**
pp.108–09

LOWER ABDOMEN
RIGHT

The end of the small intestine and start of the large intestine sit in the lower right side of the abdomen. Here also is the appendix as well as (in women) the right ovary and right fallopian tube. Pain is a common symptom that can be caused by appendicitis, an appendix abscess, and infection, as well as irritable bowel syndrome.

➕ **SEEK URGENT MEDICAL ATTENTION IF:**

PAIN IS **PERSISTENT** OR **SEVERE**

Mesenteric adenitis *(p.188)* ➕ ➕
Pain and associated viral illness (usually a sore throat). May have swollen lymph nodes. Common in children under 15 years old.

Appendix abscess *(p.205)* ➕ ➕
Pain in centre of abdomen that may come and go. Pain may disappear for a long time but then recur. May progress to appendicitis (below).

Appendicitis *(p.205)* ➕ ➕ ➕
Pain in centre of abdomen that may come and go. Within hours, the pain travels to lower right-hand side and becomes constant and severe. Often with fever and vomiting and feeling unwell.

Meckel's diverticulum *(pp.203)* ➕ ➕ ➕
Symptoms can be similar to those of appendicitis: pain that develops over 6–24 hours. May start around the belly button and then move to right lower abdomen. Associated with fever and vomiting and feeling unwell.

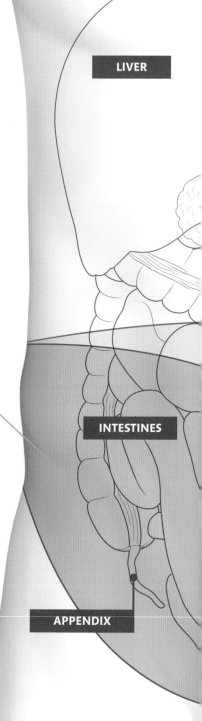

LIVER

INTESTINES

APPENDIX

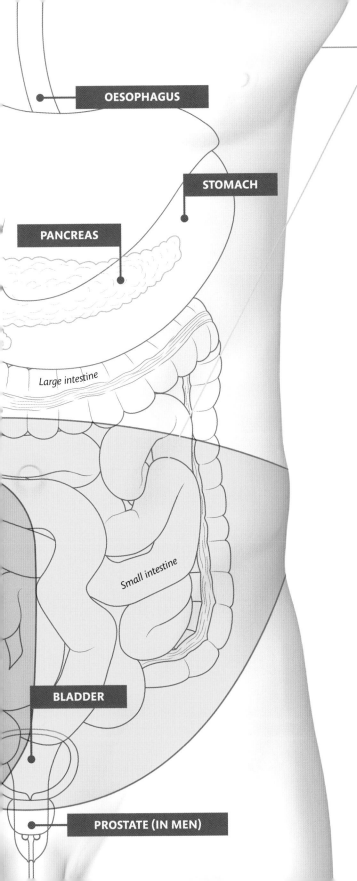

OESOPHAGUS

STOMACH

PANCREAS

Large intestine

Small intestine

BLADDER

PROSTATE (IN MEN)

Gastroenteritis *(p.196)*
General lower abdominal pain or pain felt specifically anywhere in abdomen. Associated with nausea and/or vomiting and diarrhoea. Seek medical advice in children or in those with persistent or very frequent vomiting.

Food poisoning *(p.197)*
General lower abdominal pain or pain felt specifically anywhere in abdomen after eating contaminated food. Associated with nausea and/or vomiting and diarrhoea.

Irritable bowel syndrome *(p.203)*
Episodes of pain anywhere in abdomen with diarrhoea and/or constipation. Can have mucus in the stools. Bloating and excessive wind.

Crohn's disease *(p.203)*
Pain anywhere in abdomen and feeling of fullness. Can cause diarrhoea mixed with blood or mucus. Weight loss, anaemia and feeling unwell. Episodic. Often with anal fissures. More common in young adults.

Diverticular disease *(p.205)*
Discomfort and tenderness, which can be all over abdomen. Associated with blood and mucus from rectum; often with diarrhoea and/or constipation.

Cholera *(p.235)*
Profuse watery diarrhoea that can quickly lead to severe dehydration and death. Often occurs following natural disasters as it is transmitted by contaminated water.

Dysentery *(p.237)*
Bloody diarrhoea often with mucus. Abdominal cramps and fever. Can cause dehydration, especially in children and elderly people, who should seek urgent medical advice.

Amoebiasis *(p.237)*
General lower abdominal pain with bloody diarrhoea. More common in warmer climates where there is limited access to good sanitation and clean water.

Bowel obstruction *(p.204)*
Pain in lower abdomen and vomiting; not passing wind nor having bowels move. Abdomen is tense (hard) and often bloated.

Volvulus *(p.204)*
Pain and symptoms of bowel obstruction (see above). Abdomen is tense (hard) and often bloated. More common in elderly people.

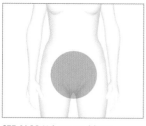

SEE ALSO Urinary problems, female *pp.112–13*, Female genitals *pp.114–15*

FEMALE LOWER ABDOMEN

The female reproductive organs, which include the ovaries, fallopian tubes, uterus, and vagina, are situated in the woman's pelvis. Abnormal bleeding, pain, and discharge are common symptoms here.

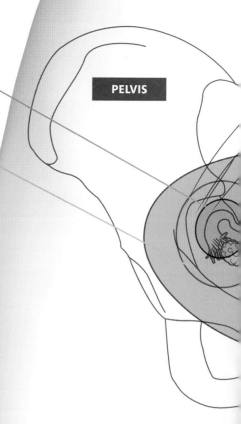

PELVIS

Mittelschmerz *(p.213)* ✚
Pain that occurs most months, usually on the side of the ovary that is releasing an egg (half-way between periods).

Ovarian cyst *(p.213)* ✚✚
Dull lower abdominal discomfort; heaviness in abdomen; pain during intercourse or bowel movements.

Ovarian cancer *(p.213)* ✚✚
Vague symptoms that include a feeling of pressure in lower abdomen; persistent bloating, and painful intercourse. Also, weight loss, generally feeling unwell, and changes to frequency of passing urine.

DURING PREGNANCY

Problems in pregnancy may be checked out by a doctor or midwife. If there is bleeding, seek medical advice straight away.

Miscarriage *(p.217)* ✚✚
Vaginal bleeding followed by abdominal pain and passing of blood clots. Seek medical advice to ascertain diagnosis and, if pregnancy is far enough along, whether infant could survive.

Ectopic pregnancy *(p.217)* ✚✚✚
Sharp lower abdominal pain that may come and go, vaginal bleeding, heavier or lighter than a normal period. May be weak and dizzy. This is a medical emergency, dial 999.

Placental abruption *(p.217)* ✚✚✚
Bleeding, continuous pain in abdomen or back, and contractions. Lack of fetal movements. More likely in late pregnancy. Medical emergency, dial 999.

Premature labour *(p.217)* ✚✚✚
Labour (signalled by regular uterine contractions) that starts before 37 weeks of pregnancy is defined as premature. Seek urgent medical advice, especially if occurs early in pregnancy.

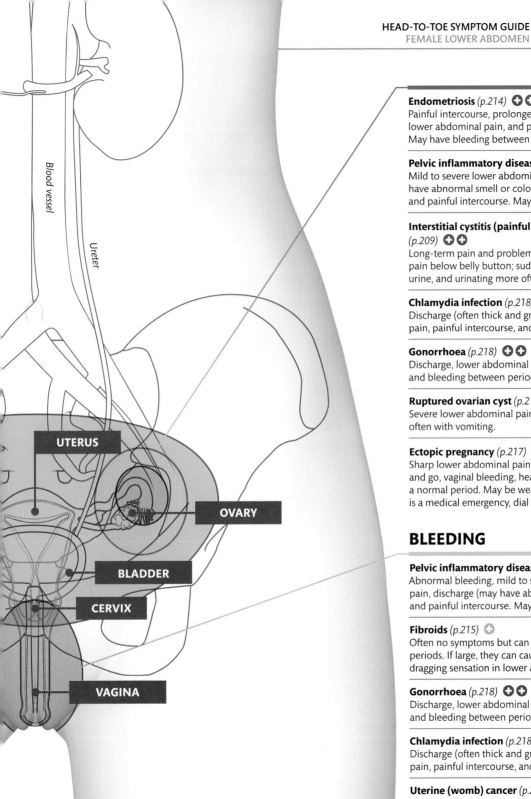

Blood vessel

Ureter

UTERUS

OVARY

BLADDER

CERVIX

VAGINA

Endometriosis *(p.214)* ⊕⊕
Painful intercourse, prolonged period pain, general lower abdominal pain, and problems conceiving. May have bleeding between periods.

Pelvic inflammatory disease *(p.213)* ⊕⊕
Mild to severe lower abdominal pain. Discharge (may have abnormal smell or colour), abnormal bleeding, and painful intercourse. May have fever and backache.

Interstitial cystitis (painful bladder syndrome) *(p.209)* ⊕⊕
Long-term pain and problems passing urine. Intense pain below belly button; sudden, strong urges to pass urine, and urinating more often than normal.

Chlamydia infection *(p.218)* ⊕⊕
Discharge (often thick and green), lower abdominal pain, painful intercourse, and bleeding between periods.

Gonorrhoea *(p.218)* ⊕⊕
Discharge, lower abdominal pain, painful intercourse, and bleeding between periods.

Ruptured ovarian cyst *(p.213)* ⊕⊕⊕
Severe lower abdominal pain if cyst twists or ruptures; often with vomiting.

Ectopic pregnancy *(p.217)* ⊕⊕⊕
Sharp lower abdominal pain that may come and go, vaginal bleeding, heavier or lighter than a normal period. May be weak and dizzy. This is a medical emergency, dial 999.

BLEEDING

Pelvic inflammatory disease *(p.213)* ⊕⊕
Abnormal bleeding, mild to severe lower abdominal pain, discharge (may have abnormal smell or colour), and painful intercourse. May have fever and backache.

Fibroids *(p.215)* ⊕
Often no symptoms but can cause heavy and prolonged periods. If large, they can cause heaviness and a dragging sensation in lower abdomen.

Gonorrhoea *(p.218)* ⊕⊕
Discharge, lower abdominal pain, painful intercourse, and bleeding between periods.

Chlamydia infection *(p.218)* ⊕⊕
Discharge (often thick and green), lower abdominal pain, painful intercourse, and bleeding between periods.

Uterine (womb) cancer *(p.214)* ⊕⊕
Abnormal bleeding. May be lower abdominal pain and bloating. More common in older women who have never had a baby or are overweight.

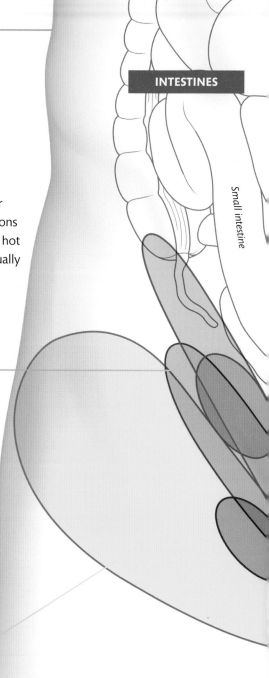

INTESTINES

Small intestine

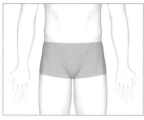

SEE ALSO Female lower abdomen
pp.108–09, **Female genitals**
pp.114–15, **Male genitals** *pp.118–19*

GROIN
MALE AND FEMALE

The groin is the hollow between the upper thigh and the lower abdomen. Skin infections are very common here as the area is often hot and sweaty. Swelling is common and is usually related to a lymph node or hernia.

SKIN CONDITIONS

Sebaceous cyst *(p.225)* ✚✚
A painless and harmless fluid filled lump. May be one or several.

Genital warts *(p.218)* ✚✚
Small, fleshy lumps in the groin area; typically firm and with a rough surface. Usually sexually transmitted.

Skin abscess *(p.228)* ✚✚
Painful lump with redness; can discharge pus.

Dermatitis *(p.222)* ✚✚
Itchy and red skin. Often associated with dermatitis or eczema in other areas.

Intertrigo *(p.224)* ✚✚
Redness and itching in skin folds that is made worse by heat and moisture. Also often occurs under breast and armpit. More common in people who are overweight.

Jock itch (tinea cruris) *(p.230)* ✚✚
Redness and itching due to fungal infection. More common in young men.

Groin strain *(p.163)* ✚✚
Pain in groin and upper thigh when moving or exercising. Usually occurs after playing sports.

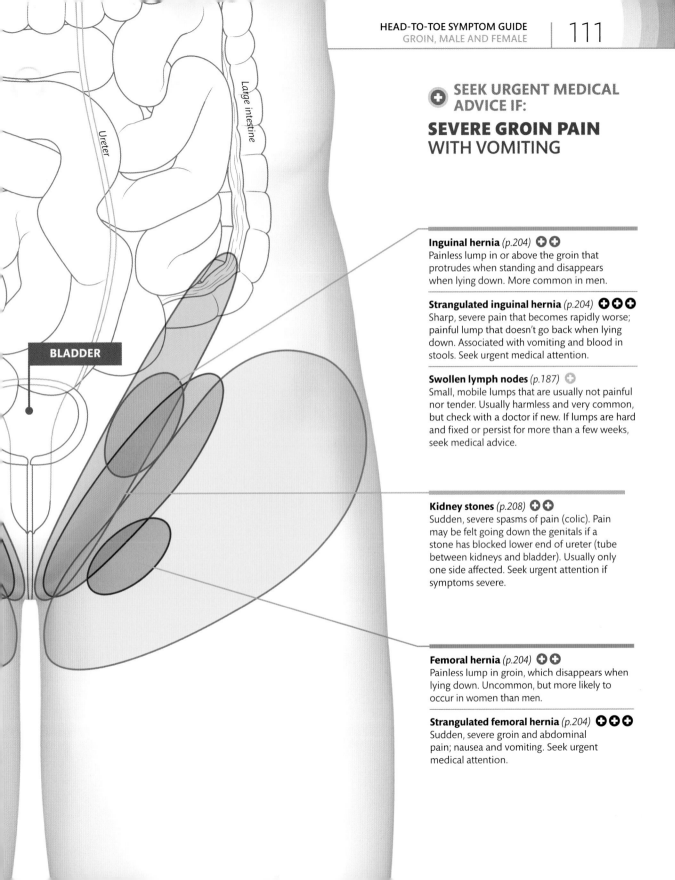

Large intestine

Ureter

BLADDER

⊕ SEEK URGENT MEDICAL ADVICE IF:
SEVERE GROIN PAIN
WITH VOMITING

Inguinal hernia *(p.204)* ⊕ ⊕
Painless lump in or above the groin that protrudes when standing and disappears when lying down. More common in men.

Strangulated inguinal hernia *(p.204)* ⊕ ⊕ ⊕
Sharp, severe pain that becomes rapidly worse; painful lump that doesn't go back when lying down. Associated with vomiting and blood in stools. Seek urgent medical attention.

Swollen lymph nodes *(p.187)* ⊕
Small, mobile lumps that are usually not painful nor tender. Usually harmless and very common, but check with a doctor if new. If lumps are hard and fixed or persist for more than a few weeks, seek medical advice.

Kidney stones *(p.208)* ⊕ ⊕
Sudden, severe spasms of pain (colic). Pain may be felt going down the genitals if a stone has blocked lower end of ureter (tube between kidneys and bladder). Usually only one side affected. Seek urgent attention if symptoms severe.

Femoral hernia *(p.204)* ⊕ ⊕
Painless lump in groin, which disappears when lying down. Uncommon, but more likely to occur in women than men.

Strangulated femoral hernia *(p.204)* ⊕ ⊕ ⊕
Sudden, severe groin and abdominal pain; nausea and vomiting. Seek urgent medical attention.

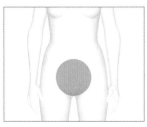

SEE ALSO Lower abdomen, left
pp.104–05, **Lower abdomen,
right** *pp.106–07*, **Female lower
abdomen** *pp.108–09*

URINARY PROBLEMS
FEMALE

Infections of the urinary tract are very common in women and cause pain (and sometimes blood) when passing urine. If the infection travels to the kidneys, it can cause fever, vomiting, and severe back pain.

PROBLEMS WITH CONTROL

Stress incontinence *(p.209)* ⊕
Urine leaks out at times when bladder is under pressure – for example, when coughing, sneezing, or exercising.

Urge incontinence *(p.209)* ⊕
A sudden, intense urge to pass urine. May leak small amounts of urine.

Overactive bladder *(p.209)* ⊕
Urge to urinate frequently; passing small amounts of urine. Often getting up in the night to urinate.

Chronic urinary retention *(p.210)* ⊕
Inability to fully empty bladder, which causes frequent leaking.

Total incontinence *(p.209)* ⊕⊕⊕
Inability to control passing urine means there may be constant leaking.

Acute urinary retention *(p.210)* ⊕⊕⊕
Failure to pass urine; can be very painful. Uncommon, but can occur after spinal damage or childbirth.

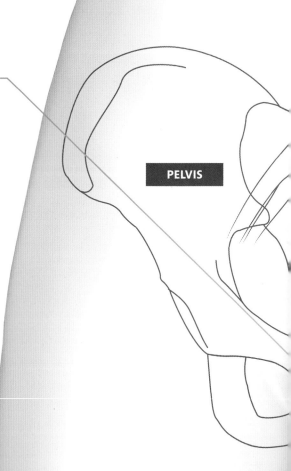

PELVIS

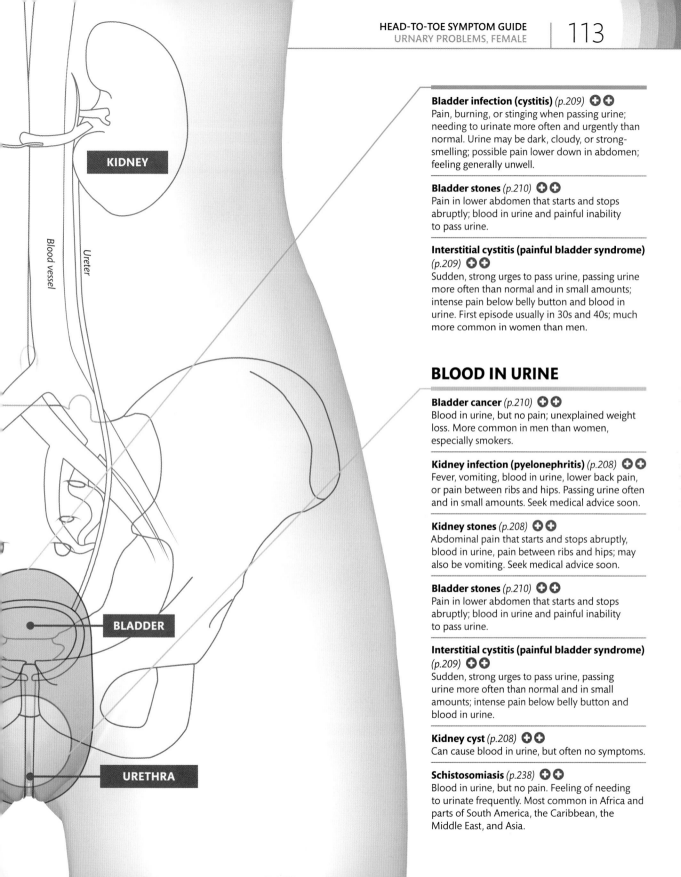

KIDNEY

Blood vessel

Ureter

BLADDER

URETHRA

Bladder infection (cystitis) *(p.209)* ✚ ✚
Pain, burning, or stinging when passing urine; needing to urinate more often and urgently than normal. Urine may be dark, cloudy, or strong-smelling; possible pain lower down in abdomen; feeling generally unwell.

Bladder stones *(p.210)* ✚ ✚
Pain in lower abdomen that starts and stops abruptly; blood in urine and painful inability to pass urine.

Interstitial cystitis (painful bladder syndrome) *(p.209)* ✚ ✚
Sudden, strong urges to pass urine, passing urine more often than normal and in small amounts; intense pain below belly button and blood in urine. First episode usually in 30s and 40s; much more common in women than men.

BLOOD IN URINE

Bladder cancer *(p.210)* ✚ ✚
Blood in urine, but no pain; unexplained weight loss. More common in men than women, especially smokers.

Kidney infection (pyelonephritis) *(p.208)* ✚ ✚
Fever, vomiting, blood in urine, lower back pain, or pain between ribs and hips. Passing urine often and in small amounts. Seek medical advice soon.

Kidney stones *(p.208)* ✚ ✚
Abdominal pain that starts and stops abruptly, blood in urine, pain between ribs and hips; may also be vomiting. Seek medical advice soon.

Bladder stones *(p.210)* ✚ ✚
Pain in lower abdomen that starts and stops abruptly; blood in urine and painful inability to pass urine.

Interstitial cystitis (painful bladder syndrome) *(p.209)* ✚ ✚
Sudden, strong urges to pass urine, passing urine more often than normal and in small amounts; intense pain below belly button and blood in urine.

Kidney cyst *(p.208)* ✚ ✚
Can cause blood in urine, but often no symptoms.

Schistosomiasis *(p.238)* ✚ ✚
Blood in urine, but no pain. Feeling of needing to urinate frequently. Most common in Africa and parts of South America, the Caribbean, the Middle East, and Asia.

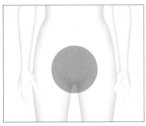

SEE ALSO Female lower abdomen pp.108–09, Urinary problems, female pp.112–13

FEMALE GENITALS

Thrush (candidiasis) is the most common problem affecting the vagina. It can be itchy and produce a white discharge. Itching is common after the menopause, when it is the result of low oestrogen levels. Bleeding from the vagina other than during menstruation is not normal, and you should seek medical advice.

SKIN CHANGES/ITCHING AND SORENESS

Thrush (candidiasis) *(p.238)* ✚✚
Vaginal soreness and itching. Thick white discharge; worse before a period.

Atrophic vaginitis *(p.215)* ✚✚
Lack of lubrication, soreness, and painful intercourse. May lead to need to pass urine more frequently, and painful urination. Common after menopause.

Genital herpes *(p.218)* ✚✚
Small blisters on the vulva. First episode very painful but recurrent episodes less so. May cause painful intercourse.

Lichen planus *(p.222)* ✚✚
Itching with red-purple bumpy skin rash.

Genital warts *(p.218)* ✚✚
Fleshy lumps in vulva. May cause soreness and irritation.

Lichen sclerosus *(p.227)* ✚✚
Pain and itching from thinning of skin in the vulva. Skin looks shiny. May cause painful intercourse.

Vulvodynia (vulval pain) *(p.215)* ✚✚
Soreness and itching in vulva. Painful intercourse. More common in young women.

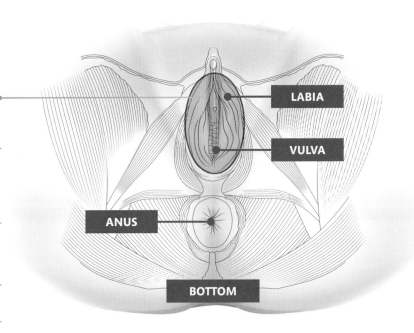

LABIA

VULVA

ANUS

BOTTOM

PAINFUL INTERCOURSE

This is common especially when a woman first begins having sex. Other causes of painful sex include insufficient lubrication, infections, endometriosis *(p.214)*, and vaginismus *(p.215)*. The following all may cause painful intercourse, usually with other symptoms too:

Thrush *(p.238)*

Chlamydia infection *(p.218)*

Gonorrhoea *(p.218)*

Trichomoniasis *(p.218)*

Genital herpes *(p.218)*

Vaginismus *(p.215)*

Prolapse *(p.214)*

Atrophic vaginitis *(p.215)*

Lichen sclerosus *(p.227)*

Vulvodynia (vulval pain) *(p.215)*

Cervical cancer *(p.215)*

Pelvic inflammatory disease *(p.213)*

DISCHARGE

Thrush (candidiasis) *(p.238)* ✚✚
Thick white discharge; worse before a menstrual period. Can cause vaginal soreness and itching, and painful intercourse.

Bacterial vaginosis *(p.215)* ✚
Fishy smelling discharge. Seek medical advice if persists or if pregnant.

Chlamydia infection *(p.218)* ✚✚
Discharge, often thick and green. Lower abdominal pain, painful intercourse, and bleeding between periods.

Gonorrhoea *(p.218)* ✚✚
Discharge, lower abdominal pain, painful intercourse, and bleeding between periods.

Pelvic inflammatory disease *(p.213)* ✚✚
Mild to severe lower abdominal pain. Discharge (may have abnormal smell or colour), abnormal bleeding, and painful intercourse. May have fever and backache.

Trichomoniasis *(p.218)* ✚✚
Frothy yellow-greeny vaginal discharge. Soreness at entrance to vagina, and painful intercourse.

Foreign body ✚✚
Very smelly and blood-stained discharge caused by a retained tampon or other object left in vagina.

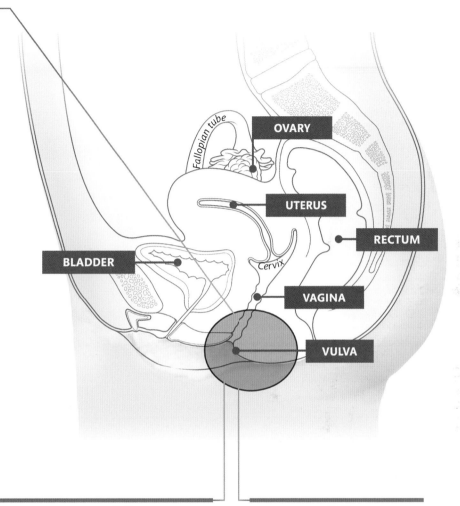

OVARY

Fallopian tube

UTERUS

RECTUM

BLADDER

Cervix

VAGINA

VULVA

ABNORMAL BLEEDING

Uterine polyps *(p.215)* ✚✚
Bleeding between periods or after intercourse, or heavy periods.

Pelvic inflammatory disease *(p.213)* ✚✚
Mild to severe lower abdominal pain. Discharge (may have abnormal smell or colour), abnormal bleeding, and painful intercourse. May have fever and backache

Fibroids *(p.215)* ✚✚
Can cause heavy and prolonged periods. Heaviness and dragging in lower abdomen.

Chlamydia infection *(p.218)* ✚✚
Discharge, often thick and green. Lower abdominal pain, painful intercourse, and bleeding between periods.

Gonorrhoea *(p.218)* ✚✚
Discharge, lower abdominal pain, painful intercourse, and bleeding between periods.

Cervical ectropion *(p.214)* ✚✚
Bleeding between periods or after intercourse. More common in young women.

Cervical cancer *(p.215)* ✚✚✚
Abnormal bleeding (postmenopausal, between periods, or after intercourse). Smelly discharge or pain on intercourse can occur. Often found on routine screening.

Uterine (womb) cancer *(p.214)* ✚✚
Abnormal bleeding. May be lower abdominal pain and bloating.

Prolapse *(p.214)* ✚✚
Feeling of something coming down or out of vagina. Can cause bleeding, discomfort, painful intercourse, needing to pass urine frequently, urinary incontinence, difficulty having bowels open and having to strain.

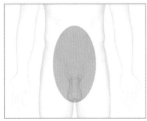

SEE ALSO Lower abdomen, left *pp.104–05,* **Lower abdomen, right** *pp.106–07,* **Male genitals** *pp.118–19*

URINARY PROBLEMS
MALE

The most common urinary problems affecting men are caused by the prostate. This gland gets larger as men age and can cause problems with passing urine (by obstructing the outflow tube called the urethra). Symptoms can occur on one or both sides unless otherwise stated.

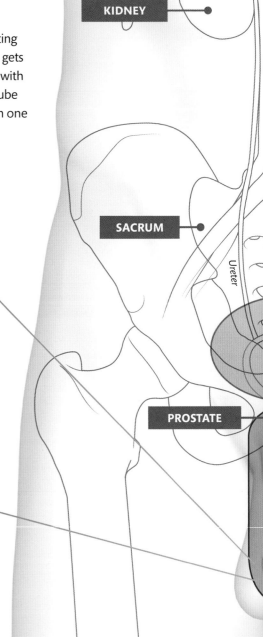

KIDNEY

SACRUM

Ureter

PROSTATE

PAIN PASSING URINE

Nongonococcal urethritis *(p.218)* ➕➕
Pain, burning, or stinging when passing urine.

Bladder infection *(p.209)* ➕➕
Pain, burning, or stinging when passing urine; needing to pass urine more often and urgently than normal. Urine may be dark, cloudy, or strong-smelling; possible pain in lower abdomen. Feeling generally unwell.

Acute urinary retention *(p.210)* ➕➕➕
Failure to pass urine, and can be very painful.

Prostatitis *(p.211)* ➕➕
Painful and frequent urination. Fever and flu-like illness. Less severe, but recurrent symptoms may occur with long-term (chronic) prostatitis.

Bladder stones *(p.210)* ➕➕
Spasmodic pain in lower abdomen; blood in urine and painful urination or inability to pass urine.

FREQUENT URGE TO URINATE

Enlarged prostate *(p.212)* ➕➕
Need to pass urine often and urgently; dribbling, poor flow and "hesitancy"; feeling of incomplete emptying of bladder. Blood in urine.

Prostate cancer *(p.212)* ➕➕
Need to pass urine often and urgently at night; dribbling, poor flow and "hesitancy"; feeling of incomplete emptying of bladder. Blood in urine.

Overactive bladder *(p.209)* ➕➕
Urge to pass urine frequently and stress incontinence (passing urine while coughing, sneezing, or running).

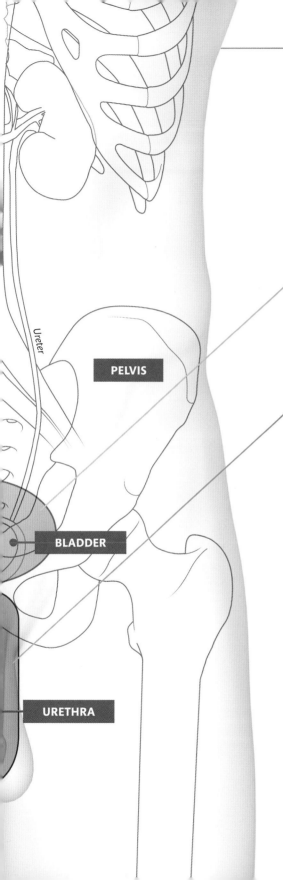

Bladder stones *(p.210)* ✚ ✚
Spasmodic pain in lower abdomen; blood in urine and painful urination or inability to pass urine.

BLOOD IN URINE

Enlarged prostate *(p.212)* ✚ ✚
Need to pass urine often and urgently at night; dribbling, poor flow and "hesitancy"; feeling of incomplete emptying of bladder. Blood in urine.

Prostate cancer *(p.212)* ✚ ✚
Need to pass urine often and urgently at night; dribbling, poor flow and "hesitancy"; feeling of incomplete emptying of bladder. Blood in urine.

Bladder cancer *(p.210)* ✚ ✚
Blood in urine, but no pain. Most commonly affects older men, smokers, and workers in rubber or dyeing industries.

Kidney infection (pyelonephritis) *(p.208)* ✚ ✚
Blood in urine, fever, vomiting, lower back pain or pain between ribs and hips. See doctor soon.

Kidney stones *(p.208)* ✚ ✚
Blood in urine, spasmodic abdominal pain, pain between ribs and hips; may also be vomiting. See doctor soon.

Kidney cancer *(p.209)* ✚ ✚
Blood in urine, but no pain. Anaemia and night sweats.

Bladder stones *(p.210)* ✚ ✚
Spasmodic pain in lower abdomen; blood in urine and painful urination or inability to pass urine. See doctor soon.

Kidney cyst *(p.208)* ✚ ✚
Can cause blood in urine, but often no symptoms.

Schistosomiasis *(p.238)* ✚ ✚
Blood in urine, but no pain. Feeling of needing to pass urine frequently. Most common in Africa, the Caribbean, the Middle East, Asia, and parts of South America.

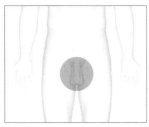

SEE ALSO: Urinary problems, male *pp.116–17*

MALE GENITALS

Problems with the penis or testicles (also called testes) can cause considerable discomfort. Some conditions are sexually transmitted; others result from more varied causes. Checking the testicles for lumps is important in spotting cancer at an early stage.

⊕ SEEK URGENT MEDICAL ATTENTION IF:
YOU HAVE **SEVERE TESTICULAR PAIN**

Erectile dysfunction *(p.211)* ⊕⊕
An inability to achieve or maintain an erection.

Genital warts *(p.218)* ⊕⊕
Small, firm fleshy growths anywhere on penis or scrotum; raised lumps with a rough surface.

Genital herpes *(p.218)* ⊕⊕
Painful red blisters that burst to produce open sores anywhere on penis.

Dermatitis *(p.222)* ⊕⊕
Redness and itching; can make intercourse painful.

Nongonococcal urethritis *(p.218)* ⊕⊕
Burning sensation when passing urine; can also cause itching and pain in the penis. White and cloudy discharge from penis.

Chlamydia infection *(p.218)* ⊕⊕
Maybe discharge from tip of penis, redness, and itching; painful urinating; can make intercourse painful. (Often no symptoms)

Gonorrhoea *(p.218)* ⊕⊕
Associated with feeling of needing to pass urine, pain when passing urine, redness at the tip of the penis, and cloudy discharge. Most common in young men and in those over 40.

Thrush (candidiasis) *(p.238)* ⊕⊕
Irritation, burning, or itching under foreskin or on tip of penis. Redness, or red patches under foreskin or on tip of penis. Discharge and difficulty pulling back foreskin.

Trichomonas infection *(p.218)* ⊕⊕
Discharge, redness, and itching; can make intercourse painful.

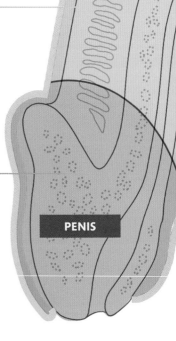

PENIS

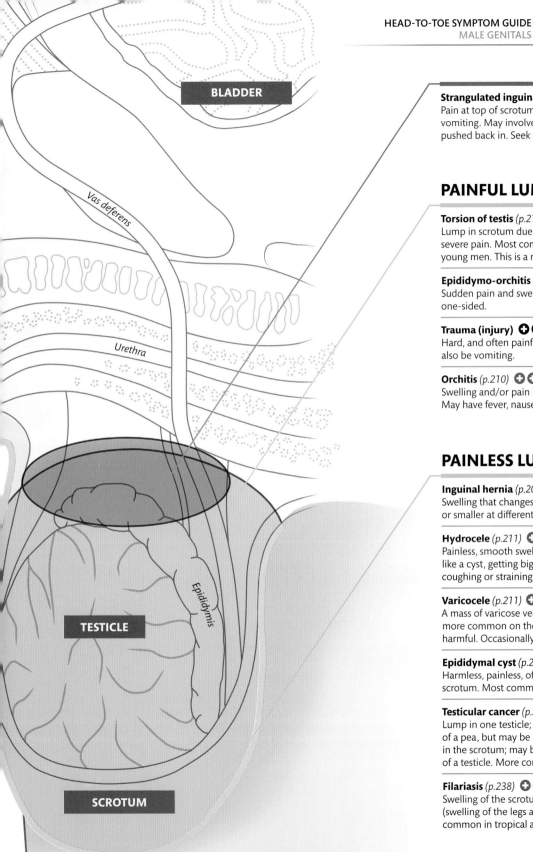

BLADDER

Vas deferens

Urethra

Epididymis

TESTICLE

SCROTUM

Strangulated inguinal hernia *(p.204)* ✚✚✚
Pain at top of scrotum, often with nausea and vomiting. May involve lump that cannot be pushed back in. Seek urgent medical attention.

PAINFUL LUMP

Torsion of testis *(p.210)* ✚✚✚
Lump in scrotum due to twisting of the testicle; severe pain. Most common in adolescents and young men. This is a medical emergency.

Epididymo-orchitis *(p.210)* ✚✚✚
Sudden pain and swelling in scrotum; usually one-sided.

Trauma (injury) ✚✚✚
Hard, and often painful lump with bruising. May also be vomiting.

Orchitis *(p.210)* ✚✚
Swelling and/or pain in one or both testicles. May have fever, nausea, and vomiting.

PAINLESS LUMP

Inguinal hernia *(p.204)* ✚✚
Swelling that changes in size, getting bigger or smaller at different times.

Hydrocele *(p.211)* ✚✚
Painless, smooth swelling in scrotum that feels like a cyst, getting bigger when upright or with coughing or straining.

Varicocele *(p.211)* ✚✚
A mass of varicose veins close to the testicles, more common on the left, not painful nor harmful. Occasionally may ache.

Epididymal cyst *(p.210)* ✚✚
Harmless, painless, often small swelling in the scrotum. Most common in men over 40.

Testicular cancer *(p.211)* ✚✚✚
Lump in one testicle; may be about the size of a pea, but may be larger; feeling of heaviness in the scrotum; may be change in firmness of a testicle. More common in young men.

Filariasis *(p.238)* ✚✚
Swelling of the scrotum. Can have elephantiasis (swelling of the legs and scarring). More common in tropical areas. Rare elsewhere.

BUTTOCKS AND ANUS

The anus is the end of the gut through which faeces are expelled from the body. Bleeding from the anus can happen as a result of constipation or haemorrhoids. It can sometimes be itchy because of threadworms or fungal infections. Lumps are common here and can be due to skin tags, warts, or abscesses.

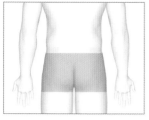

SEE ALSO Bowels, diarrhoea *pp.122–23*, **Bowels, constipation** *pp.124–25*, **Bowels, abnormal stools** *pp.126–27*

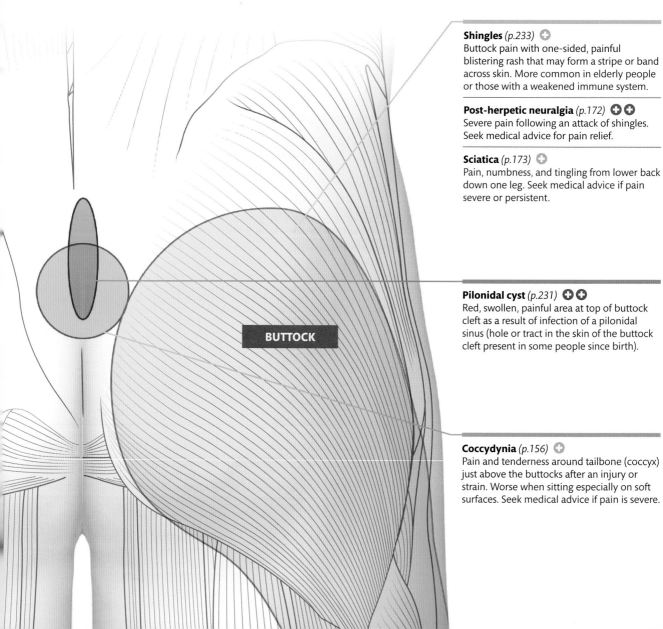

BUTTOCK

Shingles *(p.233)* ⊕
Buttock pain with one-sided, painful blistering rash that may form a stripe or band across skin. More common in elderly people or those with a weakened immune system.

Post-herpetic neuralgia *(p.172)* ⊕ ⊕
Severe pain following an attack of shingles. Seek medical advice for pain relief.

Sciatica *(p.173)* ⊕
Pain, numbness, and tingling from lower back down one leg. Seek medical advice if pain severe or persistent.

Pilonidal cyst *(p.231)* ⊕ ⊕
Red, swollen, painful area at top of buttock cleft as a result of infection of a pilonidal sinus (hole or tract in the skin of the buttock cleft present in some people since birth).

Coccydynia *(p.156)* ⊕
Pain and tenderness around tailbone (coccyx) just above the buttocks after an injury or strain. Worse when sitting especially on soft surfaces. Seek medical advice if pain is severe.

ANAL PAIN

Proctitis *(p.206)* ⊕⊕
Soreness and pain with bleeding from anus; mucus and pus discharge.

Anal fissure *(p.207)* ⊕
Pain and bright red bleeding when having a bowel movement. Common in pregnancy and after delivery. May lead to constipation. If symptoms persist, seek medical advice.

Proctalgia fugax *(p.206)* ⊕
Episodes of severe cramping pain around the anus, often at night. Seek treatment if severe.

Haemorrhoids *(p.207)* ⊕⊕
Swollen veins may protrude causing lumps around anus; possible bleeding, itching, and pain when having a bowel movement. May be very painful if blood clots develop inside.

Rectal cancer *(p.206)* ⊕⊕
Rectal bleeding and diarrhoea or constipation. Pain is a late symptom. Most common in those aged 50–70.

Anal fistula *(p.207)* ⊕⊕
Swelling, redness, and irritation around anus. Throbbing pain that may worsen when sitting. Most common in inflammatory bowel disease.

ANAL LUMPS

Haemorrhoids *(p.207)* ⊕⊕
Swollen veins may protrude causing lumps around anus; possible bleeding, itching, and pain when having a bowel movement.

Anal warts *(p.218)* ⊕⊕
Fleshy lumps around the anus that can be itchy.

Ano-rectal abscess *(p.228)* ⊕⊕
Throbbing pain with a hard tender lump. May be associated with small cracks around anus. An abscess may lead to constipation; may be pus.

Anal cancer *(p.207)* ⊕⊕⊕
Pain, bleeding, small lumps around anus, ulceration, and lack of control over bowel movements.

Rectal prolapse *(p.207)* ⊕⊕
When part of the rectum or its lining hangs out of the anus. Can be associated with constipation and rectal bleeding. More common in elderly people.

ANAL ITCHING

Haemorrhoids *(p.207)* ⊕⊕
Swollen veins in lining of anus. May protrude causing lumps; possible bleeding, itching, and pain when having a bowel movement.

Threadworms *(p.238)* ⊕⊕
Anal itching, which may disturb sleep. More common in children. Seek treatment from pharmacist or doctor.

Thrush (candidiasis) *(p.238)* ⊕⊕
Anal itching. Seek treatment from doctor or pharmacist.

Skin tags *(p.226)* ⊕
Small, painless, often on a stalk. Harmless, but may cause itching.

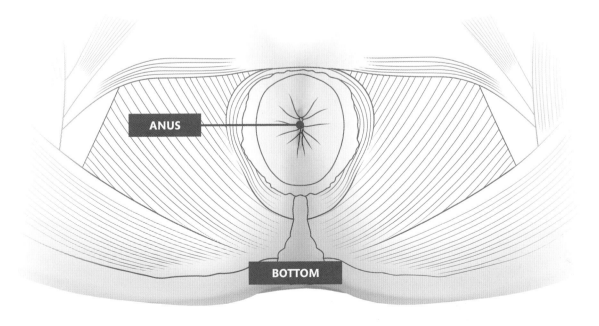

ANUS

BOTTOM

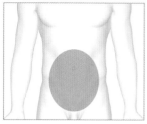

SEE ALSO, Lower abdomen, left *pp.104–05,* **Lower abdomen, right** *pp.124–25,* **Bowels, abnormal stools** *pp.126–27*

BOWELS
DIARRHOEA

Diarrhoea is defined as the passage of frequent (more than three times a day), loose stools (faeces). Usually, sudden and short-lived diarrhoea is as result of infection caused by eating or drinking contaminated food or water. Dehydration is a danger with severe diarrhoea. Always seek medical advice with long-term diarrhoea (lasting more than four weeks) or if a child.

LONG TERM

Coeliac disease *(p.204)* ✚✚
May have diarrhoea or constipation, bloating, and wind. In babies and infants, failure to put on weight. Caused by immune reaction to gluten in diet.

Crohn's disease *(p.203)* ✚✚
Pain, bleeding, and diarrhoea. Fever and feeling generally unwell.

Ulcerative colitis *(p.203)* ✚✚
Blood-stained diarrhoea, lower abdominal pain, weight loss, and fever. Can be associated with joint pains and eye problems.

Irritable bowel syndrome *(p.203)* ✚
Constipation and/or diarrhoea. Abdominal bloating, wind, and burping. More common in women and in the West.

Bile acid diarrhoea *(p.196)* ✚✚
Watery diarrhoea with no blood. Can be continuous or intermittent. Associated with conditions like Crohn's disease (p.203), pancreatitis (p.202), after surgery, or following gallbladder removal.

Diverticular disease *(p.205)* ✚✚
Diarrhoea and/or constipation; passing blood or mucus in stools.

Diverticulitis *(p.205)* ✚✚✚
Abdominal discomfort and tenderness; blood and mucus from rectum; often with diarrhoea and/or constipation.

Bowel cancer *(p.206)* ✚✚✚
Weight loss, diarrhoea (with or without blood) and sometimes constipation. May also have anaemia and abdominal pain.

Lactose intolerance *(p.203)* ✚✚
Frothy diarrhoea and stools that float. Abdominal pain and failure to put on weight (in babies and young children); weight loss.

Pancreatitis *(p.202)* ✚✚✚
Diarrhoea and stools that float, abdominal pain, often unwell; jaundice (yellowing of skin and eyes).

Cancer of pancreas *(p.202)* ✚✚
Weight loss, diarrhoea, and jaundice (yellowing of skin and eyes); abdominal pain. Stools may be pale and float.

Hyperthyroidism *(p.220)* ✚✚
Diarrhoea with weight loss, feeling hot, palpitations (sensation of heart beating or skipping), and sweating.

Bowel infection *(p.203)* ✚✚
Persistent diarrhoea with weight loss due to infection, such as amoebiasis (p.237), hookworm (p.238), Cryptosporidium (p.237), and giardiasis (p.237). Most common where access to clean water is limited.

Diabetes *(p.219)* ✚✚
Diarrhoea that is often continuous and difficult to control.

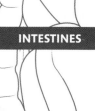

LIVER

INTESTINES

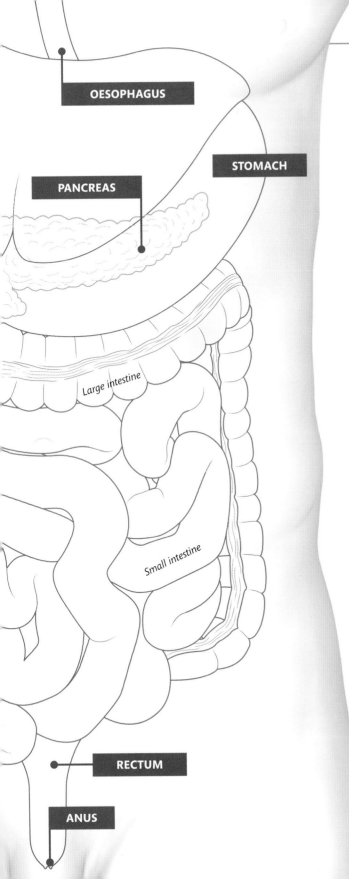

OESOPHAGUS

STOMACH

PANCREAS

Large intestine

Small intestine

RECTUM

ANUS

DIARRHOEA IN CHILDREN

Young children may become severely dehydrated if they have severe or prolonged diarrhoea, and you should seek urgent medicical advice. Sometimes diarrhoea is a longer-term condition.

Toddler's diarrhoea *(p.196)* ➕➕
Loose stools often with food in it. The child is usually otherwise well. Cause usually unknown.

Cow's milk allergy *(p.189)* ➕➕
Diarrhoea and/or constipation and may be blood or mucus in stools. Often associated with eczema (p.222), asthma (p.193), or other food allergies (p.189). Follows minutes or hours after drinking milk. Can have bloating, failure to gain weight, and weight loss. May also be wheezy.

SHORT TERM

Infective gastroenteritis *(p.196)* ➕
Sudden and often profuse diarrhoea. Can be associated with vomiting and fever, colicky (spasmodic) abdominal pain and can have blood in the diarrhoea. In adults usually lasts a few days and resolves spontaneously.

Overflow diarrhoea *(p.196)* ➕➕
Constipation followed by uncontrollable diarrhoea. Abdominal pain, often colicky (severe and spasmodic). Common in elderly and immobile people.

Anxiety disorders *(p.240)* ➕
Usually short-lived episode of diarrhoea that resolves without treatment.

Appendicitis *(p.205)* ➕➕➕
Abdominal pain starting in the centre of the abdomen and settling in the right lower side. Can be associated with diarrhoea and fever.

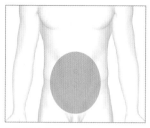

SEE ALSO Abdomen, lower left *pp.104–05*, **Abdomen, lower right**, *pp.106–07*, **Buttocks and anus** *pp.120–21*

BOWELS
CONSTIPATION

Constipation – either infrequent bowel movement or passing hard and dry stools (faeces) infrequently – is common in the West, where people are likely to have a low-fibre diet. Constipation is also more common in older people and in children. If accompanied by blood or weight loss, or if it persists, seek medical advice.

WITH BLOOD

Diverticulitis *(p.205)* ✚✚✚
Diarrhoea and/or constipation, lower left-sided pain and passing blood or mucus in faeces. Can be quite unwell.

Bowel cancer *(p.206)* ✚✚✚
Constipation and/or diarrhoea for more than three weeks, often with blood in faeces, weight loss; poor appetite; anaemia.

LIVER

INTESTINES

ANAL PROBLEMS

Any problem that affects the anus can lead to constipation indirecty, as a result of pain when having a bowel movement. See also *pp.120–21*.

Anal fissure *(p.207)* ✚✚
Small tear in anus that causes pain on passing stools and bright red bleeding. Often leads to constipation.

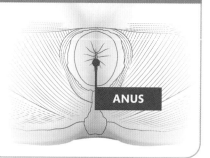

ANUS

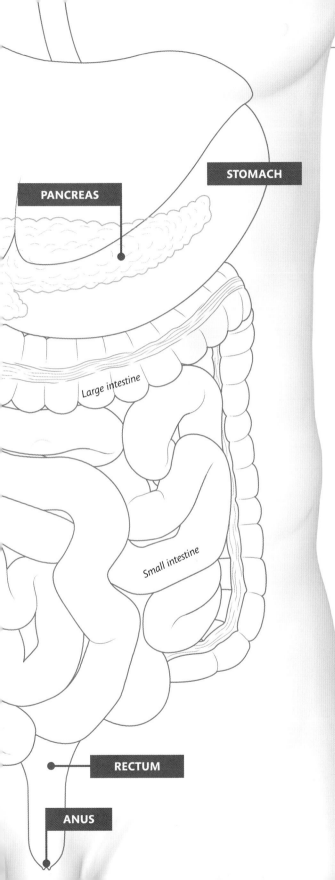

PANCREAS

STOMACH

Large intestine

Small intestine

RECTUM

ANUS

Irritable bowel syndrome (IBS) *(p.203)* ⊕
Constipation and/or diarrhoea with bloated abdomen, wind, and burping. More common in women and in the West.

Coeliac disease *(p.204)* ⊕ ⊕
May have constipation or diarrhoa; bloating and wind. In children, failure to thrive. Worse with gluten in diet.

Diverticular disease *(p.205)* ⊕ ⊕
Constipation and abdominal pain; passing blood or mucus in stools.

Bowel cancer *(p.206)* ⊕ ⊕ ⊕
Constipation and/or diarrhoea for more than three weeks, often with blood in stools, weight loss; poor appetite; anaemia.

Intestinal obstruction *(p.204)* ⊕ ⊕ ⊕
Constipation with severe spasmodic abdominal pain. Lots of bowel noises but no wind; vomiting. Associated with conditions such as bowel cancer *(p.206)*, diverticulitis *(p.205)* andCrohn's disease *(p.203)*, and after bowel surgery.

Hypothyroidism *(p.220)* ⊕ ⊕
Constipation, weight gain, dry skin and hair; feeling cold; generally sluggish metabolism. More common in women.

Hypercalcemia *(p.187)* ⊕ ⊕
Constipation, painful bones, severe spasmodic abdominal pain. May have psychiatric issues, such as depression, anxiety, difficulty thinking, and insomnia.

CONSTIPATION IN CHILDREN

Constipation is common in children. It is often related to withholding, toilet-training issues, and changes in diet or routine. Rarely, it can result from an underlying serious medical condition. Seek advice if the constipation persists, the child is very young, or passes blood in the stools.

Hirschsprung's disease *(p.205)* ⊕ ⊕ ⊕
Constipation that doesn't respond to treatment, possibly with "overflow" diarrhoea. May be weight loss and failure to grow and put on weight, bloated abdomen, and discomfort.

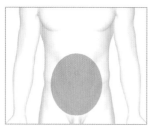

SEE ALSO Bowels, diarrhoea *pp.122–23,* Bowels, constipation *pp.124–25*

BOWELS
ABNORMAL STOOLS

Stools (faeces) are usually light to dark brown in colour depending on diet. If stools are very pale or smelly and frothy, this can be a sign of problems with absorption in the bowel. Black, sticky, and tarry stools can be a sign of bleeding from the stomach. In either case you should visit your doctor.

PALE/FATTY STOOLS

Gallstones *(p.202)* ✚✚
Fatty, oily, pale stools. Severe spasmodic abdominal pain and jaundice. Seek medical advice if have fever or pain is severe.

Pancreatitis *(p.202)* ✚✚✚
Pale smelly loose stools that may float. Abdominal pain and jaundice.

Cancer of pancreas *(p.202)* ✚✚✚
Weight loss, diarrhoea, loose fatty pale stools that floats. Abdominal pain.

Cystic fibrosis *(p.194)* ✚✚✚
Pale, loose, fatty and/or smelly stools. In infants, associated with failure to grow and gain weight and recurrent chest infections. Usually diagnosed in childhood.

Lactose intolerance *(p.203)* ✚✚
Smelly, pale, and frothy stools after drinking milk. May follow an episode of gastroenteritis (p.196).

Primary biliary cholangitis *(p.201)* ✚✚✚
Tiredness, itchy skin, smelly and pale diarrhoea, nausea and bloating.

BLACK STOOLS

Peptic ulcers *(p.200)* ✚✚✚
Black and smelly faeces with abdominal pain. May have vomiting and nausea.

Stomach cancer *(p.200)* ✚✚✚
Dark blood mixed in with the stools. Weight loss, anaemia, and loss of appetite. Nausea/vomiting and abdominal pain.

LIVER

INTESTINES

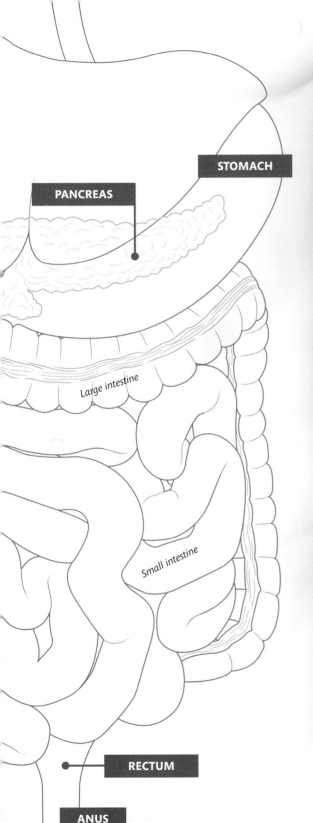

BLOOD MIXED IN WITH STOOLS

Crohn's disease (p.203)
Pain, bleeding, and diarrhoea. Fever and feeling
generally unwell.

Ulcerative colitis (p.203)
Blood-stained diarrhoea, lower abdominal pain, weight
loss, and fever. Can be associated with joint pains and
eye problems.

Bowel cancer (p.206)
Blood, either bright red or mixed in with the stools.
Associated with weight loss and change in bowel habits
– especially persistent diarrhoea – and anaemia.

Diverticulitis (p.205)
Diarrhoea and/or constipation, lower left-sided pain
and passing blood or mucus in stools. Can be
quite unwell.

Proctitis (p.206)
Soreness around anus and bleeding. Sometimes with
mucus or pus discharge.

Polyp (p.204)
Bright red bleeding and change in bowel habits.

BRIGHT RED BLEEDING

Haemorrhoids (p.207)
Bright red bleeding not mixed in with the stools.

Anal fissure (p.207)
Bright red blood usually on the toilet paper. Often with
constipation (as a result of pain having a bowel motion).

Anal fistula (p.207)
Localized pain, discomfort, mucus or pus discharge,
and itching around the anus. Can be accompanied by
bright red blood.

Proctitis (p.206)
Soreness around anus, and bleeding. Sometimes with
mucus or pus discharge.

Rectal prolapse (p.207)
Pain, constipation, and faecal incontinence (leaking of
faeces), often with straining. Bright red bleeding is a sign
of ulceration. See doctor soon.

Bowel infections
Diarrhoea, wind, and bright bleeding due to infections
such as amoebiasis (p.237). Can have fever and be unwell.

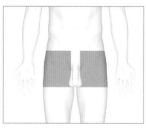

SEE ALSO Groin, male and female *pp.110–11*, Hip, back *pp.130–31*

HIP
FRONT

The hips support and balance the body in standing, walking, and running. Fractures of the femoral head (the hip) are common, especially in elderly people. Unless otherwise stated, symptoms can affect one or both hips.

Paget's disease of bone *(p.155)* ➕➕
Pelvic bones are painful, weaker, and misshapen with fractures and arthritis in nearby joints. More common in men than women, and rare under 55 years of age.

Osteoarthritis *(p.157)* ➕
Activity-related joint pain and impaired function, with morning stiffness lasting less than 30 minutes. The most common form of arthritis affecting hips, especially in people over 45 years of age.

Hip fracture *(p.156)* ➕➕➕
Pain in upper thigh or in groin, but may also be felt in knee. Much worse with bending or turning leg, and unable to bear weight. Far more common in elderly people, those with osteoporosis, or with cancer metastases to bone. This is a medical emergency, dial 999.

Stress fracture *(p.156)* ➕➕
Activity-related hip, groin, or thigh pain that can be reproduced by hopping on affected leg. A stress fracture may progress to a full fracture.

Septic arthritis *(p.157)* ➕➕➕
Increasing hip, groin, or thigh pain, worse with movement; hip area may be swollen. Inability to bear weight; often with fever and generally unwell. More likely in elderly people and those with diabetes and/or pre-exisiting joint damage.

Avascular necrosis *(p.154)* ➕➕
Hip pain from death of bone tissue in hip joint. Occurs most commonly between 30 and 60 years old. Associated with trauma, steroid use, excess alcohol use, as well as certain medications and medical treatments.

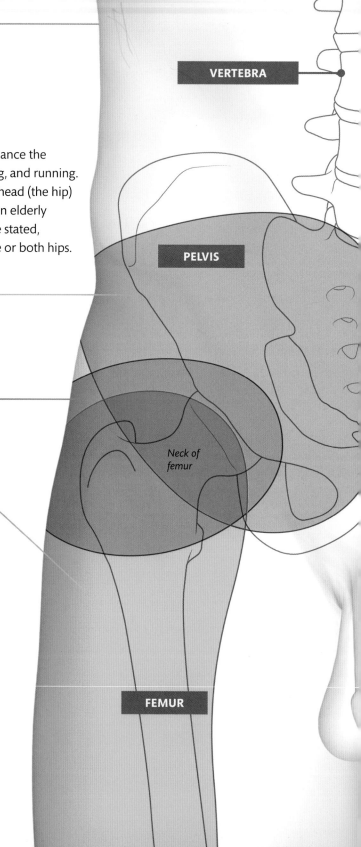

VERTEBRA

PELVIS

Neck of femur

FEMUR

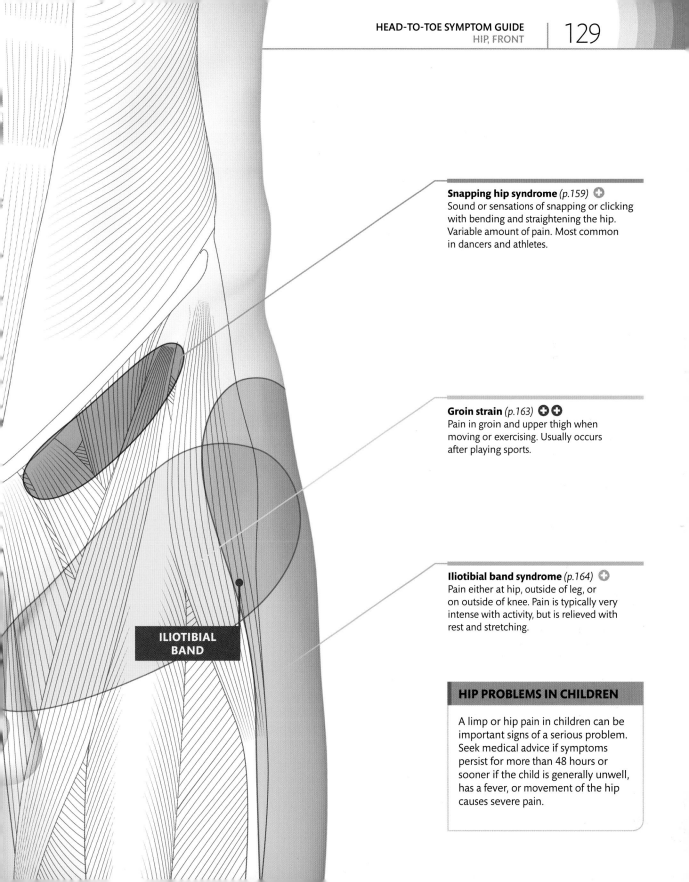

Snapping hip syndrome *(p.159)* ⊕
Sound or sensations of snapping or clicking with bending and straightening the hip. Variable amount of pain. Most common in dancers and athletes.

Groin strain *(p.163)* ⊕ ⊕
Pain in groin and upper thigh when moving or exercising. Usually occurs after playing sports.

Iliotibial band syndrome *(p.164)* ⊕
Pain either at hip, outside of leg, or on outside of knee. Pain is typically very intense with activity, but is relieved with rest and stretching.

ILIOTIBIAL BAND

HIP PROBLEMS IN CHILDREN

A limp or hip pain in children can be important signs of a serious problem. Seek medical advice if symptoms persist for more than 48 hours or sooner if the child is generally unwell, has a fever, or movement of the hip causes severe pain.

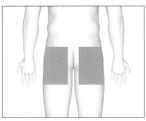

HIP
BACK

The gluteus muscles form the characteristic prominance of the buttocks. The muscles help maintain our upright posture. Some lower back problems and kidney stones can cause pain in the hip area, but this is not made worse by moving the hip.

Sciatica *(p.173)* ✚
Progressive burning pain in buttock, and which may go down leg to back of thigh, knee, even into the foot. Pain, numbness, and tingling from lower back down one leg. Seek medical advice if pain severe or persistent.

Piriformis syndrome *(p.163)* ✚✚
Tingling and numbness in the hip, buttocks, and back of thigh, similar to the pain of sciatica. Pain is eased by walking with foot pointing outwards.

Polymyalgia rheumatica *(p.161)* ✚✚
Stiffness, pain, and aching of large buttock muscles. Also affects other large muscles. May cause difficulty getting up and climbing stairs. Worst first thing in the morning. Mainly affects people over 65, and more common in women than men.

Cauda equina syndrome *(p.171)* ✚✚✚
Severe lower back pain with numbness or "pins-and-needles" sensation of perineum (area between genitals and anus) and inner thighs; reduced bladder and bowel control; sciatica-type pain on one or both sides. This is a medical emergency, dial 999.

Pressure sores *(p.225)* ✚✚
Inflamed, painful red areas from local pressure and friction damage to the skin and tissue over a bone. Common sites include base of the spine and the hip. More likely if bedridden and in wheelchair users.

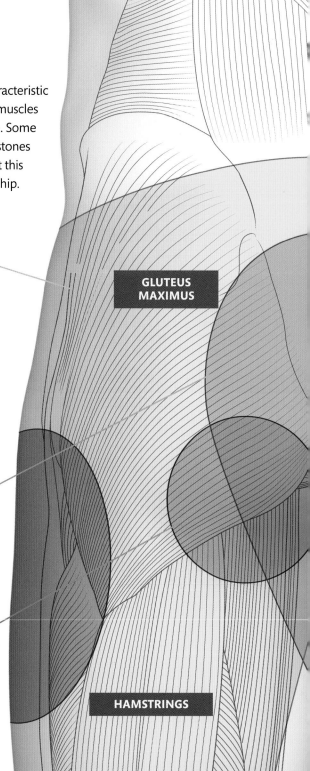

GLUTEUS MAXIMUS

HAMSTRINGS

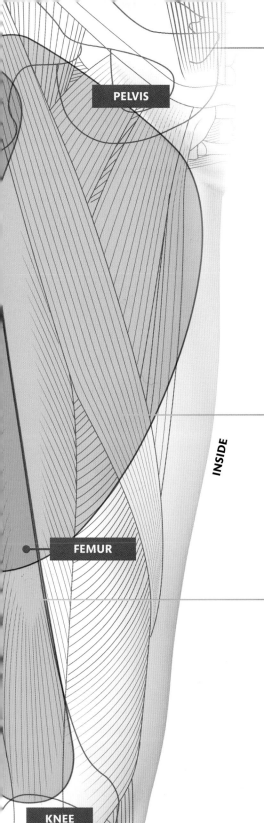

PELVIS

INSIDE

FEMUR

KNEE

Polymyalgia rheumatica *(p.161)* ✚ ✚
Stiffness, pain, and aching of muscles. Also affects other large muscles, such as the buttocks. May cause difficulty getting up from sitting and climbing stairs. Worse first thing in the morning. Mainly affects people over 65.

Osteoid osteoma *(p.155)* ✚ ✚
Small bony, hard, lump, fixed to the thigh bone. Usually causes continuous deep aching and intense pain, especially at night. Affects children and young adults; more common in males than females.

Femoral fracture (thigh bone fracture) *(p.156)* ✚ ✚ ✚
Sudden severe pain and swelling, and possible deformity. Usually due to obvious violent injury. This is a medical emergency, dial 999.

Ewing's sarcoma *(p.155)* ✚ ✚
Pain worse at night. Tender, warm swelling. May also cause a limp. Fever and weight loss are usually later signs. Affects teenagers and young adults. See doctor soon.

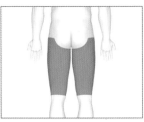

THIGH
BACK

The three hamstring muscles make up the bulk of the back of the thigh. They attach to the pelvis under the buttock muscles and pass on either side of the knee to the lower leg bones (tibia and fibula). Most conditions involve these muscles, but the thigh bone (femur) and sciatic nerve can also give problems.

BUTTOCK

Cramp *(p.161)* ⊕
Sudden, involuntary, sustained (seconds to several minutes) contraction of a muscle, causing severe pain and temporary incapacity. More likely in fatigued muscles, or when at rest at night.

Hamstring injury *(p.163)* ⊕
Sudden pain and tenderness in back of thigh during maximum activity. May be painful to move leg. Loss of strength, with bruising above and behind knee visible.

Polymyalgia rheumatica *(p.161)* ⊕⊕
Stiffness, pain, and aching muscles. Also affects other large muscles elsewhere in the body. May cause difficulty getting up and climbing stairs. Worse first thing in the morning. Mainly affects people over 65, and more common in women than men.

Sciatica *(p.173)* ⊕
Progressive burning pain from buttock, all the way down thigh and may include knee. May also go down into foot. If symptoms persist, seek medical advice.

INSIDE

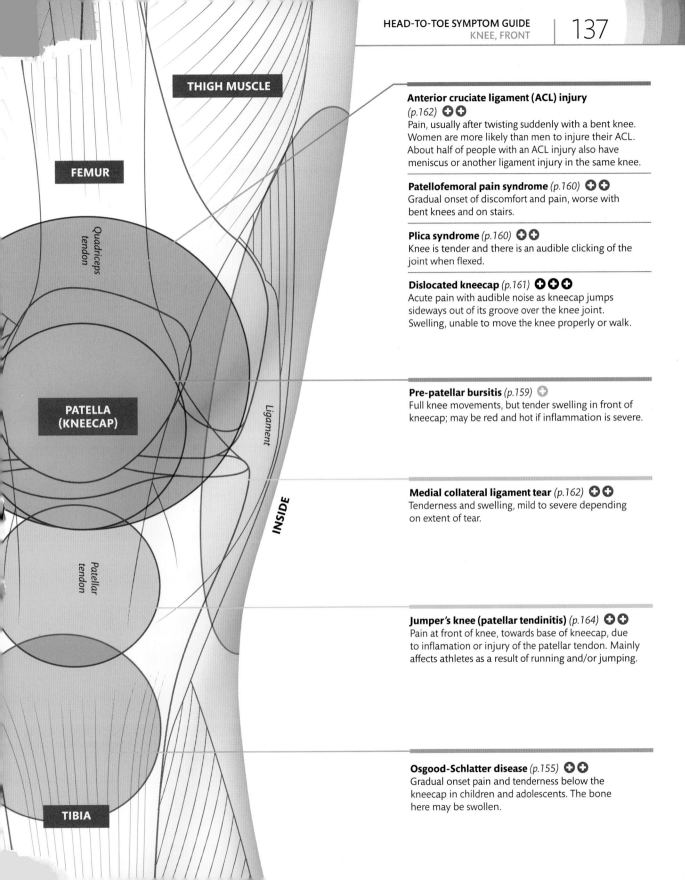

THIGH MUSCLE

FEMUR

Quadriceps tendon

PATELLA (KNEECAP)

Ligament

Patellar tendon

INSIDE

TIBIA

Anterior cruciate ligament (ACL) injury
(p.162) ⊕ ⊕
Pain, usually after twisting suddenly with a bent knee. Women are more likely than men to injure their ACL. About half of people with an ACL injury also have meniscus or another ligament injury in the same knee.

Patellofemoral pain syndrome *(p.160)* ⊕ ⊕
Gradual onset of discomfort and pain, worse with bent knees and on stairs.

Plica syndrome *(p.160)* ⊕ ⊕
Knee is tender and there is an audible clicking of the joint when flexed.

Dislocated kneecap *(p.161)* ⊕ ⊕ ⊕
Acute pain with audible noise as kneecap jumps sideways out of its groove over the knee joint. Swelling, unable to move the knee properly or walk.

Pre-patellar bursitis *(p.159)* ⊕
Full knee movements, but tender swelling in front of kneecap; may be red and hot if inflammation is severe.

Medial collateral ligament tear *(p.162)* ⊕ ⊕
Tenderness and swelling, mild to severe depending on extent of tear.

Jumper's knee (patellar tendinitis) *(p.164)* ⊕ ⊕
Pain at front of knee, towards base of kneecap, due to inflamation or injury of the patellar tendon. Mainly affects athletes as a result of running and/or jumping.

Osgood-Schlatter disease *(p.155)* ⊕ ⊕
Gradual onset pain and tenderness below the kneecap in children and adolescents. The bone here may be swollen.

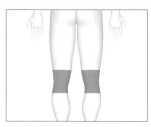

SEE ALSO Knee, front
pp.136–37

KNEE
BACK

Problems in the back of the knee may include
ligament sprains, muscle or tendon strains,
or more severe ligament and joint injuries.
The blood vessels here are close to the surface
and can produce complications. The skin
behind the knee is a common site for eczema.

Eczema *(p.222)* ⊕
Itchy, dry, inflamed skin. May become infected from
scratching. Skin becomes oozy, crusting, swollen,
and sore, and may also become thickened and darker
over time.

Posterior cruciate ligament (PCL) injury *(p.162)* ⊕ ⊕
Initially few symptoms, apart from instability and pain
walking up or down stairs. Occurs following a fall or
direct blow to bent knee.

INSIDE

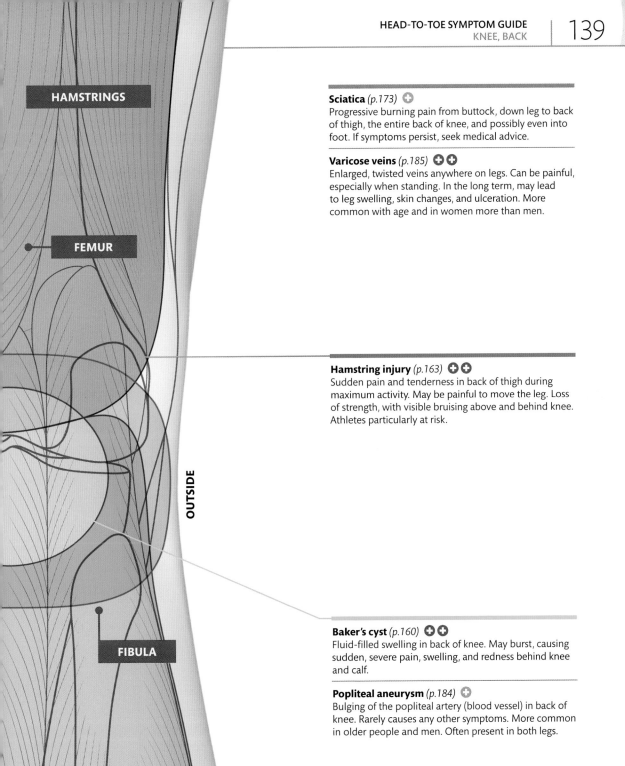

HAMSTRINGS

FEMUR

OUTSIDE

FIBULA

TIBIA

Sciatica *(p.173)* ⊕
Progressive burning pain from buttock, down leg to back of thigh, the entire back of knee, and possibly even into foot. If symptoms persist, seek medical advice.

Varicose veins *(p.185)* ⊕ ⊕
Enlarged, twisted veins anywhere on legs. Can be painful, especially when standing. In the long term, may lead to leg swelling, skin changes, and ulceration. More common with age and in women more than men.

Hamstring injury *(p.163)* ⊕ ⊕
Sudden pain and tenderness in back of thigh during maximum activity. May be painful to move the leg. Loss of strength, with visible bruising above and behind knee. Athletes particularly at risk.

Baker's cyst *(p.160)* ⊕ ⊕
Fluid-filled swelling in back of knee. May burst, causing sudden, severe pain, swelling, and redness behind knee and calf.

Popliteal aneurysm *(p.184)* ⊕
Bulging of the popliteal artery (blood vessel) in back of knee. Rarely causes any other symptoms. More common in older people and men. Often present in both legs.

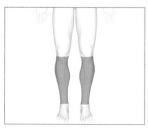

SEE ALSO Knee, back *pp.138–39*, Lower leg, back *pp.142–43*

LOWER LEG
FRONT

The lower leg has two bones, the tibia and fibula. The tibia supports most of the body weight and is an important part of both the knee and ankle joints. Lower leg injuries are common sports injuries. Sprains (stretched ligaments) and strains (stretched or torn muscles) are the most common injuries, and normally get better of their own accord.

Shin splints (medial tibial stress syndrome) *(p.163)*
Dull, achy pain after starting exercise, easing on rest. There can be some swelling. Pain may become severe, preventing exercise. Being overweight and low fitness levels are risk factors.

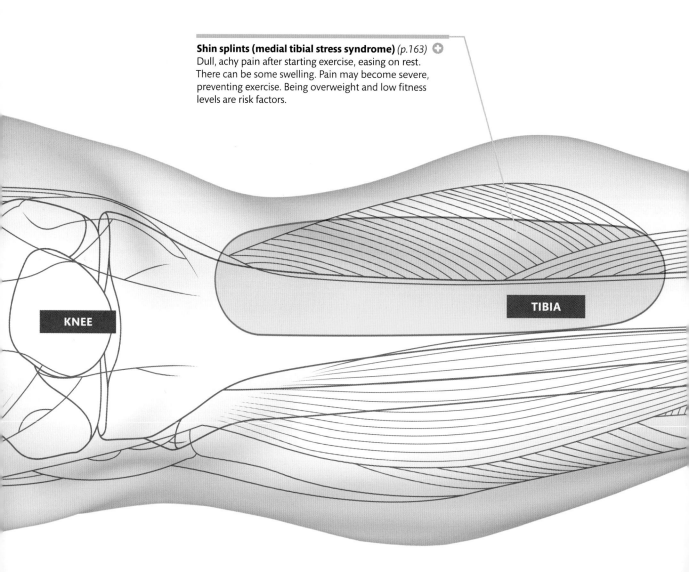

KNEE

TIBIA

Fracture *(p.156)* ✚✚✚
Severe pain, swelling, an odd shape, and bruising. Walking may be impossible. Follows trauma such as car accident or sports impact. The shinbone (tibia) is the most commonly fractured long bone; 75 per cent of fractures involve the fibula too. This is a medical emergency, dial 999.

Stress fracture *(p.156)* ✚✚
Pain with weight bearing, increasing with exercise or activity, improving with rest. Localized tenderness on the bone; tapping it produces the symptoms. Athlete's overuse injury; occurs in weight-bearing bones such as tibia (shin bone) and bones of ankles and feet.

Restless legs syndrome *(p.162)* ✚
An unpleasant feeling in the legs with urge to move them. Worse at rest, so difficulty sleeping. May be limb twitching during sleep. More likely if have anaemia, kidney failure, Parkinson's disease, diabetes mellitus, rheumatoid arthritis, or are pregnant.

Lymphoedema *(p.188)* ✚
Swollen area or swelling of whole lower leg. If press on skin, doesn't leave an imprint. Seek medical advice if painful or persists.

SKIN SYMPTOMS

Oedema ✚
Swelling caused by excess fluid in tissues. Usually also affects feet and ankles. Leg may keep imprint of a pressed finger for a short while. Associated with skin discolouration, aching, and weight gain. Seek medical advice if painful or persists for more than 48 hours.

Cellulitis *(p.228)* ✚✚
Red, hot, and painful area resulting from infection. More likely after recent injury or local surgery, insect bites, skin rashes. More common in pregnancy, diabetes, and people who are obese.

Lymphangitis *(p.187)* ✚✚✚
Red skin, warmth, and often a raised border around the affected area. May also affect arms at same time. May have chills and fever with pain as a result of infection. Characteristic thin red line on skin towards groin (or armpit). Associated with tender lumps in groin or armpit.

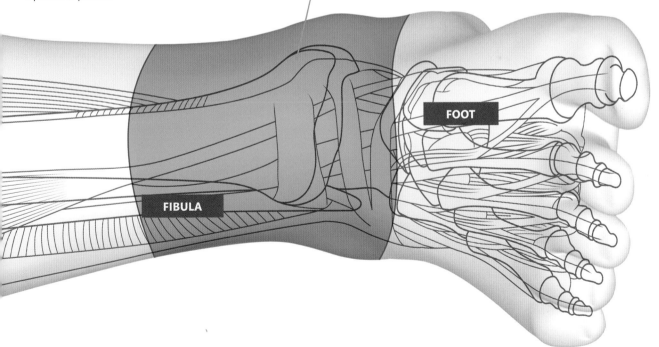

FOOT

FIBULA

LOWER LEG
BACK

The back of the lower leg has large muscle groups that are susceptible to injury and strain. Sprains (stretched ligaments) and strains (stretched or torn muscles) are the most common types of injury, and normally get better on their own. Symptoms affecting the skin can be a sign of a more serious disorder.

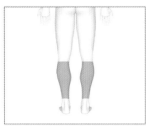

SEE ALSO Knee, back *pp.138–39*, **Lower leg, front** *pp.140–41*

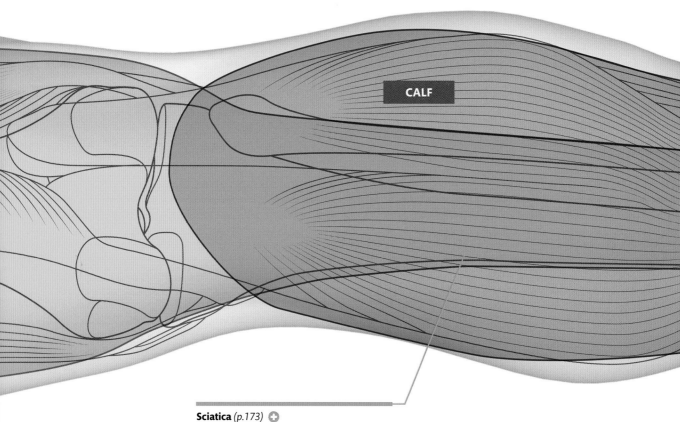

CALF

Sciatica *(p.173)* ⊕
Progressive burning pain from buttock, down back of thigh, into the leg and foot. See doctor if persists or for pain relief.

Muscle strain *(p.163)* ✚
Pain, usually from muscle overuse (such as excessive running or jumping) and from sudden stretching if ankle forced upwards. May be acutely painful and disabling.

Cramp *(p.161)* ✚
Sudden, involuntary, sustained (seconds to several minutes) contraction of a muscle, causing severe pain and temporary incapacity. More likely in tired muscles, although 75 per cent of cramps occur at night. Muscle soreness remains for a while once cramp has ceased.

Compartment syndrome *(p.163)* ✚✚✚
Severe pain and tightness triggered by exercise and eased by stopping. Pain if muscle stretched. Affected muscles feel hard and tense. Muscle weakness, numbness and/or tingling, and difficulty walking. Typically affects athletes aged under 40.

Deep vein thrombosis *(p.184)* ✚✚✚
Pain and tenderness that is worse on stretching calf; heavy, aching feeling; warm red skin; one calf more swollen than other. More likely if over age 40, previous DVT or family history of DVT.

Growing pains ✚
Non-specific aches and pains in both legs. Common in children, usually occurring in the evening or night. Also affects shins, ankles, and front lower thigh. Not harmful, but seek advice if diagnosis in doubt.

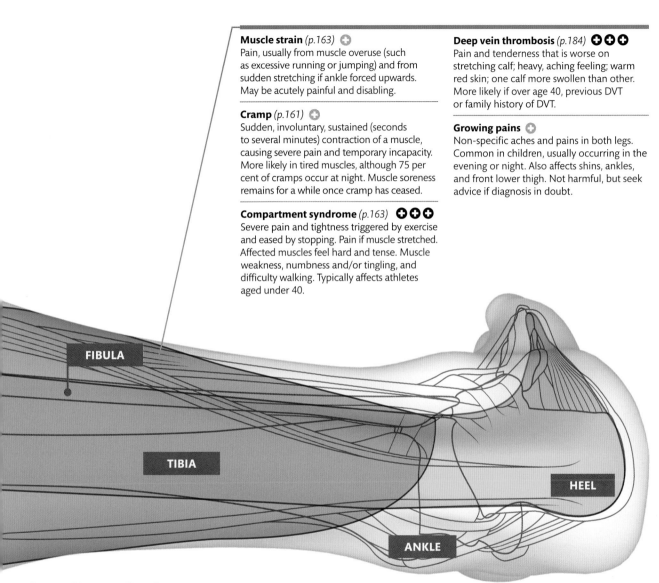

FIBULA

TIBIA

HEEL

ANKLE

SKIN SYMPTOMS

Varicose veins *(p.185)* ✚
Enlarged, twisted surface veins mainly behind the knee into the calf and ankle. Ache, especially when standing. May lead to leg swelling and skin changes, including ulceration. More common in women.

Cellulitis *(p.228)* ✚✚
Red, hot, and painful area resulting from infection. More likely after recent injury or local surgery, insect bites, or with a skin rash. More common in pregnancy, diabetes, and people who are obese.

Venous leg ulcer *(p.225)* ✚✚
Skin changes, with redness and ulcers. May be painful.

Restless legs syndrome *(p.162)* ✚
An unpleasant feeling in legs with urge to move them. Worse at rest, so difficulty sleeping. May be limb twitching during sleep. More likely if have anaemia, kidney failure, Parkinson's disease, diabetes mellitus, rheumatoid arthritis, or if pregnant.

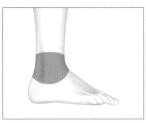

SEE ALSO Lower leg, front *pp.140–41*, Lower leg, back *pp.142–43*, Foot, general *pp.146–47*

ANKLE

The ankle is a complicated joint and frequently injured as walking on two legs, rather than four like other animals, causes the ankle extra work in weight-bearing and balance. It is liable to sprains (stretched ligaments), strains (stretched or torn muscles), and sometimes fracture.

JOINT CONDITIONS

Osteoarthritis *(p.157)* ⊕
May affect ankle after previous fracture or injury. Variable pain and stiffness, worse with activity. Reduced range of movement and grating sensation. Usually affects one ankle only.

Rheumatoid arthritis *(p.157)* ⊕⊕
Pain, swelling, stiffness and reduced function. Usually affects both ankles. Other joints, such as in hands and feet, may be affected.

Rheumatic fever *(p.184)* ⊕⊕
Fever, painful joints (including ankle), involuntary muscle movements, and a non-itchy rash, 2–4 weeks after bacterial sore throat (p.192). Mostly affects children aged 5–14 years.

Ankle sprain *(p.162)* ⊕⊕
Pain, swelling, bruising, and tenderness, difficulty moving the ankle, and limping.

Fracture *(p.156)* ⊕⊕⊕
Severe pain, swelling, and bruising. Walking may be impossible. Follows trauma such as car accident or sports impact. An abnormal joint position may indicate dislocation.

Gout *(p.159)* ⊕⊕
Intense pain with red, warm, very tender swelling of a joint such as the ankle, but more commonly affects big toe. Walking may be impossible. May also be hard, painless chalk-like lumps (tophi) on back of heel.

Septic arthritis *(p.157)* ⊕⊕⊕
Increasing pain, swelling, redness, and heat in ankle after a recent injury or surgery; worse with movement. Inability to bear weight; often with fever and feeling generally unwell.

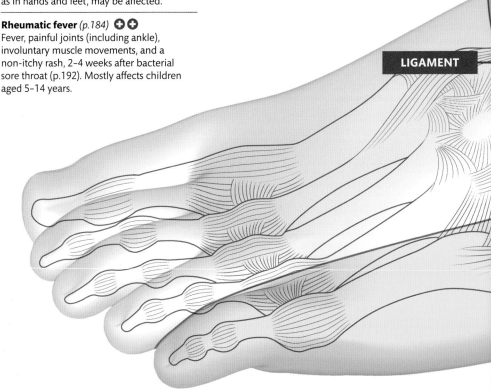

LIGAMENT

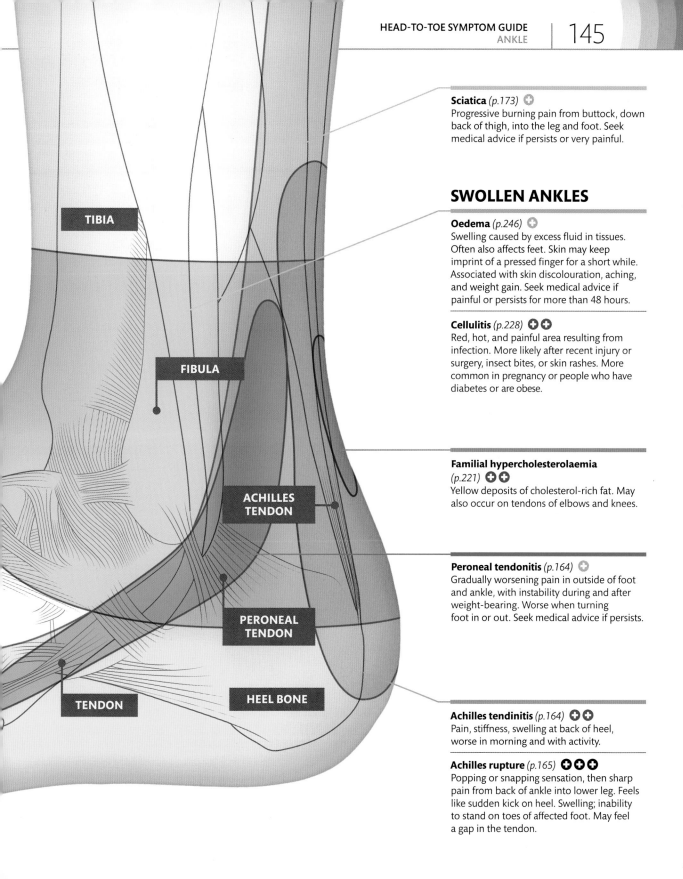

TIBIA

FIBULA

ACHILLES TENDON

PERONEAL TENDON

TENDON

HEEL BONE

Sciatica *(p.173)* ⊕
Progressive burning pain from buttock, down back of thigh, into the leg and foot. Seek medical advice if persists or very painful.

SWOLLEN ANKLES

Oedema *(p.246)* ⊕
Swelling caused by excess fluid in tissues. Often also affects feet. Skin may keep imprint of a pressed finger for a short while. Associated with skin discolouration, aching, and weight gain. Seek medical advice if painful or persists for more than 48 hours.

Cellulitis *(p.228)* ⊕⊕
Red, hot, and painful area resulting from infection. More likely after recent injury or surgery, insect bites, or skin rashes. More common in pregnancy or people who have diabetes or are obese.

Familial hypercholesterolaemia *(p.221)* ⊕⊕
Yellow deposits of cholesterol-rich fat. May also occur on tendons of elbows and knees.

Peroneal tendonitis *(p.164)* ⊕
Gradually worsening pain in outside of foot and ankle, with instability during and after weight-bearing. Worse when turning foot in or out. Seek medical advice if persists.

Achilles tendinitis *(p.164)* ⊕⊕
Pain, stiffness, swelling at back of heel, worse in morning and with activity.

Achilles rupture *(p.165)* ⊕⊕⊕
Popping or snapping sensation, then sharp pain from back of ankle into lower leg. Feels like sudden kick on heel. Swelling; inability to stand on toes of affected foot. May feel a gap in the tendon.

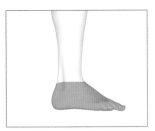

SEE ALSO Ankle *pp.144–45*,
Foot, upper *pp.148–49*,
Foot, underside *pp.150–51*

FOOT
GENERAL

The human foot is a strong, complex mechanical structure with 26 bones. Feet are prone to a variety of infections and injuries, which can be aggravated by high heels and poorly fitting shoes.

EFFECT OF COLD TEMPERATURES

Frostbite *(p.239)* ✚✚
Initially just numb, swollen skin with a reddened border. Later, formation of more ice crystals may damage the tissues irreversibly.

Frostnip *(p.239)* ✚
Similar to frostbite, but without ice-crystal formation in skin. Whitening of skin and numbness reverse quickly after rewarming.

Chilblains (pernio) *(p.225)* ✚
Localized inflammatory skin lumps on exposed extremities of the body, aggravated by cold. Redness, itching, inflammation, and sometimes blisters.

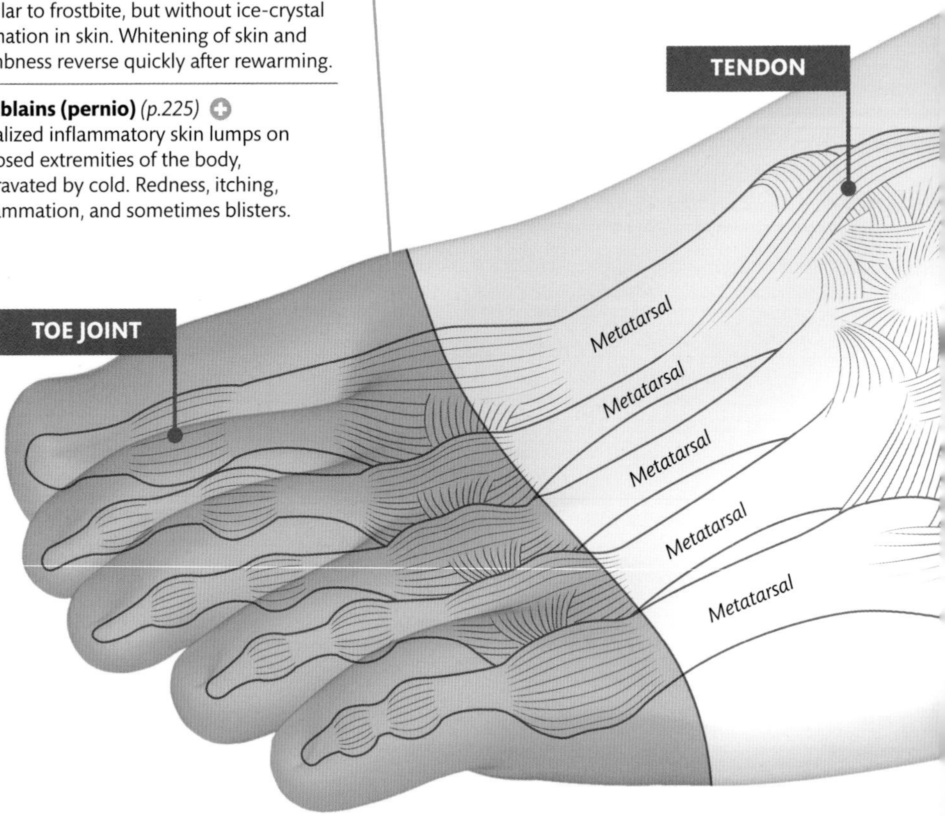

TENDON

TOE JOINT

Metatarsal

Metatarsal

Metatarsal

Metatarsal

Metatarsal

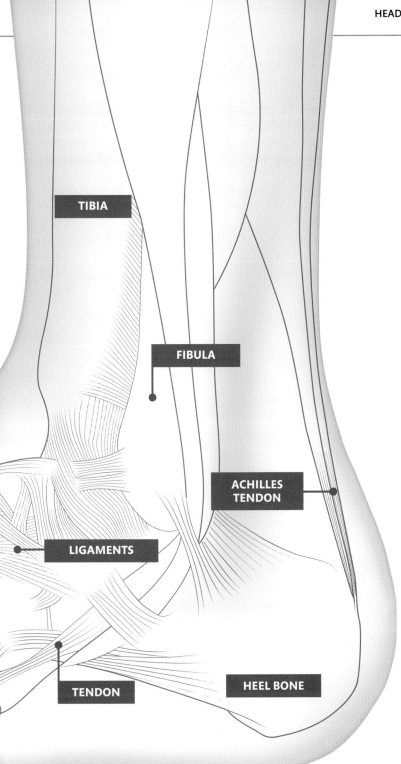

TIBIA

FIBULA

ACHILLES
TENDON

LIGAMENTS

TENDON

HEEL BONE

JOINT PROBLEMS

Gout (p.159) ⊕ ⊕
Intense pain with red, warm, very tender swelling of joints. Mostly affects big toe but can affect any joint in foot. Walking may be impossible. May also have hard, painless chalk-like lumps (tophi) on toes and heels.

Osteoarthritis (p.157) ⊕
Variable pain and stiffness, worse with activity. Reduced range of movement.

Rheumatoid arthritis (p.157) ⊕ ⊕
Pain, swelling, and stiffness in joints. Usually affects joints symmetrically (such as both big toes); and may affect several joints of the body. More general symptoms include mild fever, aches, tiredness, and weight loss.

Psoriatic arthritis (p.157) ⊕ ⊕
Tender, inflamed area where tendon inserts onto bone (such as Achilles to heel bone). End joint of toe(s) may be inflamed. May occur with or without typical psoriasis skin rash (p.222).

Diabetic foot ulcers (p.219) ⊕ ⊕
Usually painless, "punched-out", smelly ulcers in areas of thick tough skin (callus), with pus, swelling, and surrounding redness.

Club foot (p.156) ⊕
A congenital (present from birth) deformity with inward rotation that leads to walking on outer ankles or sides of feet.

Bone cancer (p.155) ⊕ ⊕
Initially may be a painless hard, fixed lump. Pain may gradually increase over time. Also fatigue, fever, weight loss, and/or unexplained bone fractures. Seek medical attention soon.

FOOT
UPPER

Upward flexion of the foot lifts the toes, helping to stretch the calf muscles and reduce stress on the tendons along the top of the foot, which can otherwise cause pain. Toe and nail problems are often the result of poorly fitting shoes.

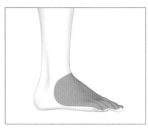

SEE ALSO Foot, general *pp.146–47*

Peroneal tendonitis *(p.164)* ➕➕
Gradually worsening pain in outside of foot and behind the ankle with instability during and after weight bearing, worse with turning the foot in or out.

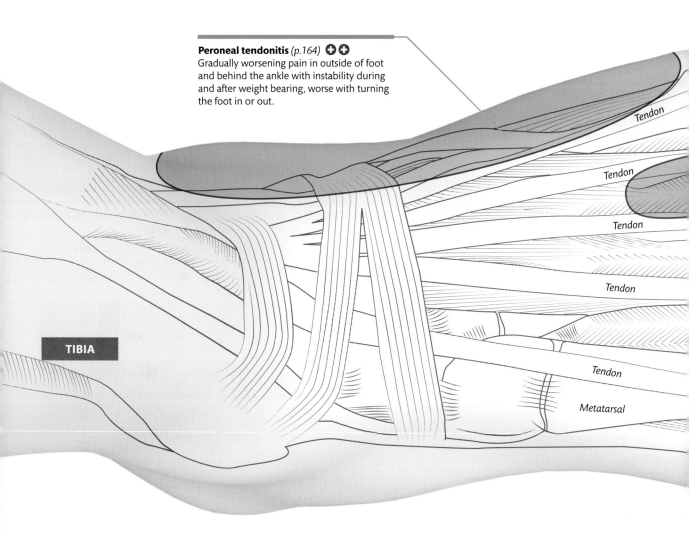

TIBIA

Tendon

Tendon

Tendon

Tendon

Tendon

Metatarsal

NAIL PROBLEMS

Stress fracture *(p.156)* ⊕
Pain in weight-bearing bone made worse with exercise. Localized bone tenderness; tapping it produces pain.

Fracture *(p.156)* ⊕⊕
Pain, tenderness, bruising, swelling, tingling, or numbness caused by trauma to (usually) a long bone of the foot.

Ingrown toenail *(p.231)* ⊕
A disorder where the nail grows up into the soft fleshy area of the toe. It results in infection with redness, pain, and swelling.

Fungal nail infection (onychomycosis) *(p.231)* ⊕
Discoloured, thickened, cracked, flaking, and even disintegrating toenail developing over several weeks.

Morton's neuroma *(p.173)* ⊕⊕
Sharp intermittent pain shooting into usually the 3rd and 4th toes when wearing shoes. Localized tenderness, partial numbness, and/or pins-and-needles sensation.

Osteoarthritis *(p.157)* ⊕⊕
Variable pain and stiffness, worse with activity. Reduced range of movement.

Bunion (hallux valgus) *(p.160)* ⊕
A deformity where the big toe points sideways to the second toe with a characteristic bump on inner side of the bottom toe joint.

TOE PROBLEMS

Hammer toe *(p.165)* ⊕
An abnormally curled toe in which the closest joint is cocked upward and the middle joint bends downwards.

Athlete's foot (tinea pedis) *(p.229)* ⊕
Itchy, scaling, weeping rash especially between toes, but can spread to most of bottom of foot. May blister.

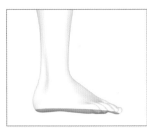

SEE ALSO Ankle *pp.144–45,*
Feet, general *pp.146–47,*
Foot, upper *pp.148–49*

FOOT
UNDERSIDE

The sole contains the thickest layers of skin on the body due to the weight placed on it. It has a high concentration of sweat glands. The bones under the sole form the arch of the foot, which may give way later in life, causing flat feet.

Plantar fasciitis *(p.165)* ⊕
Pain under heel or in arch. From first steps out of bed, improves after a while but may return after prolonged standing.

Heel spur *(p.155)* ⊕⊕
A hard bony lump under tender area of heel and/or arch.

Sever's disease *(p.162)* ⊕⊕
Heel pain in active children, causing limping, or running awkwardly with pain in one or both heels worse if rising onto tiptoes.

HEEL BONE

PLANTAR FASCIA

Flat feet *(p.156)* ⊕
Generally painless, flattening of the long arch of the foot.

High arches *(p.156)* ⊕
Foot pain under ball of foot, arch, and even ankle.

Big toe tendinitis *(p.164)*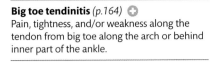
Pain, tightness, and/or weakness along the tendon from big toe along the arch or behind inner part of the ankle.

Tarsal tunnel syndrome *(p.173)*
Burning pain, tingling, and pins-and-needles sensation along inner ankle and/or into bottom of foot. Pain worse with extended periods of time spent walking or standing.

Tendon

Tendon

Tendon

Tendon

Tendon

SKIN PROBLEMS

Callus *(p.246)*
Thick, tough layer of skin. If the middle of a callus becomes harder and more separate, it is known as a corn.

Blister *(p.225)*
Small pocket of body fluid within the upper layers of skin caused by too much friction too rapidly for the skin to develop a protective callus.

Pressure sores *(p.225)*
Ranging from patches of discoloured skin to open wounds exposing underlying bone or muscle. Seek medical advice if severe.

Warts (verrucas) *(p.229)*
Small, thick, whorled skin lumps caused by a virus infection. Flattened into ball of foot by walking on them. Can be contagious, especially in children aged 5–15 years.

Cramp *(p.161)*
Sudden, involuntary, sustained (seconds to several minutes) contraction of a muscle, causing severe pain and temporary incapacity. More likely in tired muscles, although 75 per cent of cramps occur at night. Muscle soreness remains for a while once the cramp has ceased.

Metatarsalgia *(p.165)*
Pain in the ball of the foot, when walking (especially on the toes) or on impact (running). Uncomfortable when wearing shoes.

Morton's neuroma *(p.173)*
Sharp, intermittent pain shooting into usually 3rd and 4th toes when wearing shoes. Localized tenderness, partial numbness, and/or pins-and-needles sensation.

PART 3
DIRECTORY OF CONDITIONS

MUSCULOSKELETAL DISORDERS

OSTEOPOROSIS

In osteoporosis, there is loss of bone tissue, making the bones thinner and weaker. It is a natural part of ageing, but women are especially vulnerable after menopause because their ovaries no longer produce oestrogen, which helps to maintain bone mass. Other risk factors for developing osteoporosis include a diet low in calcium; disorders such as rheumatoid arthritis, hyperthyroidism, and chronic kidney disease; long-term corticosteroid treatment; prolonged immobility; and smoking.

The first sign of osteoporosis is typically a fracture, often at the wrist or top of the thigh bone near the hip joint. Sometimes, one or more vertebrae may fracture and crumble, leading to pain and progressive loss of height.

Treatment is with calcium and vitamin D supplements, regular exercise to build up and maintain bone strength, and medication to help prevent bone loss and reduce the risk of fractures. Hormone replacement therapy may also be suggested for some postmenopausal women, but it is not generally recommended because of the increased risk of adverse effects from long-term use, such as breast cancer.

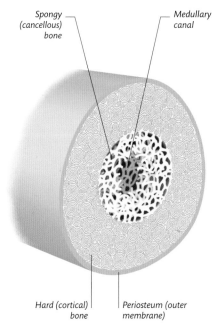

Spongy (cancellous) bone — Medullary canal

Hard (cortical) bone — Periosteum (outer membrane)

Normal bone
The inner layer is spongy (cancellous) bone, often with a central channel called the medullary canal. Around the layer of cancellous bone is a layer of hard (cortical) bone, which is covered by a membrane called the periosteum.

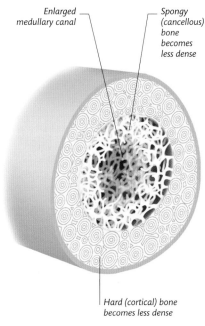

Enlarged medullary canal — Spongy (cancellous) bone becomes less dense

Hard (cortical) bone becomes less dense

Bone in osteoporosis
In osteoporosis, the medullary canal is enlarged and the spongy and cortical bone become less dense. The result is a loss of bone mass and increased brittleness and fragility of the bone.

OSTEOMYELITIS

Osteomyelitis is infection of a bone, usually due to injury, surgery, or the spread of infection from elsewhere in the body. Often, the infection is with *Staphylococcus aureus* bacteria; other possible causes include tuberculosis and fungal infection.

In acute osteomyelitis, symptoms develop suddenly and may include fever and severe pain in the affected bone. In chronic osteomyelitis, symptoms develop gradually and may include mild fever and persistent pain in the affected bone.

Treatment is with antibiotics or antifungal drugs. Surgery to remove the affected area of bone may also be necessary.

SPONDYLOLYSIS

Spondylolysis is a disorder of the spine in which part of the fifth (or, rarely, the fourth) lumbar vertebra in the lower back consists of soft, fibrous tissue instead of normal bone. As a result, the affected vertebra is weak and vulnerable to damage under stress, which may produce spondylolisthesis (forward slippage of the vertebra over the one below it, p.158).

If spondylolisthesis does occur, it may produce symptoms such as pain and stiffness and require treatment. Otherwise, spondylolysis usually produces no symptoms and treatment is not needed.

AVASCULAR NECROSIS

Avascular necrosis is death of part of a bone due to disruption of its blood supply, usually as a result of an injury to the bone, such as a fracture. It most commonly affects the shoulder, hip, or knee. It may not produce any obvious symptoms in the early stages, but later there is often persistent, gradually worsening pain in the affected area.

Treatment of avascular necrosis depends on the amount of bone damage, but may include medication, or, if there is extensive damage to the bone, surgery, such as a bone graft or joint replacement.

PAGET'S DISEASE OF BONE

Also called osteitis deformans, Paget's disease is the disruption of the process of bone renewal, leading to weakened and sometimes distorted bones. Normally, bone is continually broken down and replaced by strong, new bone, but in Paget's disease the new bone is weak. The cause of the disease is not known.

The most common sites affected by this condition are the skull, spine, pelvis, and legs. Symptoms may include bone and joint pain; bone deformities, such as bow legs; fractures after only a minor injury; numbness, tingling, or weakness in the affected area; and hearing loss. There is no cure for Paget's disease but medication can relieve symptoms.

BONE CANCER
Ewing's sarcoma

Malignant bone tumours may originate in the bone itself (primary bone cancer) or occur as a result of cancer spreading from elsewhere in the body (secondary, or metastatic, bone cancer).

The main types of primary cancer are known medically as osteosarcoma, Ewing's sarcoma, and chondrosarcoma. Their cause is unknown. Symptoms for all types of bone cancer may include persistent, gradually worsening bone pain; swelling and inflammation over the affected area of bone; fever; fatigue; and weight loss. Treatment is usually with a combination of surgery to remove the cancerous part of the bone, chemotherapy, and radiotherapy. Sometimes, amputation is necessary.

Secondary bone cancer most commonly affects the spine, pelvis, ribs, or skull. It is most often due to the spread of breast (p.216), lung (p.195), prostate (p.212), thyroid, or kidney cancer (p.209). The main symptom is gnawing bone pain. Cancer affecting the spine may also cause a collapse of the vertebrae, which may lead to weakness or paralysis of a limb. Treatment is directed primarily at the underlying primary cancer.

OSGOOD-SCHLATTER DISEASE

Osgood-Schlatter disease is painful swelling of the bony prominence of the shin (called the tibial tuberosity) just below the knee. It occurs most commonly in teenagers who play a lot of sport and is thought to be caused by excessive, repetitive pulling of the quadriceps muscle at the front of the thigh, which is transmitted to the tibial tuberosity. The pain is usually worse during physical activity and eases with rest. Usually, only one leg is affected.

Treatment is not usually needed, apart from rest and painkillers, and the condition typically clears up within a few weeks or months.

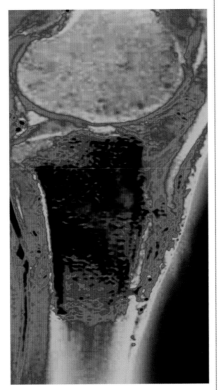

Bone cancer
This coloured scan of the lower leg shows an osteosarcoma (dark blue area) at the top of the shin bone. This type of malignant tumour most commonly affects children and people under 20.

BONE SPURS

Also known as osteophytes, bone spurs are bony lumps that grow on bones, around joints, or on the vertebrae (spinal bones). Bone spurs often develop in osteoarthritis (p.157), cervical spondylosis (osteoarthritis of the neck, p.158), and ankylosing spondylitis (inflammation of the vertebrae, p.158). They commonly affect the neck, shoulder, knee, lower back, fingers, or toes. Heel spurs are often caused by repeated damage to foot muscles and ligaments. They are common in athletes.

Bone spurs do not always cause symptoms. If they do, symptoms may include pain, restricted movement, and tingling, numbness, or weakness in the affected area.

Treatment is usually with painkillers; if movement is restricted, physiotherapy may be helpful. In severe cases, surgery to remove the spur may be offered.

NONCANCEROUS BONE TUMOURS
Osteoid osteoma

Noncancerous bone tumours may affect any bone, but are most common in the long bones of the limbs or the vertebrae, or the bones of the hands. The main types are osteoid osteomas, osteochondromas, and chondromas. They usually develop during childhood or adolescence. Their cause is not known.

The presence of a tumour normally causes no symptoms, although sometimes the affected bone may become enlarged and deformed. Occasionally, a tumour may press on a nerve, causing tingling or numbness. In some cases, movement may be restricted or painful if the tumour presses on nearby tendons.

A noncancerous bone tumour that is not causing problems may just be monitored. One that is causing symptoms or growing rapidly may be removed by surgery, often followed by a bone graft to replace the removed section of bone.

COCCYDYNIA

Coccydynia is severe, sharp pain in the coccyx (tailbone), the small triangular bone at the base of the spine. It may result from an injury (for example, due to a fall, for example; prolonged pressure from sitting with a poor posture; or a baby pushing against the mother's coccyx during childbirth. However, often there is no obvious cause.

Coccydynia can usually be relieved by over-the-counter painkillers and usually clears up by itself within a few weeks. Persistent coccydynia may be treated with an injection into the lower back of a corticosteroid drug, often in combination with an anaesthetic. Usually, no further treatment is needed.

FOOT DEFORMITIES
Club foot | Flat feet | High arches

Flat feet are normal in children until the age of about two or three years, when the arch starts to develop. Sometimes this fails to happen, resulting in flat feet (pes planus). In adults, flat feet are due to fallen arches, which sometimes occurs as a result of weight gain. Flat feet sometimes ache, but this can usually be alleviated by using arch supports. Rarely, corrective surgery may be advised.

High arches (pes cavus) may be an inherited condition or may develop as a result of a muscle or nerve disorder. It may sometimes cause foot pain, which can usually be relieved by using orthotic inserts (special inserts that support the arches). In severe cases, corrective surgery may be advised.

Club foot (talipes) is an inward twisting of one or both feet and is present from birth. It may be treated by repeated manipulation of the foot and special footwear. If this method is unsuccessful, corrective surgery may be necessary.

BONE FRACTURE
Cheek-bone fracture | Collarbone fracture | Femoral fracture | Hip fracture | Humerus fracture | Rib fracture | Stress fracture | Vertebral fracture

A fracture can be a complete break, a crack, or a split part of the way through a bone. Most fractures are due to a trauma (sudden, strong impact), although stress fractures result from repeated jarring. Osteoporosis (p.154) may lead to cracks in the vertebrae (compression fractures) or to femoral (thigh bone) fractures near the hip joint.

Symptoms of a fracture may include pain, which may be severe; swelling and bruising; deformity in the affected area; and, in some cases, bone protruding through the skin. There is also often bleeding, which may sometimes be severe. Traumatic vertebrae (spinal) fractures may also damage the spinal cord or spinal nerves, which may lead to paralysis of part of the body.

Treatment usually involves immobilizing the affected part in a cast until the bone heals. If the bone ends are displaced, they will first be realigned, which may involve surgery. A bone broken near a joint may sometimes be replaced with an artificial substitute, comprising either part of the bone or the entire joint. Compression fractures are usually treated primarily with painkillers. Traumatic fractures require specialist treatment.

Fractured radius
This coloured X ray shows a fracture of the radius (a bone of the forearm). This is a closed (simple) fracture, because the bone ends remain beneath the skin. In an open (compound) fracture, one or both bone ends pierce the skin.

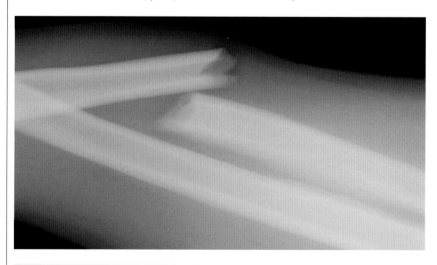

ABNORMAL SPINAL CURVATURES
Kyphosis | Scoliosis

In kyphosis, there is excessive outward curvature of the spine in the chest area, sometimes causing back pain. Kyphosis is common in children and usually corrects itself as the child grows. In adults, kyphosis is typically due to poor posture, weakening of the vertebrae usually caused by osteoporosis (p.154), or obesity. In scoliosis, the spine is curved to the left or right, most commonly in the chest area or lower back region. It may cause leaning to one side and sometimes back pain. Scoliosis usually starts in childhood or adolescence and tends to become progressively worse until growth stops.

Treatment is similar for all types of spinal curvature. Mild cases can often be treated with painkillers and physiotherapy. Severe cases may be treated with a spinal brace and surgery to straighten the spine.

OSTEOARTHRITIS

Osteoarthritis is a common joint disease in which there is gradual degeneration of the cartilage that covers the bone ends in joints, causing pain and stiffness. In a normal joint, the bone ends are protected by a smooth layer of cartilage and lubricated by synovial fluid. In osteoarthritis, the cartilage becomes worn or frayed, causing friction between the bone ends, which results in inflammation, pain, and excess fluid production. Bony growths (osteophytes) may also develop around the joint, further increasing friction and limiting the range of movement. Eventually, the cartilage becomes so worn that bone grinds on bone.

There is no cure for osteoarthritis. Treatment involves painkillers, medications to reduce inflammation, exercise, and physiotherapy. In severe cases, surgery may be necessary to repair or replace the joint.

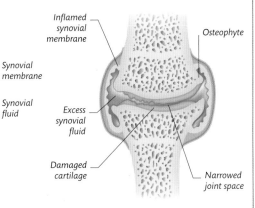

Healthy joint
The bone ends are covered with a smooth, intact layer of cartilage, and the whole joint capsule (the tissue enclosing the joint) is lined with synovial membrane, which produces lubricating fluid.

Early osteoarthritis
Changes begin with damage and degeneration of the cartilage. This leads to narrowing of the joint space, increased friction, and excess synovial fluid production, resulting in swelling and pain.

PSORIATIC ARTHRITIS

Psoriatic arthritis is a type of arthritis (joint inflammation) that occurs in some people with the skin condition psoriasis (p.222). In mild cases, only a few joints are affected, often those at the ends of the fingers or toes. In severe cases, many joints are involved, including those of the spine. Often, the symptoms – joint pain, swelling, and stiffness – flare up at the same time as those of psoriasis. Untreated, psoriatic arthritis may lead to permanent joint damage.

Treatment may involve nonsteroidal anti-inflammatory drugs and corticosteroids to reduce pain and inflammation, and medications such as disease-modifying anti-rheumatic drugs to slow the progress of the condition.

REACTIVE ARTHRITIS

Formerly known as Reiter's syndrome, reactive arthritis is joint inflammation due to an abnormal immune response to a recent infection, usually a bacterial infection of the genital tract or intestine.

The main symptom is joint pain, swelling, and stiffness. The condition may also affect the eyes, causing conjunctivitis or blurred vision, or urethra, causing painful urination and a discharge from the urethra.

Treatment may include antibiotics if the infection is still present. The arthritis itself is usually treated with painkillers, corticosteroids to reduce inflammation, and sometimes disease-modifying anti-rheumatic drugs to block the abnormal immune response.

SEPTIC ARTHRITIS

Septic arthritis is inflammation of a joint caused by bacterial infection. It is usually due to bacteria entering through a nearby open wound or travelling through the bloodstream from an infection elsewhere.

Symptoms usually appear suddenly and may include swelling, redness, and warmth around the affected joint; severe joint pain; restricted movement of the joint; and fever. Treatment is with antibiotics, painkillers, and rest. The joint may also be drained if pus has built up inside it.

RHEUMATOID ARTHRITIS

Rheumatoid arthritis is a long-term autoimmune disorder in which the immune system attacks the joints, causing pain, stiffness, and swelling in affected joints. Sometimes, small, painless lumps may develop around affected joints, and there may also be general symptoms, such as tiredness, fever, and weight loss. Symptoms may flare up then diminish before flaring up again. In some cases, other body tissues may also be affected, such as the lungs, heart, eyes, or blood vessels.

Treatment typically involves disease-modifying anti-rheumatic drugs or other medications to slow progression of the disease; painkillers; corticosteroids to reduce inflammation; and physiotherapy. Surgery to remove damaged joint tissue or replace an affected joint may also be recommended.

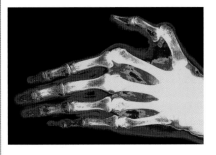

Rheumatoid hand
This coloured X ray shows rheumatoid arthritis in the thumb and hand joints, which have become swollen and distorted as a result.

SPONDYLOLISTHESIS

In spondylolisthesis, a vertebra (bone of the spine) slips forward over the one below it. The condition usually affects vertebrae in the lower back. It may be present from birth or develop during growth in mid-to-late childhood. However, most cases occur in adults and result from a degenerative joint disorder, such as osteoarthritis (p.157), or, more rarely from a spinal injury, such as a stress fracture of the spine (p.156). In most cases, there are no symptoms, although some people have pain, stiffness, or sciatica. Treatment may include medication and special exercises or physiotherapy. In severe cases, surgery may be needed.

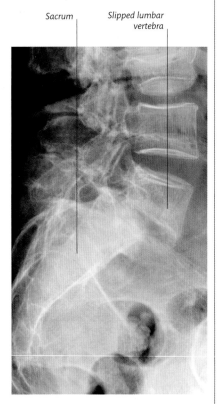

Sacrum   Slipped lumbar
                  vertebra

Spondylolisthesis
The lower back is the area most commonly affected by spondylolisthesis, as shown in this coloured X-ray, which reveals that the fifth (lowest) lumbar vertebra has slipped over the sacrum.

CERVICAL SPONDYLOSIS

Cervical spondylosis is the medical term for osteoarthritis (p.157) of the neck. In this disorder, the cervical vertebrae thicken, bony outgrowths develop on the vertebrae, and the joints between the vertebra may become inflamed. These changes cause pressure on nerves or blood vessels in the neck, leading to symptoms such as neck

SLIPPED DISC

Known medically as a prolapsed disc, a slipped disc is when one of the soft discs that separate the vertebrae becomes damaged and the disc's core protrudes. The protruding core may press on a spinal nerve, causing pain and other symptoms. Most commonly, the lower back is affected, causing sciatica – pain, numbness, or tingling along the back of the leg. A prolapsed disc in the neck may cause neck pain, and weakness in the arm and hand.

Symptoms usually improve on their own but may be relieved with painkillers and physiotherapy. Keeping as active as possible can help to speed recovery. In severe cases, surgery to remove part or all of the damaged disc may be necessary to relieve pressure on a spinal nerve.

ANKYLOSING SPONDYLITIS

In ankylosing spondylitis (AS), there is persistent inflammation of the sacroiliac joints (between the spine and back of the pelvis) and vertebrae (spinal bones). The cause of AS is not known, but it tends to run in families.

The symptoms usually start gradually, with pain and stiffness in the hips and lower back, which are worse after resting and are especially noticeable in the early morning. Other symptoms may include chest pain, painful heels, tiredness, and redness and pain in the eyes. Over time, the spinal inflammation may lead to permanent stiffness and spinal curvature. Treatment involves special exercises, physiotherapy, and medication to relieve symptoms.

pain and stiffness, headaches, pain that travels from the shoulders to the hands, numbness, tingling, and weakness in the hands, and sometimes dizziness. In severe cases, the spinal cord may be significantly compressed, which may cause weakness in the legs or sometimes incontinence.

Treatment is usually with medication and special exercises or physiotherapy. In severe cases, surgery may be advised.

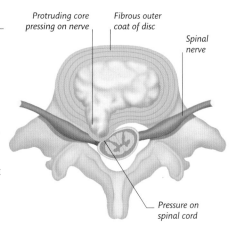

Protruding core   Fibrous outer
pressing on nerve   coat of disc

                              Spinal
                              nerve

                         Pressure on
                         spinal cord

Disc prolapse
A prolapsed disc may push into the centre of the spine, pressing on the spinal cord and the roots of the nerves leading from it. In the lower spine this can affect nerves to the legs, causing sciatica.

COSTOCHONDRITIS

In costochondritis, the cartilage that joins the breastbone to the ribs is inflamed, causing pain in the chest. Typically, the pain is made worse by deep breathing, sneezing, or coughing, pressure on the chest, exercise, moving the arms, or sometimes a particular body position, such as lying down.

The condition usually clears up without treatment, although symptoms may persist for months. The symptoms can be managed by painkillers and self-help measures, such as avoiding activities that make the pain worse.

BURSITIS
**Olecranon bursitis (student's elbow) |
Pre-patellar bursitis | Trochanteric bursitis**

Bursitis is inflammation of a bursa – one of the small, fluid-filled pads that cushion the joints. Some of the most important bursae are the pre-patellar bursa at the front of the knee, the olecranon bursa over the point of the elbow, and the trochanteric bursa at the outside point of the hip.

Bursitis is most commonly caused by prolonged or repeated stress, such as frequent kneeling, but may also result from injury or excessive exercise. Certain joint diseases – gout and rheumatoid arthritis (p.137), for example – increase the risk of developing bursitis. Occasionally, it may be caused by a bacterial infection.

The main symptoms are pain, swelling, tenderness, and restricted movement of the affected joint. Bursitis due to infection may also cause fever. Treatment may involve resting the affected joint; medication, such as corticosteroid injections to reduce inflammation or antibiotics to treat an infection; or draining the affected bursa. If bursitis is persistent or recurrent, surgery to remove the bursa may be recommended.

GOUT
Gouty tophus

Gout is a type of arthritis in which crystals form in joints, Usually, only one joint is affected, most commonly the base of the big toe, but gout can occur in several joints, and any joint can be affected. Gout results from high levels of uric acid (a waste product formed by the breakdown of cells and proteins) in the blood. The acid is deposited as crystals in the joints, causing sudden attacks of severe pain and inflammation. In longstanding gout, deposits of the acid may build up around joints, in the earlobes, and in other soft tissues and form small lumps known as tophi.

The underlying cause of gout is unknown but symptoms may be triggered by various factors, including certain foods

SNAPPING HIP SYNDROME

In snapping hip syndrome, there is a snapping sensation or snapping sound when walking, swinging the leg, or getting up from a sitting position. The snapping is usually caused by movement of a muscle or tendon over a bony part of the hip. Snapping hip syndrome is often due to tightness of the muscles and tendons

FROZEN SHOULDER

In frozen shoulder, the tissue around the shoulder joint becomes inflamed and thickened, causing pain and stiffness. The cause is not known, but in some cases it develops after a shoulder injury or is associated with other disorders, such as other inflammatory or joint disorders or diabetes. Typically, symptoms develop over three stages: a slow, painful "freezing" of the shoulder over several weeks or months; a "frozen" stage lasting for months, when there is less pain but severe stiffness; and a "thawing" stage, which may last from months to years, when symptoms ease. Treatment may involve medication, physiotherapy, or, rarely, surgery.

(such as red meat, offal, and oily fish), alcohol (especially beer, spirits, and fortified wines), and some medications. Treatment involves medication and avoiding triggers.

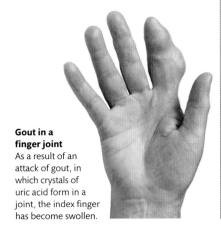

**Gout in a
finger joint**
As a result of an attack of gout, in which crystals of uric acid form in a joint, the index finger has become swollen.

around the hip. It is more common in those involved in activities that require frequent bending at the hip, such as athletes and dancers.

Treatment is not needed unless the condition causes pain. Then treatment may include rest, medication to relieve the pain, and physiotherapy. If these treatments are ineffective, surgery may be recommended.

TEMPOROMANDIBULAR JOINT DYSFUNCTION

In this condition, the chewing muscles and the joints between the skull and lower jaw do not work together properly, causing symptoms such as jaw pain, facial pain, headaches, unusual noises (such as clicks) when chewing or opening or closing the mouth, and earache. Possible causes include spasm of the chewing muscles, often due to clenching the jaw or grinding the teeth, a poor bite (known as malocclusion), a jaw injury, or certain diseases (such as osteoarthritis, p.157). Treatment involves correcting any underlying abnormality (such as a poor bite), medication, or, rarely, surgery.

SACROILIAC JOINT DYSFUNCTION

Sacroiliac joint dysfunction is a general term for pain and inflammation in the sacroiliac joint. The sacroiliac joints are located on either side of the spine and connect the sacrum (the fused bones at the base of the spine) with the ilia (pelvic bones). The joints can be strained by pregnancy, childbirth, or overstriding when running, or they may be affected by various disorders, such as arthritis.

The main symptom is pain in the lower back, hip, buttocks, thigh, or groin. Treatment may involve therapy for any underlying disorder, rest, medication, and physiotherapy.

TORN KNEE CARTILAGE
Meniscus tear

The knee contains two pads of cartilage (menisci) that act as shock-absorbers between the femur (thigh bone) and tibia (shinbone). Tearing of the cartilage (a meniscus tear) usually occurs as a result of a sudden twisting of the leg and it is a common sports injury. Symptoms typically include sudden pain in the knee, swelling of the knee, and difficulty in straightening the leg.

A mild tear may be treated with rest and nonsteroidal anti-inflammatory drugs. A severe tear may require surgery to repair or remove the damaged cartilage.

PATELLOFEMORAL PAIN SYNDROME

Patellofemoral pain syndrome is the medical term for pain around the front of the knee that is not associated with any signs of damage or problems in the knee. Typically, the pain is worse when walking up or down stairs: there may also be swelling around the kneecap and a grating sensation when the knee is bent or straightened. It is common in people who do sports.

Treatment is with rest, painkillers, and physiotherapy. It make take several months to recover fully, and sometimes the condition persists for years.

PLICA SYNDROME

The plica is a fold of membrane in the knee that is thought to be tissue that normally disappears during fetal development but persists after birth in some people. Its presence or absence makes no difference to the functioning of the knee. In plica syndrome, the plica becomes inflamed, causing pain at the inside front of the knee. The pain is usually associated with bending the knee and becomes worse during and after exercise.

Treatment is with rest, painkillers, and corticosteroid injections to reduce inflammation. If this treatment is unsuccessful, surgery may be suggested.

BAKER'S CYST

A Baker's cyst is a fluid-filled swelling that develops at the back of the knee. It may be a feature of disorders such as osteoarthritis (p.157) and rheumatoid arthritis (p.157) and it may also be caused by a knee injury. Most cysts are painless. Occasionally a cyst may rupture, causing pain in the calf.

In many cases, the cyst disappears by itself. A large or painful cyst may be treated with painkillers and corticosteroids to reduce inflammation. Rarely, a cyst may need to be drained or surgically removed.

GANGLION

A ganglion is a fluid-filled cyst that develops under the skin near a joint or tendon, most commonly on the wrist or back of the hand but sometimes on the foot. Ganglia are not harmful and may be present for years without causing problems, although some cause pain or restrict movement. If they cause no symptoms, they can be left to disappear by themselves. If they cause pain or impede movement, they can be drained or removed surgically.

BUNION

A bunion is a thickened lump at the base of the big toe. The underlying cause is a minor bone deformity, called hallux valgus, in which the joint at the base of the big toe projects outwards, forcing the toe to turn inwards. Pressure on the projecting bone causes the surrounding tissues to thicken, forming a bunion. A bunion may be painful and may become inflamed and callused.

Small bunions may be remedied by using a bunion splint to straighten the big toe. For a large or troublesome bunion, surgery to remove the protruding area of bone and straighten the big toe may be recommended.

Bunion
An abnormal outward projection of the joint at the base of the big toe leads to thickening of the soft tissues around the joint, resulting in a bunion.

Soft tissue becomes thickened

Protruding part of joint

JOINT INSTABILITY
Shoulder instability

Normally, the bones, ligaments, and muscles of a joint work together to support the various parts of the joint in their correct positions while also allowing the full range of movement of the joint. In joint instability, there is lack of support, with the result that the joint may not move correctly or may be dislocated easily. In shoulder instability, for example, the shoulder joint feels abnormally loose, and there may also be symptoms such as tingling, numbness, or weakness in the arm. In extreme cases, the shoulder may dislocate.

Treatment may involve physiotherapy and anti-inflammatory medication or surgery to stabilize or repair the joint. If the joint has dislocated, it will need to be manipulated back into position.

DISLOCATED JOINT
**Dislocated kneecap |
Shoulder dislocation**

In a joint dislocation, the bones of a joint become displaced, usually as a result of injury. A dislocation is often accompanied by tearing of the joint ligaments and damage to the membrane encasing the joint. There may also be damage to nearby nerves, tendons, and blood vessels. Symptoms typically include severe pain in the affected area, deformity of the joint, and swelling and bruising around the joint. Treatment usually involves manipulating the joint back into place, followed by immobilization in a splint or cast. In some cases, surgery to reposition the joint and repair any damage may be needed.

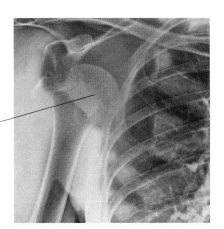

Dislocated head of humerus

Dislocated shoulder joint
In this coloured X-ray, the head of the humerus (upper arm bone) has come out of the joint socket at the end of the shoulder blade.

WHIPLASH

Whiplash is a neck injury caused by a sudden, violent back-and-forth or sideways movement of the neck. It commonly occurs in road traffic accidents – for example, due to sudden deceleration or acceleration in a vehicle collision.

The severity of a whiplash injury varies from small strains to major trauma in which neck ligaments are torn. The sudden pull of muscles and tendons on bones may break pieces off the ends of the vertebrae. Nerves and blood vessels may also be damaged, causing pain in the neck, shoulders, and arms, and possibly dizziness and vision problems. There may be muscle spasms, swelling, and stiffness in the affected area. It may take several hours for symptoms to develop after the injury, and they may become worse over the next few days.

Whiplash usually gradually improves on its own over several weeks with measures such as ice-packs to reduce inflammation, painkillers, and keeping the neck as mobile as possible. If symptoms persist, physiotherapy may be recommended.

MUSCLE CRAMPS

Sudden muscle spasms in which a muscle or group of muscles becomes hard, painful, and tight often occur during physical exercise. Another common cause is sitting or lying in an awkward position. Certain medications may also cause cramps, and cramps may sometimes be a symptom of an underlying disorder. Often, however, there is no apparent cause.

Stretching or massaging the affected muscle usually relieves cramps. For severe or recurrent cramps, a doctor may prescribe quinine (an antimalarial drug that can also relieve cramp) or a muscle relaxer and investigate possible causes.

POLYMYALGIA RHEUMATICA

Polymalgia rheumatica is an inflammatory disorder that mainly affects muscles of the hips, thighs, shoulders, and neck, causing pain, stiffness, and inflammation. The cause is unknown. The main symptoms are painful, stiff muscles in the morning; fever and night sweats; tiredness; weight loss; and depression. Symptoms may be accompanied by those of giant cell arteritis (p.183), such as headaches and scalp tenderness.

Treatment is with corticosteroids to reduce inflammation and relieve symptoms. Often, treatment needs to be continued for about two years, or sometimes longer, to prevent symptoms recurring.

Cervical spine | Disc

Ligament

Sudden acceleration
A sudden force from behind (for example, due to a collision from behind in a traffic accident) causes the head to jerk backwards, hyperextending the neck. The head then rebounds forwards.

Ligament tear

Disc pinched between vertebrae

Sudden deceleration
A sudden violent force from the front (for example, due to colliding with a stationary vehicle) causes the head to jerk forwards, flexing the neck. The head then rebound backwards.

LIGAMENT SPRAINS AND TEARS

Ankle sprain | Anterior cruciate ligament (ACL) injury | Chronic ankle instability (CAI) | Medial collateral ligament injury | Posterior cruciate ligament (PCL) injury

Ligaments are bands of tissue that hold bones together at a joint. They are not very stretchy and are prone to tearing, especially when subjected to sudden forceful twisting. The injury may range from a minor tear, called a sprain, to complete rupture of a ligament. The most commonly injured ligaments are those in the knee – the medial collateral ligament, anterior cruciate ligament (ACL), or posterior cruciate ligament (PCL) – and ankle.

Symptoms include sudden pain in the injured joint; swelling; and restricted movement of the joint. Most minor injuries can be treated with self-help measures such as PRICE (Protection, Rest, Ice, Compression, Elevation, p.246) and painkillers. A severe injury should receive medical attention as it may require surgery to repair or replace the ligament.

Sprained ankle
The ankle is prone to sprains if the foot twists suddenly. A common injury is a sprain of the lateral ligaments, due to the foot twisting inwards.

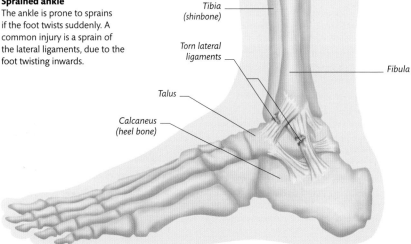

Tibia (shinbone)

Torn lateral ligaments

Fibula

Talus

Calcaneus (heel bone)

SPINAL MUSCULAR ATROPHY

Spinal muscular atrophy (SMA) is an inherited disorder that causes muscle wasting (atrophy), muscle weakness, and loss of movement.

Symptoms may include weakness in the limbs; movement problems, such as difficulty walking; tremors; swallowing problems; and breathing difficulties. The most severe type of SMA affects babies less than six months old and is usually fatal within the first few years. The least severe type begins in early adulthood, tends to cause relatively mild symptoms, and does not affect life expectancy. There is no cure for SMA. Treatment is aimed at managing the symptoms.

TORTICOLLIS

Also known as wry neck, torticollis is twisting of the neck, causing the head to tilt to one side. There may also be neck pain and stiffness. Torticollis is commonly due to a minor neck injury or sleeping or sitting in an awkward position. Less common causes include certain nerve disorders or cervical spondylosis (arthritis of the neck, p.158).

Torticollis can usually be treated with painkillers, heat treatment, massage, and gentle neck exercises. Muscle relaxants may be prescribed for persistent or severe cases.

RESTLESS LEGS SYNDROME

Restless legs syndrome is characterized by an irresistible urge to move the legs, and unpleasant tickling, burning, prickling or aching sensations in the leg muscles. The symptoms tend to come on at night and can interrupt sleep. They may also be triggered by prolonged sitting. The cause is unknown.

Mild cases may be alleviated by self-help measures, such as cooling or warming the legs, walking around, or relaxation exercises. More severe cases may be treated with medication, such as the anti-Parkinson drug levodopa or anticonvulsants.

FIBROMYALGIA

Fibromyalgia is a long-term condition that causes widespread muscle pain. The cause is unknown but the condition often develops during periods of stress. In addition to pain, other symptoms may include tiredness, headache, difficulty sleeping, diarrhoea, constipation, difficulty concentrating, anxiety, depression, and in women, painful periods.

Treatment is aimed at relieving symptoms. It includes medication, such as painkillers, muscle relaxants, and antidepressants; psychological therapy; and relaxation techniques.

SEVER'S DISEASE

Sever's disease is a painful inflammation of the bottom of the heel that affects children between about 8 and 14 years old. At this age, the heel bone is not fully developed and repeated stress on it (for example, from playing sports) can cause inflammation of the part of the heel bone that is still growing.

Treatment for Sever's disease involves avoiding any activities that cause the pain, nonsteroidal anti-inflammatory drugs to reduce pain and inflammation, and heel supports in shoes. Physiotherapy may also sometimes be recommended.

MYASTHENIA GRAVIS

In myasthenia gravis, the immune system attacks the receptors in muscles that receive nerve signals, resulting in muscle weakness. The condition is sometimes associated with a tumour of the thymus (an immune gland in the neck).

Symptoms may include drooping eyelids, double vision, slurred speech, difficulty chewing and swallowing, weakness in the legs and arms, and breathing difficulty.

Treatment may include medication to improve transmission of nerve signals, immunosuppressants, and sometimes surgery to remove the thymus. If symptoms suddenly become severe, urgent medical treatment is needed.

ROTATOR CUFF DISORDERS

The rotator cuff is a group of muscles and tendons around the shoulder joint that keep the head of the humerus (upper arm bone) in the shoulder socket and are also involved in shoulder movements.

Repeated overhead arm movements may cause inflammation or a tear in the rotator cuff, producing pain in the shoulder and restricted arm movement. A minor tear or inflammation can usually be treated with rest, ice-packs to reduce inflammation, and over-the-counter painkillers. A doctor may also sometimes recommend corticosteroid injections and physiotherapy. A severe tear may need to be repaired surgically.

PIRIFORMIS SYNDROME

The piriformis muscle is a located in the buttocks, near the top of the hip joint. In piriformis syndrome, the muscle spasms and presses on the sciatic nerve, which runs from the buttocks down the leg. This causes pain, tingling, or numbness in the buttocks and sometimes down the back of the leg.

Treatment for piriformis syndrome typically involves reducing pain by relaxing the muscle using heat or cold, massage, and physiotherapy; painkillers may also sometimes be prescribed. When symptoms have subsided, special exercises may be recommended to help prevent the condition from recurring.

COMPARTMENT SYNDROME

Compartment syndrome occurs when excessive pressure builds up within an enclosed group of muscles (called a compartment), usually as a result of bleeding or inflammation. Acute compartment syndrome develops rapidly, is usually due to an injury such as a fracture, and causes intense pain. It requires urgent surgery to relieve the pressure. Chronic compartment syndrome develops gradually, is often due to excessive exercise, and typically causes cramping pain that begins during exercise and disappears with rest. It can usually be treated by avoiding exercise, physiotherapy, and nonsteroidal anti-inflammatory drugs.

SHIN SPLINTS

Known medically as medial tibial stress syndrome, shin splints is pain in the shin, usually caused by exercise such as running. The pain tends to affect both shins. It typically starts soon after beginning exercise, becomes increasingly severe while exercising, then gradually disappears with rest. It can usually be treated by avoiding the exercise that caused the condition and by using ice-packs and painkillers to reduce pain.

MUSCLE STRAINS AND TEARS
Hamstring injury | Groin strain | Stiff neck

Muscle injuries range from a mild strain (sometimes referred to as pulling a muscle), in which the muscle fibres are overstretched, to a complete tear. Strains and tears often occur as a result of heavy physical work or overstrenuous activity during sports. Almost any muscle can be strained or torn; those commonly affected include muscles in the lower back, legs, and groin. Typical symptoms may include pain in the affected muscle during use and sometimes also at rest; swelling and bruising in the affected area; and muscle spasms (painful muscle contractions).

Most cases can be treated with PRICE (Protection, Rest, Ice, Compression, Elevation, p.246) and painkillers. A doctor may also recommend physiotherapy or immobilizing the affected area with a splint, brace, or cast. A severe injury may require surgery to repair the damaged muscle.

Torn hamstring
The hamstrings are the muscles at the back of the thigh that bend the knee and pull the leg back. Hamstring injuries are common in sportsmen and sportswomen who do a lot of sprinting or jumping.

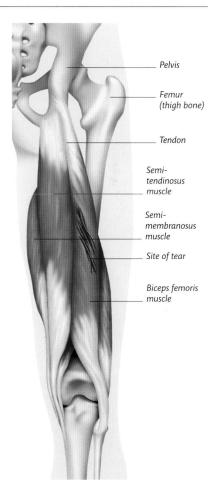

Pelvis

Femur (thigh bone)

Tendon

Semi-tendinosus muscle

Semi-membranosus muscle

Site of tear

Biceps femoris muscle

ILIOTIBIAL BAND SYNDROME

The iliotibial band is a thick band of tissue that runs from the pelvis down the outside of the femur (thigh bone) to just below the knee, where it connects to the tibia (shinbone). In iliotibial band syndrome (ITBS), the band becomes inflamed and painful at the outside of the knee due to rubbing against the knee joint when repeatedly bending and straightening the knee – movements typically made while running or cycling.

Treatment for ITBS is with rest and with ice-packs and painkillers to reduce inflammation and pain.

DEAD LEG

Dead leg is the bruising of the quadriceps muscles at the front of the thigh due to a blow that crushes the muscles against the underlying femur (thigh bone).

There is usually pain at the time of the injury and sometimes swelling and tingling. Later, the pain and swelling become worse, a bruise appears, and the injured muscle may become stiff, restricting movement.

Treatment for dead leg is with PRICE (Protection, Rest, Ice, Compression, Elevation, p.246). A doctor may also recommend physiotherapy.

REPETITIVE STRAIN INJURY

Repetitive strain injury (RSI) refers to symptoms caused by prolonged repetitive movements of one part of the body, as may occur during long sessions using a computer keyboard, for example.

RSI mainly affects the neck, shoulder, arms, and hands. Symptoms may include pain, tingling, throbbing, stiffness, weakness, and cramp in the affected area. Treatment may include painkillers, physiotherapy, and wearing a support on the affected area. Modifying the activity that causes symptoms is also important; if RSI is job-related, the employer should be informed.

TENDINITIS AND TENOSYNOVITIS

**Achilles tendinitis | Biceps tendinitis | Big toe tendinitis | De Quervain's tenosynovitis |
Patellar tendinitis (jumper's knee) | Peroneal tendinitis | Tendon inflammation |
Trigger finger or thumb**

Tendinitis (also called tendonitis) is inflammation of a tendon, the fibrous cord that attaches a muscle to bone. Tenosynovitis is inflammation of the sheath of tissues that encloses a tendon. These conditions usually occur together and are most commonly caused by overuse – for example, due to playing sports. Occasionally, they may be due to an infection or a disorder such as rheumatoid arthritis.

The areas most commonly affected are the shoulder, elbow, wrist, fingers, knee, and back of the heel. Symptoms in the affected area may include pain and swelling;

stiffness and restricted movement; warm, red skin over the tendon; and a lump over the tendon. Occasionally, there may be a crackling sensation when the tendon moves, or a joint may stick in one position.

In most cases, the conditions can be treated with rest, ice-packs to reduce inflammation, painkillers, and a bandage, splint, or brace to support the affected area. A doctor may also recommend corticosteroid injections to reduce inflammation. Physiotherapy may also be recommended. Any underlying disorder may also need treatment.

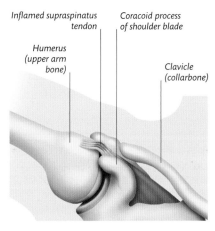

Tendinitis
Tendons transmit the pull of muscles to bones. Injury or overuse can cause inflammation or a tear in a tendon, resulting in pain and sometimes a crackling sensation when the tendon moves.

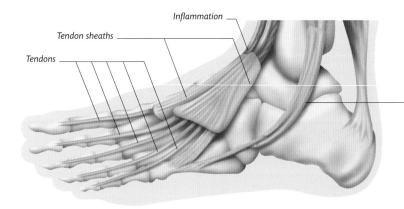

Tenosynovitis
The synovium, the protective sheath of tissue that covers some tendons, produces fluid to keep the tendon moving smoothly. Inflammation of this tissue causes pain and tenderness.

TENNIS ELBOW AND GOLFER'S ELBOW

Tennis elbow and golfer's elbow both occur when the tendon attachment of the muscle to the bone at the elbow becomes damaged. This causes inflammation, which results in pain and tenderness. In tennis elbow, the tendon on the outer side of the elbow is affected. Golfer's elbow affects the tendon on the inner side. Both conditions are caused by overuse of the forearm involving repeated twisting movements.

In tennis elbow and golfer's elbow, the pain is made worse by using the affected arm. Both conditions usually clear up with self-help measures to relieve symptoms, such as rest, ice-packs, and painkillers. In severe cases, a doctor may recommend physiotherapy or corticosteroid injections into the affected area.

RUPTURED TENDON
Achilles rupture | Biceps rupture

A ruptured tendon is a complete tear in a tendon, most commonly as a result of vigorous exercise, such as playing sports. A rupture may also be the result of an injury or may occur as a complication of a long-term joint disorder, such as rheumatoid arthritis (p.157). Tendons in the limbs are most susceptible to rupture.

Symptoms typically include a snapping sensation and severe pain when the tendon ruptures; rapid swelling; and an inability to use the affected part.

In some cases, a tendon may heal with rest and immobilization in a brace or cast. Painkillers may also be given. In more severe cases, surgery may be needed to repair the tendon, followed by immobilization while healing occurs.

PLANTAR FASCIITIS

The plantar fascia is a band of tissue that runs under the sole of the foot from the heel bone to the base of the toes. Inflammation of this tissue – plantar fasciitis – is most commonly caused by repeated overstretching the tissue during physical activity.

The main symptom is pain under the heel, which is usually worst after periods when no weight is placed on the foot. Treatment includes rest, ice-packs, and painkillers. Exercises to stretch the tissues and special shoe inserts may also be recommended. Severe cases may be treated with an injection of corticosteroids.

METATARSALGIA

Pain in the ball of the foot – metatarsalgia – is commonly due to excessive pressure on the ball of the foot from high-impact sports, poorly fitting footwear, or being overweight. Other causes include a foot deformity, such as high arches, a bunion, or hammer toe; a stress fracture of the metatarsals (the bones between the ankle and toes); and conditions such as rheumatoid arthritis (p.157), gout (p.159), diabetes (p.219), or Morton's neuroma (irritation of a nerve between the toe bones, p.173).

The pain may be relieved by rest, losing weight, if necessary, shoe inserts, and painkillers. Other treatment depends on the underlying cause.

DUPUYTREN'S CONTRACTURE

In Dupuytren's contracture, the fibrous tissue in the palm of the hand becomes thickened and forms lumps (nodules) under the skin. The nodules form cords of tissue that gradually shorten, causing one or more fingers to bend in towards the palm. The condition may occur in one or both hands and most commonly affects the fourth and fifth fingers. It is usually painless. The tissue changes usually develop slowly, over months or years.

The cause of Dupuytren's contracture is unknown, although the condition sometimes runs in families.

In many cases, the condition is mild, has little impact on the function of the hand, and does not need treatment. If treatment is needed, it may involve radiation therapy to the hand, injections of an enzyme into the thickened tissue, or cutting the thickened tissue by inserting a needle or blade though the skin. In severe cases, open surgery to cut or remove the thickened tissue may be necessary.

HAMMER TOE

Hammer toe is a deformity of the second, third, or fourth toe in which the toe is permanently bent at the middle joint. A common cause is poorly fitting footwear, but the condition can also result from injury, bunions, or rheumatoid arthritis. A hammer toe often develops a painful corn or callus on the bent joint and can also cause stress on the ball of the foot, which may lead to metatarsalgia (pain in the ball of the foot).

A protective pad over the bent joint can ease pressure on the toe and relieve pain. Surgery to straighten the toe may be recommended in severe cases.

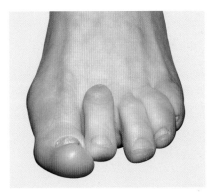

Hammer toe
In hammer toe, the middle joint of a toe is fixed in a bent position. The condition can affect any of the middle toes but most commonly occurs in the second toe, as shown here.

NERVOUS DISORDERS

HEADACHE
Medication-overuse headache | Tension-type headache

A very common type of pain, a headache is rarely a symptom of a serious underlying disorder. Most headaches are tension-type headaches, due to tightening of the muscles in the face, head, and neck. Other types include migraine (below) and cluster headaches.

Common causes of headaches include hangovers, stress, changes in sleep or eating habits, or poor posture. Food additives may be a cause in susceptible people. Headaches can also result from overusing painkillers (called medication-overuse headaches), or from conditions such as an inflammation of the sinuses (sinusitis, p.191), toothache, arthritis affecting the neck (cervical spondylosis, p.158), and head injury. Among the rare causes are inflammation of the membranes around the brain (meningitis, p.168), high blood pressure, a brain tumour, inflammation of blood vessels in the head (giant cell arteritis), or a ballooning of a blood vessel in the brain (brain aneurysm).

Most headaches do not need medical treatment. However, if a headache is severe, lasts for more than 24 hours, or is accompanied by other symptoms such as drowsiness, vomiting, a rash, or abnormal sensitivity to light, immediate medical help should be sought.

MIGRAINE

Migraine is a recurrent, often severe headache that usually occurs on one side of the head and may be accompanied by symptoms such as nausea and visual disturbances. The underlying cause is not known, but it is thought to be due to abnormal brain activity, changes in brain chemicals, and changes in the brain's blood vessels. Various factors may trigger an attack, including stress, tiredness, low blood sugar, dehydration, bright or flickering lights, caffeine, alcohol, the food additive tyramine, or particular foods, such as cheese or chocolate. Menstruation, the combined oral contraceptive pill, or hormone replacement therapy may also trigger an attack.

There are two main types of migraine: with aura and without aura. In migraine without aura, there is a headache, usually on one side of the head and typically accompanied by nausea, vomiting, and sensitivity to light and noise. Migraine with aura causes similar symptoms but the headache is preceded by warning signs (the aura), such as flashing lights or numbness on one side of the body. Some people also have very early signs (known as a prodrome), such as mood or appetite changes, before the aura or headache begins. Migraine can usually be controlled by avoiding triggers, and by medication to prevent or limit attacks or relieve symptoms.

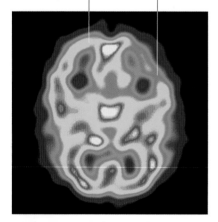

Area of high brain activity   Area of low brain activity

Brain during a migraine attack
This brain scan shows the different levels of activity during a migraine: red and yellow indicate high activity; green and blue are areas of low activity.

CLUSTER HEADACHES

Cluster headaches are excruciating attacks of pain around one eye or temple, due to widening of blood vessels in the brain. Attacks begin suddenly, affect only one side of the head, and may be accompanied by watering of the eye, drooping of the eyelid, and a blocked or runny nostril. Individual episodes may last from minutes to hours and may occur several times a day. Attacks happen in clusters, with periods when attacks occur, typically every day for weeks, followed by attack-free periods, which may last months or years, before attacks recur.

The condition may be treated with medication, by breathing pure oxygen, or by nerve stimulation (using a hand-held device to stimulate a nerve in the neck).

CHRONIC FATIGUE SYNDROME

Also sometime known as myalgic encephalomyelitis (ME), chronic fatigue syndrome is a condition that causes extreme fatigue over a prolonged period. The cause is not known, although it sometimes develops after an infection or psychological trauma. The main symptom is persistent, overwhelming tiredness. Other symptoms may include difficulty concentrating, poor short-term memory, muscle or joint pain, headaches, and sleeping problems.

The syndrome is also often associated with anxiety or depression. The severity of symptoms can vary from day to day, or even during the same day. There is no specific treatment for this condition, but options that may be offered include cognitive behavioural therapy (CBT), graded exercise therapy, or medication to relieve symptoms. Chronic fatigue syndrome is a long-term condition, but it may clear up after several years.

HEAD INJURY

Many bumps and bruises to the head are minor, but a severe injury carries the risk of brain damage and may even be fatal. A blow to the head may shake or bruise the brain, and if the skull is fractured, material may enter the brain and cause infection. A blow or penetrating injury may cause swelling of the brain or bleeding in or around the brain.

If a head injury is minor, there may only be a headache, or sometimes concussion (brief unconsciousness due to disturbance of brain function). A more severe injury may result in significant brain damage, prolonged unconsciousness or coma, and may potentially be fatal. After a severe injury, there may be muscular weakness or paralysis and loss of sensation. There may also be memory loss (amnesia). A serious head injury may require surgery and may result in long-term disability.

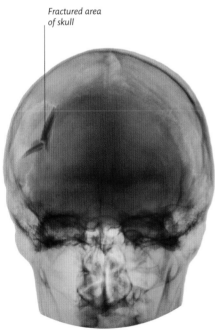

Fractured area of skull

Skull fracture
This coloured X-ray shows a fracture at the back of the skull. Injuries such as this can cause brain damage and, if severe, may be fatal.

EPILEPSY

Epilepsy is typified by recurrent seizures ("fits") as a result of abnormal electrical activity in the brain. In many people, the underlying cause is unknown. In other cases, epilepsy results from disease or damage to the brain. In people with epilepsy, seizures may be triggered by things such as flashing lights, stress, or lack of sleep.

There are various forms of epileptic seizure. Partial seizures involve only one side of the brain. Simple partial seizures, confined to a small area, produce symptoms such as twitching of one part of the body and abnormal sensations. Complex partial seizures produce loss of awareness and strange behaviour or body movements. Generalized seizures affect most or all of the brain. They typically cause loss of consciousness, collapse, and muscle spasms, followed by a period of altered consciousness and tiredness. Many people also have a warning "aura", with abnormal sensations just before a seizure. A type of generalized seizure called an absence seizure produces short periods of altered consciousness, but there are no abnormal body movements.

Epilepsy can usually be controlled with medication. Occasionally, a seizure may be very prolonged, or repeated seizures may occur without a break. Known as status epilepticus, this requires urgent medical attention.

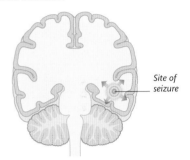

Site of seizure

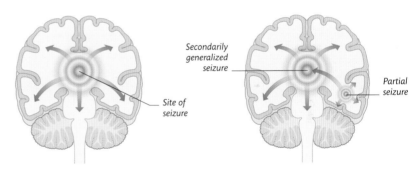

Site of seizure

Secondarily generalized seizure

Partial seizure

Generalized seizure
Abnormal activity spreads throughout the brain. Symptoms vary but typically include uncontrolled movements of the whole body, with loss of consciousness lasting up to several minutes.

Partial seizure
The abnormal activity originates in one part of the brain. Usually, it remains confined to this area (upper diagram), but may sometimes spread and become generalized (lower diagram).

NARCOLEPSY

Narcolepsy is characterized by persistent daytime sleepiness, with repeated episodes of sleep throughout the day, even at inappropriate times, such as while eating. Attacks may last from a few minutes to more than an hour. Other symptoms may include the inability to move while falling asleep or waking up (called sleep paralysis), hallucinations before falling asleep, and the temporary loss of muscle strength (cataplexy), causing the person to fall down.

In many cases, narcolepsy is due to lack of a brain chemical that regulates sleep, possibly as a result of an immune system problem. Treatment of narcolepsy involves regular naps and medication.

MENINGITIS

In meningitis, the meninges (membranes that surround the brain and spinal cord) become inflamed. It is most commonly the result of a viral or bacterial infection, but it may also sometimes be caused by a fungal or parasitic infection or result from certain drug reactions. People with reduced immunity are particularly at risk.

The main symptoms of meningitis are fever, severe headache, nausea, vomiting, sensitivity to bright light, and a stiff neck. In meningococcal meningitis (a type of bacterial meningitis), there may also be a purplish-red rash that does not fade when briefly pressed. A person with any of these symptoms should seek urgent medical advice. In viral meningitis, the symptoms develop gradually and tend to be mild. In bacterial meningitis, they may develop within hours. Untreated, it may lead to seizures, drowsiness, and coma, and may be life-threatening.

Viral meningitis often clears up without treatment. Bacterial, fungal, and parasitic meningitis are usually treated with medication. Occasionally, meningitis may lead to long-term problems, such as hearing loss or brain damage. Vaccines are available to help protect against some types of viral and bacterial meningitis.

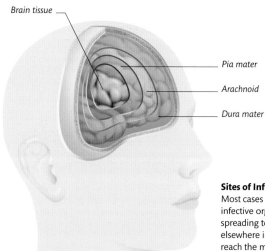

Brain tissue

Pia mater
Arachnoid
Dura mater

Meninges
The meninges consist of the pia mater (inner layer), arachnoid (middle layer), and dura mater (outer layer)

Sites of Infection
Most cases of meningitis are caused by infective organisms, such as bacteria, spreading to the meninges from elsewhere in the body. They can also reach the meninges directly due to injury, a brain abscess, or surgery.

ENCEPHALITIS

This inflammation of the brain is usually due to infection with a virus, but occasionally it occurs as a result of an immune system problem. It may be due to infection by bacteria or other organisms, or it can be a complication of meningitis or a brain abscess. Encephalitis causes flu-like symptoms, fever, and headache; more severe cases may progress rapidly to cause confusion, seizures, and coma. A person with any of these symptoms needs urgent medical attention. Treatment is with medication. Some people recover fully but others are left with long-term problems due to brain damage.

BRAIN ABSCESS

This is a pus-filled swelling in the brain. Most cases are due to infection spreading from elsewhere in the body. Occasionally an abscess results from infection after a head injury. Although rare, brain abscesses can be life-threatening or cause long-term problems, such as epilepsy or brain damage. Symptoms may include fever, nausea, headache, vomiting, and seizures. A person with any of these symptoms should seek urgent medical advice.

Other symptoms, such as speech or vision problems, may occur depending on the area of brain affected. Treatment is with medication, and sometimes surgery.

BRAIN TUMOUR

Most brain tumours (abnormal growths) are metastases – secondary tumours from the spread of cancer elsewhere in the body. Primary brain tumours, originating in the brain itself, are less common.

Malignant tumours typically grow fast and spread through the brain. Non-malignant tumours tend to grow slowly and remain in one area. Both types can compress brain tissue, impair brain function, and cause brain damage. Symptoms vary according to the part of the brain affected but may include severe headaches, blurred vision, paralysis of part of the body, difficulty in speaking or understanding speech, personality changes, and seizures ("fits"). In some cases, there may be sudden pain and loss of consciousness. Treatment may involve medication, radiotherapy, or surgery.

Brain tumour
This brain scan shows a large, non-malignant tumour in the brain. It may be possible to remove a non-malignant tumour surgically, depending on its location.

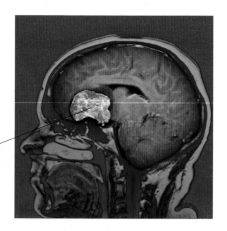

Tumour

TRANSIENT ISCHAEMIC ATTACK

Commonly called a mini stroke, a transient ischaemic attack (TIA) is a brief interruption to the brain's blood supply. It may cause temporary impairment of vision, speech, sensation, or movement. Symptoms typically last from a few minutes to several hours, but disappear completely within 24 hours. (Symptoms that last longer indicate a stroke). There are no permanent after-effects, although a TIA can be a prelude to a stroke.

The process of TIA is similar to that of a clot-related stroke (below), except that in a TIA the blockage in the blood vessel is temporary.

Risk factors for a TIA include high blood pressure, an unhealthy diet, smoking, and disorders such as diabetes, hyperlipidaemia (high levels of fat in the blood), and certain heart conditions.

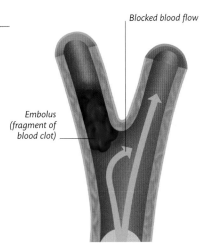

Temporary blockage
A TIA begins when a fragment of blood clot (an embolus) breaks off from a blood vessel and lodges in one of the blood vessels in the brain.

Blocked blood flow

Embolus (fragment of blood clot)

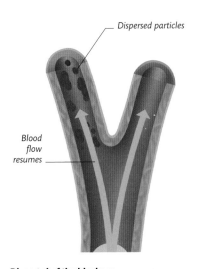

Dipsersal of the blockage
The blockage is dispersed by the pressure of blood building up behind it. Blood can then reach the part of the brain that was previously deprived of it.

Dispersed particles

Blood flow resumes

STROKE

A stroke produces sudden brain damage due to a disturbance of the brain's blood supply. The most common type (called an ischaemic stroke) is due to blockage of an artery supplying the brain caused by a clot. A stroke can also be caused by bleeding in the brain, due, for example, to a ruptured balloon-like swelling in a blood vessel (which is called an aneurysm). This is known as a haemorrhagic stroke.

Risk factors for a stroke include high blood pressure, not getting enough exercise, an unhealthy diet, smoking, and disorders such as hyperlipidaemia (high levels of fat in blood), diabetes, and certain heart conditions. Typical symptoms are facial weakness, which may cause drooping of the face, mouth, or eye on one side; weakness or numbness of the arms; and speech problems, such as slurred speech. A severe stroke may cause unconsciousness and coma, which may be life-threatening. A stroke requires urgent medical help. Treatment varies according to the type of stroke. Some people make a good recovery, but many are left with long-term problems.

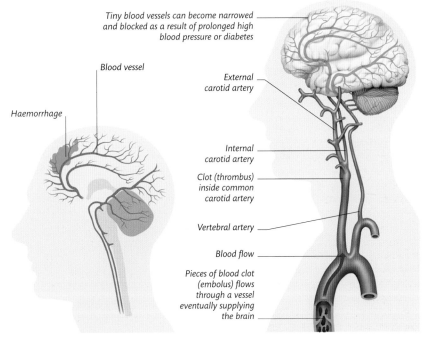

Tiny blood vessels can become narrowed and blocked as a result of prolonged high blood pressure or diabetes

Blood vessel

Haemorrhage

External carotid artery

Internal carotid artery

Clot (thrombus) inside common carotid artery

Vertebral artery

Blood flow

Pieces of blood clot (embolus) flows through a vessel eventually supplying the brain

Bleeding in the brain
Rupture of blood vessels in the brain is known as an intracerebral haemorrhage and is the cause of a haemorrhagic stroke. This type is often associated with high blood pressure.

Blocked blood vessels
Blockages may be due to a clot formed in a blood vessel itself (a thrombus) or a piece of clot (embolus) from elsewhere in the body. They may also occur when blood vessels are narrowed by disease.

SUBARACHNOID HAEMORRHAGE

Subarachnoid haemorrhage is a type of stroke in which a blood vessel ruptures and blood leaks into the space between the inner two of the three layers of membrane covering the brain (called the meninges, p.168). In most cases, it is due to rupture of an aneurysm – a swollen, weakened area at the junction between two arteries in the brain. In some people, bleeding is due to malformed blood vessels. Either problem may be present from birth. A subarachnoid haemorrhage may also occur spontaneously or after unaccustomed exercise.

The bleeding typically causes a sudden, violent headache, with vomiting, stiff neck, and sensitivity to bright light. A person with these symptoms should seek urgent medical attention. These symptoms may be followed by confusion, seizures ("fits"), unconsciousness, and coma. Treatment is with medication and surgery. However, full recovery does not always occur, and many cases are fatal.

DEMENTIA
Alzheimer's disease

Dementia is a condition in which there is gradual, progressive deterioration in mental function. It most commonly affects older people and is usually caused by diseases of the brain or blood vessels in the brain. The most common form is Alzheimer's disease, in which brain cells degenerate and abnormal deposits of protein build up in the brain. Another form is vascular dementia, in which the blockage of small blood vessels in the brain causes numerous small areas of brain damage. In dementia with Lewy bodies, tiny nodules (called Lewy bodies) collect in the brain and impair brain function. Dementia can occasionally occur in younger people, as a result of a brain injury or diseases such as Parkinson's disease. Treatment of dementia is aimed at relieving or slowing the progress of the symptoms.

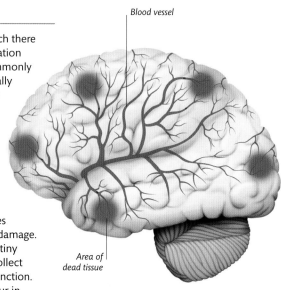

Blood vessel

Area of dead tissue

Vascular dementia
In this form, a series of transient ischaemic attacks (mini-strokes) over time leads to damage or death of brain tissue in areas supplied by blocked blood vessels. The disease becomes progressively worse as more areas of the brain become affected.

SUBDURAL HAEMATOMA

A subdural haematoma occurs when there is bleeding into the space between the outer two of the three membranes covering the brain. This produces a pocket of clotted blood (a haematoma) that presses on the brain. The bleeding may be slow (chronic) or rapid (acute). Chronic bleeding may result from an apparently trivial head injury, and it may take up to several months before symptoms develop. These typically include headaches, and gradual confusion, weakness, and decline in consciousness. Rapid bleeding usually follows a severe head injury and typically causes rapid loss of consciousness. A person who develops any of these symptoms should seek urgent medical attention. Treatment is usually with surgery. Many people make a good recovery, although some residual symptoms may persist. A large, severe haematoma may be fatal.

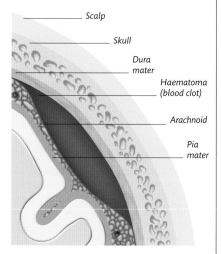

Scalp

Skull

Dura mater

Haematoma (blood clot)

Arachnoid

Pia mater

Subdural haematoma
The haematoma (collection of clotted blood) between the outer two meninges (dura mater and arachnoid) exerts pressure on the brain. The haematoma may enlarge rapidly within hours or may take weeks or months to increase in size.

EXTRADURAL HAEMATOMA

This is a collection of clotted blood (haematoma) between the skull and outer surface of one of the three membranes covering the brain. It is most commonly caused by a head injury that ruptures a blood vessel. Typically, symptoms develop within hours of the injury. They may include headache, vomiting, drowsiness, paralysis affecting one side of the body, and seizures ("fits"). Anyone with these symptoms should seek urgent medical advice. A haematoma may occur after a person briefly loses consciousness at the time of an injury and then loses consciousness again hours later. In a few cases, bleeding occurs relatively slowly and symptoms may not develop for days.

Treatment is with surgery. With prompt treatment, many people make a good recovery, although there may be long-term residual problems, such as weakness. In severe cases, it may be fatal.

MULTIPLE SCLEROSIS

In multiple sclerosis (MS), nerve cells in the brain and spinal cord become progressively damaged, causing problems with a wide range of body functions. Electrical signals pass between the brain and body along the nerves. Healthy nerves are covered by a protective sheath of a substance called myelin, which facilitates the passage of nerve signals. MS involves progressive destruction of the myelin sheaths, disrupting the transmission of signals. MS is an autoimmune disease, in which the body's immune system attacks the myelin sheaths. The underlying cause is not known, although genetic and environmental factors may play a role.

Typically, symptoms first appear between the ages of about 20 and 40. They may include problems with speech, balance, and coordination, numbness, tingling, weakness, muscle spasms, pain, fatigue, incontinence, and mood changes. In some people, symptoms come and go, while in others they get progressively worse. There is no cure but medication may relieve symptoms.

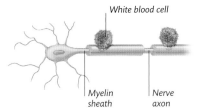

White blood cell

Myelin sheath *Nerve axon*

Early stage MS
White blood cells (cells from the immune system) attack the myelin sheaths on the nerves. Some repair may occur in the early stages.

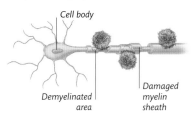

Cell body

Demyelinated area *Damaged myelin sheath*

Late stage MS
As the disorder progresses, there is increasing damage to myelin sheaths and more nerves become affected. Nerve damage is irreversible.

PARKINSON'S DISEASE

Parkinson's disease is a progressive disorder that causes tremor (involuntary trembling movements, usually of the hands), slow movement, and stiffness. It results from degeneration of cells in a part of the brain that produces dopamine, a chemical that helps to fine-tune muscle movements. In Parkinson's disease, the cells produce much less dopamine, resulting in impaired muscle control.

In most people, there is no obvious cause of the condition, although genetic factors may be involved in some cases. It can also result from an inflammation of the brain (encephalitis) or from damage to the basal ganglia from drugs or repeated head injuries. The main symptoms are trembling of one hand, arm, or leg, which may progress to affect limbs on the opposite side; muscle stiffness, making it difficult to begin moving and making movements slower; and problems with balance. Other symptoms may include a stooped posture, shuffling walk, problems speaking, loss of facial expression, and difficulty swallowing. Some people also develop dementia (opposite) or depression (p.242).

Treatment may include supportive therapies, such as physiotherapy, and medication to improve symptoms. In some cases, surgery may be an option.

HUNTINGTON'S DISEASE

Huntington's disease (also known as Huntingdon's chorea) is an inherited brain disorder that causes involuntary, rapid, jerky movements and dementia (opposite). It is caused by an abnormal gene, and if a person inherits the gene from either parent, he or she will develop the disorder. In most cases, symptoms do not appear until age 35 to 50. The condition usually progresses for about 10 to 25 years until the person eventually dies. There is no cure for the condition, but medication may relieve some of the symptoms. Those at risk can be tested to see if they have the abnormal gene.

CAUDA EQUINA SYNDROME

In this condition, nerves at the base of the spinal cord – the cauda equina, a "spray" of nerves resembling a horse's tail – become compressed, causing symptoms such as back pain, bowel and bladder problems, numbness, leg weakness, and erectile dysfunction. The cause is usually a disc prolapse (slipped disc, p.158), but cauda equina syndrome may also sometimes be caused by infection, a spinal injury, or bone cancer. Urgent treatment is usually with emergency surgery to relieve the pressure on the affected nerves.

MOTOR NEURON DISEASE

In motor neuron disease (MND), there is progressive degeneration of so-called motor nerves (nerves that control movement) in the spinal cord. The disorder also affects muscles: as the motor nerves lose the ability to stimulate muscle activity, the muscles weaken and waste away. Motor neuron disease usually begins after the age of about 50, although rarely it may occur in childhood or adolescence. The cause is unknown, although in a few people there is a genetic susceptibility.

Initially, symptoms develop over a few months, with weakness and wasting in the hands, arms, and legs. Other early symptoms of MND may include twitching, stiffness, and muscle cramps, and sometimes speech problems.

As the disease progresses, symptoms worsen and cause problems with everyday activities, such as holding objects, climbing stairs, and walking. Mental abilities are usually not impaired, although control of emotions may be affected and some people become depressed. Eventually, the muscles that control breathing are affected and become weakened and the person dies.

There is no cure for motor neuron disease, although treatment may relieve some of the symptoms and slow progression of the disease.

PERIPHERAL NEUROPATHY

Neuropathy is a general term for disease, damage, or malfunctioning of the peripheral nerves, which connect the brain and spinal cord to the rest of the body. Causes include diabetes; certain dietary deficiencies (nutritional neuropathy), such as deficiency of B vitamins; excessive alcohol consumption; liver or kidney disease; immune system disorders, such as rheumatoid arthritis; certain infections, such as HIV or Hansen's disease (leprosy); some cancers, such as lymphoma (cancer of the lymphatic system); poisoning by heavy metals, such as lead; and drug overdose. Symptoms depend on which nerves are affected. In general, they may include numbness, tingling, pain, loss of balance and coordination, muscle weakness, blurred vision, dizziness, bladder or bowel problems, and erectile dysfunction.

NEURALGIA
Post-herpetic neuralgia

Neuralgia is pain caused by damage to, or irritation of, a nerve. The pain usually occurs in brief bouts and may be severe. Some types of neuralgia are features of a specific disorder. In migraine, there may be a form that consists of intense, radiating pain around one eye. Post-herpetic neuralgia is a burning pain that may occur at the site of an attack of shingles (herpes zoster, p.233) for months or even years after the illness.

Other types of neuralgia result from disturbance of a particular nerve. For example, in trigeminal neuralgia, pain affects one side of the face supplied by the trigeminal nerve.

Treatment for neuralgia is usually with medication. Surgery may also sometimes be recommended.

TRIGEMINAL NEURALGIA

Trigeminal neuralgia is a sudden, excruciating pain on one side of the face due to a disorder of the trigeminal nerve, which provides sensation from parts of the face and controls some muscles used for chewing. The cause is usually pressure on the nerve from a blood vessel or, rarely, from a tumour. Attacks may last for a few seconds to several minutes, and may be so severe that the person is unable to do anything during them. Afterwards, the pain usually disappears completely. An attack may occur spontaneously, or may be triggered by actions such as chewing, talking, or touching the face. Attacks may be frequent, though in some cases there may be long periods of remission.

Treatment for this condition is usually with medication, although surgery may sometimes be an option.

CARPAL TUNNEL SYNDROME

Carpal tunnel syndrome is numbness, tingling, and pain in the fingers and hand due to pressure on the median nerve in the wrist. The median nerve passes down the forearm to the hand, where it controls muscles at the base of the thumb and sensation in the thumb half of the palm. En route to the hand, the nerve passes through the carpal tunnel, a space between the wrist bones and the ligament that lies over them; in addition to the nerve, tendons pass through the space.

Carpal tunnel syndrome occurs when the nerve is compressed, which may be due to swelling of the tendons or a build up of fluid in the carpal tunnel as a result of overuse, arthritis, diabetes, or thyroid problems. It can also occur with hormonal changes during pregnancy or around the menopause. The pressure on the nerve results in numbness, tingling, pain, and loss of grip in the thumb, first two fingers, and half of the ring (third) finger.

Carpal tunnel syndrome is usually treated with rest, splinting, or medication. Sometimes, surgery is needed.

Carpal tunnel
The carpal tunnel is a narrow space formed by the bones of the wrist and the carpal ligament over them. The median nerve runs through this space.

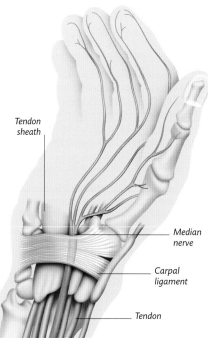

Tendon sheath

Median nerve

Carpal ligament

Tendon

COMPLEX REGIONAL PAIN SYNDROME

Formerly known by various names, including causalgia and Sudeck's atrophy, complex regional pain syndrome is a condition in which there is long-lasting pain, usually in an arm or leg, but sometimes affecting other areas of the body as well. It is most often triggered by an injury, but the pain is more severe and long-lasting than would be expected from the severity of the injury. The skin over the painful area may be red and tender, or blue, cold, and clammy. It may be so sensitive that even a light touch may provoke intense pain.

Complex regional pain syndrome may develop after either a minor or more serious injury, including fractures, sprains or strains, burns, or cuts. However, it is not known why some people develop the condition after such injuries whereas others do not.

There is no cure for complex regional pain syndrome, but symptoms may be controlled with a combination of medication, psychological therapy, and physical rehabilitation.

TARSAL TUNNEL SYNDROME

Tarsal tunnel syndrome is pain, tingling, or numbness in the sole of the foot due to pressure on the tibial nerve, which runs down the back of the leg, around the ankle, and into the foot. At the ankle, the nerve passes through the tarsal tunnel, a space formed by the ankle bones and bands of supporting tissue.

Tarsal tunnel syndrome occurs if the space is constricted and the nerve is compressed, commonly as a result of overuse, injury, or arthritis. Tarsal tunnel syndrome is also more common in people with a condition known as flat feet. Treatment is with rest, medication, or sometimes surgery.

MERALGIA PARAESTHETICA

In meralgia paraesthetica, there are abnormal sensations, such as burning pain, numbness, and tingling, in the outer thigh. Symptoms are often made worse by standing or walking. The condition is due to a specific nerve being trapped under a ligament in the groin. In many cases, the cause is unknown, although sometimes it can result from injury or overuse. It can also be associated with pregnancy and obesity.

Treatment for this condition is with rest and medication, or rarely surgery.

MORTON'S NEUROMA

In this condition, a nerve between the toe bones becomes irritated and thickened. Usually, the nerve affected is between the third and fourth toes, but sometimes the nerve between the second and third toes can be the cause. The condition typically causes a tingling sensation between the toes, and pain in the ball of the foot or base of the toes. The pain is often worse when walking or wearing tight shoes. Wearing wider shoes, rest, and painkillers may relieve symptoms. Surgery may be advised to treat severe cases.

CERVICAL RADICULOPATHY
Trapped nerve

Commonly called a trapped nerve, cervical radiculopathy is a condition that results when a nerve in the neck is irritated or compressed where it branches away from the spinal cord. It is mostly due to a ruptured disc in the neck region of the spine, or a spur (bony outgrowth) on a spinal vertebra. The condition usually affects one side and typically causes pain that radiates from the neck to the shoulder and arm, tingling in the fingers and hand, muscle weakness in the shoulder, arm, or hand, and numbness. Treatment may include medication or, in some cases, surgery.

SCIATICA

Sciatica is nerve pain caused by pressure on, or damage to, the sciatic nerve, which runs from the base of the spinal cord down the legs and into the feet. The pain usually affects only one side, and most commonly occurs in the buttock or thigh, although it may extend down to the foot. There may also be numbness or weakness in the affected area.

Sciatica is most commonly caused by a prolapsed disc – the rupture of a disc in the spine (commonly also called a slipped disc, p.158) – pressing on the sciatic nerve. Other causes include a muscle spasm, sitting awkwardly for long periods, a spinal injury or infection, or, rarely, a tumour that presses on the nerve. It may also develop during pregnancy, due to posture changes causing pressure on the sciatic nerve. In many cases, symptoms resolve on their own. When treatment is needed, it is usually with medication. Rarely, surgery may be advised.

Course of the sciatic nerve
The sciatic nerve is formed where nerves from the lower spinal cord combine to form one large nerve. The nerve and its branches extend along the length of the leg and into the ankle and foot.

FACIAL NERVE PALSY

Facial nerve palsy, also known as Bell's palsy, is weakness of the facial muscles due to damage or inflammation of the facial nerve, which controls certain muscles in the face. It affects only one side of the face, causing drooping of an eyelid and corner of the mouth. There may also be other symptoms, such as earache, increased sensitivity to sound, and an altered sense of taste. The cause is often unknown, but sometimes palsy may be due to damage to the nerve caused by a tumour or surgery, or the palsy may be associated with a viral infection. Facial nerve palsy may be treated with medication or, if the palsy is due to damage, with surgery.

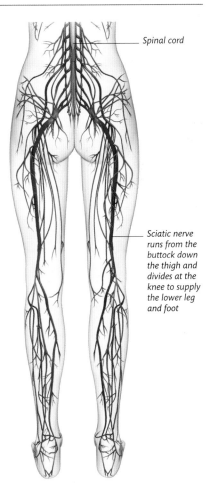

Spinal cord

Sciatic nerve runs from the buttock down the thigh and divides at the knee to supply the lower leg and foot

EAR AND EYE DISORDERS

OTITIS EXTERNA

In otitis externa, the outer ear canal becomes inflamed, usually due to bacterial, viral, or fungal infection. It is sometimes called "swimmer's ear", because persistent moisture in the ear increases the risk of infection. The condition may also occur as part of a general skin disorder, such as eczema (p.222).

Symptoms of otitis externa include swelling, discharge of pus from the ear, itchiness or pain in the ear canal, and sometimes temporary hearing loss. Often the only treatment needed is to keep the ear clean and dry until the infection clears up. If it persists or is severe, medication to treat the infection and relieve symptoms may be prescribed.

AURICULAR CHONDRITIS

Auricular chondritis is inflammation of the cartilage of the auricle (outer flap of the ear), usually as a result of a bacterial infection after a cut to the outer ear or ear piercing. The infection causes inflammation, swelling, and pain in the outer ear. Treatment with antibiotics usually clears up the infection.

OTOSCLEROSIS

In otosclerosis, there is abnormal growth of bone around the stapes, one of the three tiny bones in the middle ear that transmit sounds to the inner ear. The stapes gradually becomes immobilized, resulting in progressive loss of hearing. Usually both ears are affected. As well as resulting in hearing loss, otosclerosis may also cause tinnitus (noises in the ear).

In many cases, hearing can be improved through the use of a hearing aid. For severe cases, hearing can usually be restored by surgery to replace the stapes with an artificial substitute.

AURICULAR HAEMATOMA
Cauliflower ear

An auricular haematoma is a collection of blood (haematoma) in the outer ear flap (auricle), causing swelling, redness, and pain. It is caused by injury to the ear that has caused bleeding in the soft cartilage, as may happen during contact sports. Severe or repeated haematomas may result in permanent deformity of the outer ear, a condition commonly called cauliflower ear.

Immediate treatment is with ice-packs to reduce swelling. In severe cases, the haematoma may be drained and a compression bandage applied. Cosmetic surgery may be needed to correct a cauliflower ear.

EARWAX

Also called cerumen, earwax is produced by glands in the outer ear canal to clean and moisten the canal. Normally, the wax emerges naturally, but sometimes it builds up and causes a blockage, producing a feeling of fullness in the ear and impairing hearing. Wax blockage can usually be treated with eardrops. Persistent blockage may need treatment to flush out the ears or suck out the wax.

SENSORINEURAL HEARING LOSS

Sensorineural hearing loss is hearing loss caused by damage to sensory nerves in the ear or the nerve that carries auditory information to the brain. It is usually due to age or prolonged exposure to noise. However, it may also sometimes be present at birth or result from various disorders. Sensorineural hearing loss is usually permanent. Hearing aids may be helpful in some cases. With profound deafness, a cochlear implant may allow hearing of sounds such as speech.

OTITIS MEDIA
Glue ear

Otitis media is inflammation of the middle ear, usually due to a bacterial or viral infection. It is more common in children, because their Eustachian tubes (which connect the middle ear to the back of the nose) are narrower and easily blocked, allowing pus and fluid to accumulate in the middle ear rather than draining away, (which is then known as otitis media with effusion, or glue ear).

Sometimes, the eardrum may rupture, causing a bloodstained discharge and decrease in pain. Treatment for otitis media is with medication to clear up the infection and relieve pain.

BAROTRAUMA

Barotrauma is damage or pain, mainly affecting the middle ear, caused by changes in pressure. Such changes are common when flying or diving, and may cause minor damage to the middle ear, producing pain, a feeling of fullness in the ears, and tinnitus (noises in the ear). Symptoms usually clear up by themselves within a few hours, but in severe cases the eardrums may be ruptured, which requires medical attention.

PRESBYCUSIS

A form of sensorineural deafness, presbycusis is progressive loss of hearing that occurs with age. It is due to the natural degeneration and death of sensory nerve cells in the ear. Both ears are usually affected. The loss of hearing causes difficulty in hearing high-pitched sounds and difficulty in hearing speech clearly, especially if there is background noise.

There is no cure for presbycusis, but in most cases hearing can be improved with hearing aids.

RUPTURED EARDRUM

Also known as a perforated eardrum, a ruptured eardrum is a hole or tear in the eardrum, typically producing sudden, intense pain, a bloodstained discharge from the ear, and impaired hearing. A ruptured eardrum most commonly results from infection of the middle ear (otitis media). It may also be caused by pressure damage (barotrauma) or injury, for example, due to a blow or poking something into the ear.

Treatment is usually with medication to eliminate the infection and relieve pain. With treatment, the eardrum usually heals within about a month although, rarely, surgery to repair the eardrum may be needed.

Ruptured eardrum
An intact, healthy eardrum (below left) transmits sounds to the middle ear. If the eardrum is ruptured (below right), transmission of sound is impaired, causing hearing loss.

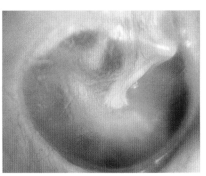

HEALTHY EARDRUM

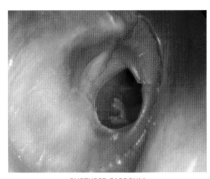

RUPTURED EARDRUM

VERTIGO
Benign paroxysmal positional vertigo

People with vertigo have the sensation that they or their surroundings are spinning or tilting, which produces unsteadiness and sometimes nausea and vomiting. The symptoms are often worsened by sudden head movements. Vertigo can be brought on simply by spinning around or drinking too much alcohol. In some people, it is triggered by heights, and it may occur as a side effect of certain medications.

Vertigo may also be a symptom of an inner ear disorder, such as infection, Ménière's disease (p.176), or benign paroxysmal positional vertigo, in which tiny crystals that are normally embedded in gel in the inner ear become dislodged, disrupting the balance system. Other possible causes include migraine, stroke, a brain tumour or an acoustic neuroma (p.176), or multiple sclerosis (p.171). Symptoms may be alleviated by drugs to relieve nausea and vomiting. Other treatment for vertigo depends on the underlying cause.

EUSTACHIAN TUBE DYSFUNCTION

The Eustachian tube, running from the middle ear to the back of the nose, acts as a drainage tube and also regulates pressure in the middle ear. In Eustachian tube dysfunction, the tube is blocked or inflamed, causing symptoms such as impaired hearing, a feeling of fullness in the ear, tinnitus (noises in the ear), and sometimes dizziness.

Most commonly, Eustachian tube dysfunction is due to a nose, sinus, ear, or throat infection, or from an allergy, such as hay fever. Children are particularly susceptible to problems of the Eustachian tubes because their tubes are shorter and narrower. Often, mild Eustachian tube dysfunction clears up by itself in a few days.

If symptoms persist or are severe, medication may be prescribed to relieve the inflammation and clear the blockage.

Structure of the ear
The Eustachian tube connects the middle ear and the nose. The middle ear contains tiny bones that transmit sound from the eardrum to the inner ear. The inner ear contains the organs of hearing (cochlea) and balance (semicircular canals).

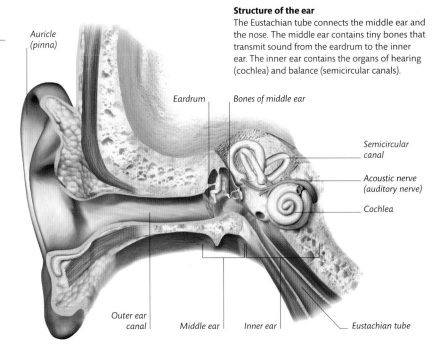

Auricle (pinna)

Eardrum

Bones of middle ear

Semicircular canal

Acoustic nerve (auditory nerve)

Cochlea

Outer ear canal

Middle ear

Inner ear

Eustachian tube

VESTIBULAR NEURITIS

Also known as vestibular neuronitis, vestibular neuritis is inflammation of the vestibular nerve in the inner ear, usually as a result of a bacterial or viral infection, such as the common cold or influenza. The main symptoms are dizziness, vertigo, nausea, vomiting, and blurred vision. Viral vestibular neuritis usually clears up by itself within a few weeks, although medication may help to relieve symptoms such as nausea and vomiting. Bacterial vestibular neuritis usually needs treatment with antibiotics.

TINNITUS

Tinnitus is the term for noises such as buzzing, ringing, or hissing that originate within the ear rather than externally. It is commonly associated with hearing loss and can also occur as a symptom of ear disorders, such as labyrinthitis, Ménière's disease, otitis media (p.174), or earwax blockage. It may also be caused by certain medications, such as aspirin.

Tinnitus may improve if the underlying cause can be treated. Otherwise, listening to background sounds, using a tinnitus masker (a device that produces white noise), counselling, psychotherapy, or tinnitus retraining (altering how the brain responds to tinnitus) may help.

LABYRINTHITIS

Labyrinthitis is inflammation of the labyrinth of the inner ear, which contains the organs of hearing and balance. It is usually caused by a bacterial or viral infection, such as the common cold, and is a possible complication of otitis media (inflammation of the middle ear, p.174). Symptoms include vertigo, nausea, vomiting, blurred vision, impaired hearing, and tinnitus (noises in the ear). Viral labyrinthitis usually clears up on its own within a few weeks, but symptoms may be relieved with medication. Bacterial labyrinthitis usually needs treatment with antibiotics.

MENIERE'S DISEASE

Ménière's disease is an inner-ear disorder characterized by recurrent attacks of vertigo, tinnitus (noises in the ear), and hearing loss. It is due to a build-up of fluid in the labyrinth, which contains the organs of balance and hearing. Usually, only one ear is affected, but both can become involved. Attacks typically come on suddenly and may last from minutes to days before subsiding.

Symptoms include vertigo, nausea, vomiting, tinnitus (noises in the ear), impaired hearing, and a feeling of pressure or pain in the ear. The time between attacks may vary from days to years, and repeated attacks often lead to progressive hearing loss or sometimes total deafness.

Treatment is primarily with medication to relieve symptoms, but in some cases drugs may be given to help to reduce the frequency of attacks. If medication is ineffective, surgery may be an option.

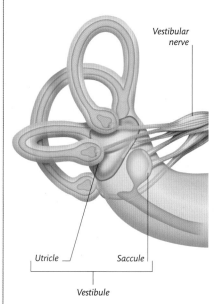

Vestibular nerve

Utricle — — Saccule

Vestibule

Normal balance mechanism
Within the bony labyrinth of the ears are the organs of balance: the semicircular canals and vestibule, which are filled with fluid. Movement of this fluid results in nerve signals being sent to the brain, which interprets the signals as motion.

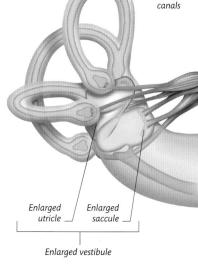

Semicircular canals

Enlarged utricle — Enlarged saccule —

Enlarged vestibule

Balance mechanism in Ménière's disease
In Ménière's disease, there is a build-up of fluid in the vestibule, causing the chambers of the vestibule to enlarge. This is thought to disrupt the normal functioning of the balance mechanism, leading to symptoms such as vertigo.

ACOUSTIC NEUROMA

An acoustic neuroma is a noncancerous tumour of the acoustic nerve (also called the vestibulocochlear nerve), which carries balance and auditory signals from the ear to the brain. Usually, only the nerve of one ear is affected. In most cases, the cause is unknown, although a minority are due to the genetic condition neurofibromatosis, in which multiple tumours grow on nerves.

A small neuroma often does not cause any significant problems. A larger neuroma may cause hearing loss, vertigo, tinnitus (noise in the ear), and sometimes headaches, pain and weakness in the face, blurred vision, and problems with coordination. If the tumour is small, regular monitoring may be all that is required. A larger or troublesome neuroma may be removed by surgery or treated with radiotherapy, or both.

CATARACT

A cataract is cloudiness of the lens in the eye, causing blurred vision. Typically, cataracts affect both eyes, but usually one eye is more severely affected. In most cases, cataracts are a result of normal ageing; most people over about 65 have some cataract formation. However, they may also sometimes be present from birth or may be due to factors such as eye injury, certain eye diseases like uveitis (inflammation of various internal

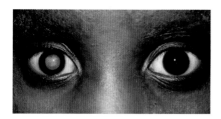

eye structures), prolonged exposure to sunlight, long-term corticosteroid treatment, or diabetes. Cataracts are also common in people with Down's syndrome. Smoking increases the risk of developing cataracts.

Typically, cataracts develop over months or years. They cause only visual symptoms, such as blurred vision, altered colour vision, and seeing haloes around bright lights. Treatment is with surgery to remove the natural lens and, in most cases, replace it with an artificial one. This usually improves vision significantly, although some people still need to wear glasses or contact lenses afterwards.

Appearance of a cataract
A severe cataract, like the one in this person's right eye, often appears as a pale, cloudy area in the eye.

TRACHOMA

Trachoma is an infectious eye disease caused by the bacterium *Chlamydia trachomatis*. Although rare in developed countries, it is a major cause of visual impairment and blindness worldwide.

The infection is spread to the eyes by contact with contaminated hands or by flies. Symptoms include a discharge from the eye and redness of the white of the eye. Repeated infections can scar the eyelids and make the eyelashes turn inwards so that they rub against the cornea, leading to it becoming scarred and eventually resulting in blindness.

In the early stages, trachoma can be treated with antibiotics. If the eyelashes have turned inwards, surgery may be needed to stop them rubbing against the cornea. If the cornea has become scarred, treatment involves corneal transplant surgery.

SUBCONJUNCTIVAL HAEMORRHAGE

A subconjunctival haemorrhage is bleeding under the conjunctiva (the clear membrane covering the white of the eye), producing a red area over the white of the eye. The condition often occurs spontaneously or may result from a minor eye injury, sneezing, coughing, or, rarely, a bleeding disorder such as haemophilia. A subconjunctival haemorrhage is usually painless and clears up in a few weeks without treatment, but medical advice should be sought if it persists or if the eye is painful.

CONJUNCTIVITIS

Conjunctivitis is inflammation of the conjunctiva (the clear membrane covering the white of the eye), causing redness – hence its common name "red eye" – discomfort, and a discharge. One or both eyes may be affected.

There are two common types of conjunctivitis: infective, caused by a bacteria or viruses, and allergic, which is an allergic response to substances such as pollen or cosmetics. Newborn babies sometimes develop conjunctivitis as a result of catching an infection from the

mother's vagina during birth. Infective conjunctivitis is contagious and can be spread by hand-to-eye contact.

Both types of conjunctivitis produce similar symptoms, but in infective conjunctivitis the discharge contains pus and may cause the eyelids to stick together. In allergic conjunctivitis, the discharge is clear and the eyelids are often swollen. Usually, infective conjunctivitis clears up without treatment within about two weeks, although if it is severe or persistent, anti-infective medication may be prescribed. Allergic conjunctivitis may be treated with medication to relieve symptoms.

PTERYGIUM

A pterygium is a wing-shaped thickening of the conjunctiva (the clear membrane covering the white of the eye) that starts on the side of the eye nearest the nose and extends inwards towards the centre. One or both eyes may be affected. Pterygium is thought to be due to prolonged exposure to bright sunlight. If it causes discomfort or threatens vision, a pterygium may be removed surgically.

UVEITIS

Uveitis is inflammation of any part of the uvea, which comprises the iris (the coloured part of the eye), ciliary body (a ring of muscle behind the iris), and the choroid (the tissue layer that supports the retina). In many cases, uveitis is thought to be due to an autoimmune disorder (in which the immune system attacks the body's own tissues), such as Crohn's disease (p.203) or ankylosing spondylitis (p.158),

or an infection, such as chickenpox (p.233), shingles (p.233), or tuberculosis (p.236). In some cases, there is no obvious cause.

Symptoms may include redness and soreness of the eye, blurred vision, small or irregularly shaped pupils, and sensitivity to bright light.

Treatment with corticosteroids is usually effective. In some cases, eye drops to relax muscles in the eye may also be given. Without prompt treatment, there is a risk of permanent visual impairment.

RETINAL BLOOD VESSEL THROMBOSIS

Blockage of a retinal artery by a thrombus (blood clot) typically affects only one eye, causing sudden blindness or loss of part of the visual field. It requires urgent treatment, which may include eye massage, draining fluid from the eye, or medication; even with treatment, loss of vision is usually permanent. Blockage of a retinal vein also usually affects only one eye and tends to cause deterioration of vision over several days, although sometimes visual loss may occur suddenly. Treatment may involve medication injected into the eye or laser surgery. Even with treatment, there is likely to be some permanent loss of vision.

RETINAL DETACHMENT
Vitreous detachment

In retinal detachment, the retina separates from the back of the eye. It may follow an eye injury, but usually occurs spontaneously. Typically, only one eye is affected. Vitreous detachment is when the inside of the eye separates from the retina.

Symptoms of retinal detachment may include flashing lights in the corner of the eye and large numbers of floaters, or a black area in the field of vision. Retinal detachment requires urgent treatment to prevent blindness. Treatment may involve laser therapy, cryotherapy (freezing), or surgery and is usually successful, although vision may not always be fully restored.

CHALAZION

A chalazion is a round, red, usually painful swelling in the upper or lower eyelid caused by blockage of one of the meibomian glands (oil-secreting glands that lubricate the eyelids). Chalazions are also known as meibomian cysts. They resemble styes but, unlike styes, do not develop on the edges of the eyelids. Warm compresses can be used to ease discomfort. Most chalazions disappear on their own within a few weeks.

MACULAR DEGENERATION

Macular degeneration (also known as age-related macular degeneration, or AMD) is a deterioration of the macula, the central area of the retina responsible for seeing detail. AMD tends to affect both eyes and causes a roughly central, circular area of blindness that gradually enlarges; peripheral vision is not affected. There are two forms of AMD. Dry AMD

STYE

A stye is a small, pus-filled swelling at the base of an eyelash, which may cause pain when blinking. It is usually due to a bacterial infection. A stye typically begins as a red lump on the edge of the eyelid. The eyelid then becomes red and swollen, and a yellow spot may form at the centre of the stye. A stye usually ruptures, drains, and heals within a few days with the application of warm compresses. One that persists or worsens may be treated with antibiotics. Styes are more common in people with the skin condition seborrhoeic dermatitis (p.222).

GLAUCOMA

Normally, fluid is continually secreted into the front of the eye by a structure called the ciliary body, to nourish the tissues and maintain the shape of the eye. Any excess fluid drains away through a gap, called the drainage angle. In glaucoma, the flow of fluid is blocked and fluid builds up, raising pressure in the eye and leading to impaired vision or even blindness.

Acute glaucoma develops quickly, causing pain and sudden loss of vision. It requires emergency treatment with drugs or surgery. Chronic glaucoma develops more slowly, is painless, and may go unnoticed for years until it eventually causes significant deterioration of vision. Both types of glaucoma are treated with medication or surgery. Treatment usually prevents further visual loss but does restore any vision already lost.

usually progresses over several months or even years. There is no treatment, although a diet rich in green, leafy vegetables may possibly slow its progression. Visual aids, such as magnifying glasses, may also help to make everyday tasks easier. Wet AMD tends to progress more rapidly, sometimes causing visual deterioration within days. The condition's progress may be slowed or halted by medication injected into the eye or by laser surgery.

SQUINT

Known medically as strabismus, a squint is where the eyes point in different directions. This is common in babies but usually disappears naturally within a few months. A squint in later childhood is usually due to a breakdown in the mechanism for aligning the eyes. In adults, a squint is usually due to an underlying disorder, such as a stroke (p.169).

Squint in children may be treated with glasses, eye exercises, injections into the eye muscles, or surgery. The treatment of squint in adults depends on the cause.

Chronic glaucoma
The ciliary body continually produces fluid, which usually flows out through the pupil and drains out through the sieve-like trabecular meshwork located between the iris and the edge of the cornea. In chronic glaucoma, the meshwork is blocked and pressure builds up in the eye.

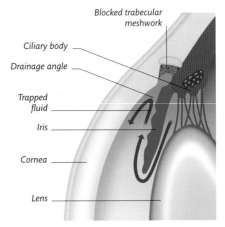

Blocked trabecular meshwork

Ciliary body

Drainage angle

Trapped fluid

Iris

Cornea

Lens

FOCUSING PROBLEMS
Longsightedness | Shortsightedness | Astigmatism

Focusing an image sharply on the retina (the light-sensitive layer at the back of the eye) depends mainly on the lens, the size of the eyeball, and the cornea. Muscles around the lens contract or relax to change the shape of the lens

(and therefore its focusing power) in order to adjust focus between near and far objects.

In longsightedness (hypermetropia), the eyeball is too short relative to the focusing power of the lens, making distant objects clear but nearby ones blurred. In shortsightedness (myopia), the eyeball is too long relative to the focusing power of the lens, so distant objects appear

blurred but nearby objects can be seen clearly. In astigmatism, the shape of the lens or cornea is irregular. As a result, all of the light rays entering the eye cannot be focused on the retina, causing vision to be distorted or blurred.

All three of these conditions can be corrected by glasses, contact lenses, or by laser surgery to reshape the cornea.

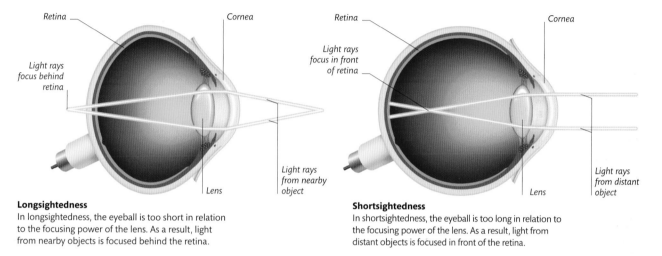

Longsightedness
In longsightedness, the eyeball is too short in relation to the focusing power of the lens. As a result, light from nearby objects is focused behind the retina.

Shortsightedness
In shortsightedness, the eyeball is too long in relation to the focusing power of the lens. As a result, light from distant objects is focused in front of the retina.

ECTROPION AND ENTROPION

Ectropion is a turning outwards of the lower eyelid. The eyelid's exposed inner surface becomes dry and sore, and the eye may water continuously. Because the eyelids cannot close fully, the cornea is exposed and vulnerable to damage or infection. Ectropion is usually due to ageing but may also be caused by damage to a facial nerve. Treatment is with surgery to tighten the eyelid.

Entropion is a turning inwards of the upper or lower eyelid, or both. As a result, the eyelashes rub against the cornea, causing pain, irritation, and eye watering. Constant rubbing may scar the cornea, leading to loss of vision. Entropion is commonly due to ageing, but may also be due to the eye infection trachoma (p.177). It can usually be corrected with surgery.

BLEPHARITIS

Blepharitis is inflammation of the eyelids, causing redness and itchiness, greasy scales at the lid margins, and crusts on the eyelashes. It may be associated with skin disorders such as seborrhoeic dermatitis (p.222), or with bacterial infection or allergy. Avoiding allergens, keeping the eyelids clean, and using an antidandruff shampoo often results in blepharitis clearing up by itself. If it persists or recurs repeatedly, antibiotics may be prescribed.

PTOSIS

Ptosis is abnormal drooping of the upper eyelid, due to weakness of the muscle that normally keeps the eyelid raised. The sagging lid may partly or totally close the eye. One or both eyes may be affected. Ptosis is occasionally present from birth

XANTHELASMA

Xanthelasmas are yellowish deposits of fatty material around the eyes. They are common in older people and are harmless, although they can be removed by surgery, if desired. In younger people, xanthelasmas may be associated with raised levels of fats in the blood (hyperlipidaemia), and measures such as dietary changes or medication may be advised to reduce the risk of a heart attack (p.180) or stroke (p.169).

but is more common in adults. It may be due to normal ageing or occur as a result of injury or a disease such as myasthenia gravis (p.163), which causes progressive muscle weakness. Ptosis can be corrected by surgery to tighten the eyelid muscle.

CARDIOVASCULAR DISORDERS

HEART ATTACK

Known medically as myocardial infarction, a heart attack is death of part of the heart muscle following a blockage in a coronary artery, or one of its branches, which supply the heart itself with blood. When a coronary artery becomes blocked, an area of heart muscle is starved of oxygen and dies.

Blockage of the coronary arteries is usually a result of coronary artery disease, in which the insides of the arteries become narrowed by fatty deposits called plaques. The plaques may rupture, leading to the formation of a blood clot (thrombus) at the site of rupture. The clot may then block blood flow, leading to a heart attack.

The typical symptom of a heart attack is sudden pain in the centre of the chest. Sometimes, the first symptom is sudden collapse. A few people have very mild or no symptoms, a condition called silent myocardial infarction. After a heart attack, the damage to the heart muscle may result in heart failure (reduced pumping efficiency) or heart rhythm problems, which in severe cases may be rapidly fatal. Urgent treatment with "clot-busting" medication or angioplasty (a procedure to widen narrowed blood vessels) can restore blood flow to the heart. Other medications may also be given to help prevent heart rhythm problems and further blood clots.

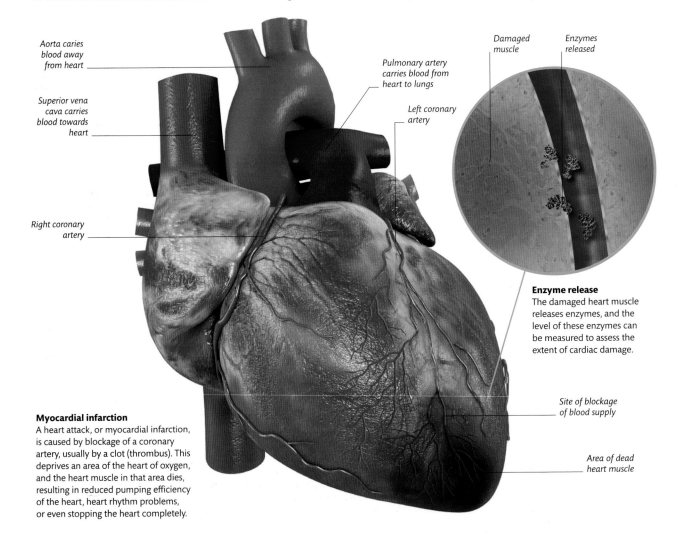

Aorta caries blood away from heart

Superior vena cava carries blood towards heart

Right coronary artery

Pulmonary artery carries blood from heart to lungs

Left coronary artery

Damaged muscle

Enzymes released

Enzyme release
The damaged heart muscle releases enzymes, and the level of these enzymes can be measured to assess the extent of cardiac damage.

Site of blockage of blood supply

Area of dead heart muscle

Myocardial infarction
A heart attack, or myocardial infarction, is caused by blockage of a coronary artery, usually by a clot (thrombus). This deprives an area of the heart of oxygen, and the heart muscle in that area dies, resulting in reduced pumping efficiency of the heart, heart rhythm problems, or even stopping the heart completely.

ANGINA

Angina is chest pain due to an inadequate blood supply to the heart. It is usually caused by coronary artery disease, in which the coronary arteries that supply blood to the heart are narrowed by fatty deposits. Other causes include coronary artery spasm, in which the blood vessels narrow suddenly for a short period of time, heart valve problems, and heart rhythm disorders. Severe anaemia, which reduces the blood's oxygen-carrying capacity, may also cause angina.

The pain of angina usually starts in the centre of the chest but it may spread to the neck, back, and arms, or between the shoulder blades. Typically, the pain is brought on by exertion and eases with rest. If the pain continues after rest, it may be due to a heart attack (opposite).

Angina can often be controlled with medication to open up blood vessels, but if attacks become more severe or frequent, angioplasty to widen or surgery to bypass narrowed arteries may be recommended.

HEART FAILURE

Heart failure is the term used when the heart is unable to pump blood around the body effectively. It may develop quickly (acute heart failure), often as a result of a heart attack, or more gradually (chronic heart failure) due to a long-term disorder such as high blood pressure, coronary artery disease, chronic obstructive pulmonary disease, or heart valve or rhythm problems.

Heart failure may be classified as left- or right-sided, according to the part of the heart affected. In left-sided failure, fluid builds up in the lungs, causing breathlessness. In right-sided failure, fluid builds up in the liver, spleen, kidneys, and tissues under the skin, causing swelling, especially of the legs and ankles.

Treatment varies according to the type, severity, and cause of the heart failure. It may include medication, surgery, an implanted device that regulates heart rhythm, or a heart transplant.

HEART RHYTHM DISORDERS

Abnormalities of the heart rate or rhythm (arrhythmias) are caused by disturbances in the electrical system that controls the heart beat. The heart has a natural pacemaker (called the sinoatrial node) in the right atrium. This node sends electrical signals through the atria (upper chambers) to another node (the atrioventricular node), from where they pass to the ventricles (lower chambers). The signals regulate the heart muscle contractions and, therefore, the heart rate and rhythm. Poor signal transmission or abnormal electrical activity can cause various arrhythmias (some of the main ones are shown below). The electrical system disturbances themselves may be due to various underlying causes, including other heart disorders (a heart attack, or heart muscle or valve problems, for example), the effects of certain drugs, or overproduction of thyroid hormones.

Treatment may include electrically shocking the heart back into normal rhythm, medication, surgery, or fitting a pacemaker or similar device to maintain or restore a normal heart rhythm.

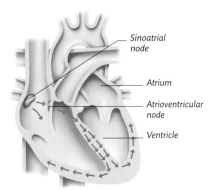

Sinoatrial node

Atrium

Atrioventricular node

Ventricle

Sinus tachycardia
In this condition, the heart rate of more than 100 beats/minute and a normal rhythm may simply be due to anxiety or exercise, but can also occur in fever, anaemia, and thyroid disease.

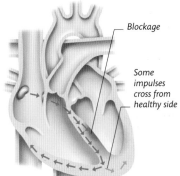

Blockage

Some impulses cross from healthy side

Bundle-branch block
The sinoatrial node impulses are partly or fully blocked, slowing ventricular contractions. In complete heart block, the ventricles contract at only 20–40 beats/minute.

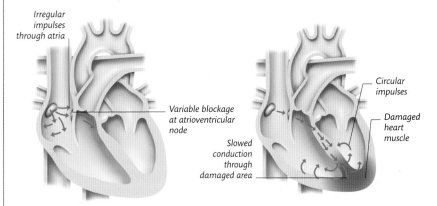

Irregular impulses through atria

Variable blockage at atrioventricular node

Atrial fibrillation
If the sinoatrial node is overridden by random electrical activity in the atria, impulses pass through the atrioventricular node erratically, causing very fast, irregular ventricular contractions.

Circular impulses

Damaged heart muscle

Slowed conduction through damaged area

Ventricular tachycardia
Abnormal electrical impulses in the ventricular muscle cause the ventricles to contract rapidly, overriding the sinoatrial signal and producing a fast, regular, but inefficient beat.

HEART VALVE DISORDERS
Heart valve incompetence | Mitral valve prolapse

The heart has four valves that ensure that blood flows in the correct direction around the heart. Their function may be impaired by changes due to ageing, infections such as endocarditis (infection of the heart lining) or rheumatic fever, or a heart attack; heart valve problems may also sometimes be present at birth.

Stiffness of a valve (known as stenosis) prevents it from opening fully, restricting the blood flow. Alternatively, a valve may be incompetent – it does not close fully and some blood leaks backwards. Incompetence is often due to a valve being floppy, a condition known as prolapse. In both cases, the heart has to work harder to pump blood around the body, which may eventually lead to heart failure; valve disorders also increase the risk of clots and stroke. In mild cases, there may be no symptoms.

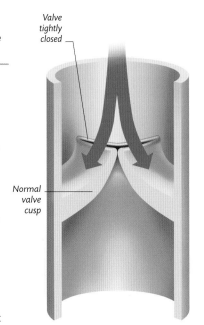

Normal heart valve closed
The pressure of blood outside the closed valve builds up, and the valve cusps snap shut so that blood cannot flow backwards.

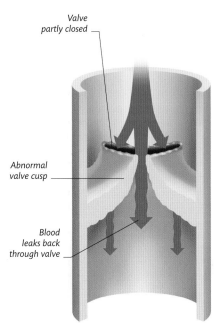

Incompetent heart valve
An incompetent valve does not close properly, allowing blood to leak back through the valve (regurgitation), forcing the heart to work harder.

PERICARDITIS

The pericardium is a two-layered membrane that surrounds the heart. In pericarditis, this membrane becomes inflamed, usually due to infection, but sometimes as a result of a heart attack, an inflammatory disease, such as rheumatoid arthritis, the spread of cancer from another site, or damage from an injury. Pericarditis may come on suddenly (acute) or may be persistent (chronic).

Acute pericarditis typically causes pain in the centre of the chest and may be mistaken for a heart attack. In chronic pericarditis, the pericardium becomes scarred and contracts around the heart, preventing the heart from beating normally. In both types of pericarditis, fluid may build up between the pericardial layers, a condition called pericardial effusion. This fluid build-up may stop the heart from beating effectively and lead to heart failure. Pericarditis may be treated with medication or surgery.

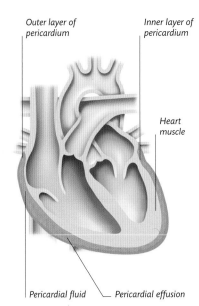

Pericardial effusion
An accumulation of fluid between the two layers of pericardium may compress the heart and restrict its action.

INFECTIVE ENDOCARDITIS

The endocardium is the membrane that lines the inside of the heart and surfaces of the heart valves. In infective endocarditis, this membrane becomes inflamed due to an infection, usually with bacteria but occasionally with other microorganisms. The infection may occur during surgery (including dental surgery) or another invasive procedure (such as insertion of a catheter), through breaks in the skin, or as a result of intravenous drug use.

People whose endocardium has previously been damaged are particularly vulnerable, as are those who have an artificial heart valve and people with reduced immunity. Symptoms of infective endocarditis, which may come on suddenly or gradually, include persistent fever, fatigue, and breathlessness. Untreated, it may lead to life-threatening complications, such as heart failure or stroke. Treatment is usually with medication, although surgery is sometimes necessary.

GIANT CELL ARTERITIS

Also called temporal arteritis, giant cell arteritis is a condition in which certain arteries become inflamed. Usually the inflamed arteries are those in the head and scalp, such as the temporal arteries, but it may also involve other arteries in the head and neck and the aorta (the main artery).

The cause of giant cell arteritis is not known, but it may occur with polymyalgia rheumatica (p.189), an inflammatory condition of the muscles, and sometimes runs in families. Giant cell arteritis typically produces severe headaches, scalp tenderness, pain when chewing, and sometimes loss of an area of vision. The condition is treated with medication to reduce inflammation.

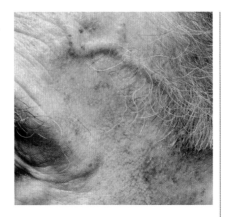

Dilated temporal artery
Giant cell arteritis most commonly affects the temporal arteries on one or both sides of the side of the forehead, causing it to become inflamed and prominent.

HYPOTENSION

Hypotension is the medical term for low blood pressure. In its most common form, known as postural hypotension, dizziness or faintness occur when a person stands or sits up suddenly. Hypotension can have many possible causes, from dehydration to the side effects of certain medications or an underlying health problem. Disorders that may cause hypotension include heart problems; hormonal conditions, such as diabetes (p.219); and nervous system conditions, such as Parkinson's disease (p.171). Severe blood loss or burns, anaphylactic shock (severe allergic reaction), septicaemia (infection in the bloodstream), and heart attack can all cause sudden, severe hypotension.

THROMBOSIS AND EMBOLISM
Pulmonary embolism

In thrombosis, a blood clot (thrombus) forms in a blood vessel. In embolism, a plug of material (embolus) travels though the bloodstream and becomes lodged in a blood vessel. In both cases, blood flow is blocked. A thrombus may form when blood is flowing sluggishly, if the blood is prone to clotting due to a genetic condition, pregnancy, taking combined oral contraceptives or hormone replacement therapy, or as a result of the build-up of fatty deposits on artery walls (atherosclerosis). Most emboli are pieces of blood clot that have broken off from a larger clot elsewhere, as may occur after a heart attack or as a result of deep vein thrombosis. Other types include an air embolus, caused by air introduced into the bloodstream, and a fat embolus, caused by fat being released from a fractured bone.

The symptoms of thrombosis or embolism depend on which blood vessels are affected. Blockage of the arteries to the brain may cause a stroke; blockage of the coronary arteries may cause a heart attack; and blockage of the pulmonary arteries to the lungs (pulmonary embolism) may cause breathing difficulty.

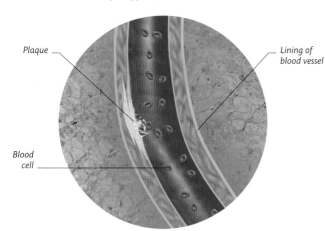

Plaque

Lining of blood vessel

Blood cell

How thrombosis begins
Thrombosis often begins with formation of a plaque on the lining of a blood vessel. The plaque is formed from fatty substances, waste products, and fibrin, a stringy substance that helps blood to clot.

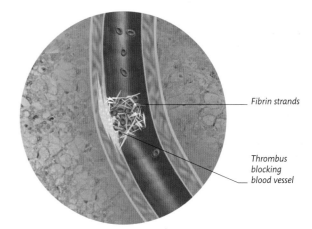

Fibrin strands

Thrombus blocking blood vessel

Clot formation
The plaque enlarges, reducing blood flow, and then ruptures. When the plaque ruptures, the fibrin from the plaque binds to platelets (a type of blood cell) to form a clot (thrombus).

DEEP VEIN THROMBOSIS

In deep vein thrombosis (DVT), a blood clot (thrombus) forms in a deep-lying vein, usually in the leg. Although not dangerous in itself, part of the clot may break off and lodge in a blood vessel supplying the lungs, causing a potentially life-threatening blockage, called a pulmonary embolism.

DVT is caused by a combination of slow blood flow, blood vessel damage, and an increased tendency of the blood to clot. Risk factors include prolonged immobility, injuries such as bone fractures, surgery, dehydration, pregnancy, certain blood disorders, hormone replacement therapy or taking the combined contraceptive pill, smoking, and being overweight. Treatment includes medication to prevent further clotting and to stop an embolism (p.183), and sometimes surgery.

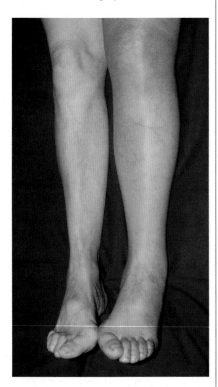

Deep vein thrombosis
This person's left leg is noticeably swollen due to deep vein thrombosis. In addition to swelling, deep vein thrombosis may cause pain and redness of the leg.

ANEURYSM
Abdominal aortic aneurysm | Popliteal aneurysm

An aneurysm is a swelling in an artery caused by the pressure of blood on a weakened area of artery wall. Most aneurysms are associated with the narrowing and weakening of arteries due to fatty deposits (atherosclerosis), but they may also sometimes be due to an injury or a genetic disorder that weakens artery walls. Aneurysms are more common in men, and the risk of developing them increases with age. Other risk factors include high blood pressure, an unhealthy lifestyle, and having a close relative who has, or has had, an aneurysm. Aneurysms can occur in any artery but they most commonly affect the aorta (the body's main artery) or cerebral arteries supplying the brain. Popliteal aneurysms, which affect the popliteal artery around the knee, are also relatively common.

Most aneurysms do not cause symptoms. However, if an aneurysm is very large, it may case pain or a pulsating sensation. If an aneurysm ruptures, it may cause massive internal bleeding. A form of aneurysm known as a dissecting aneurysm is particularly prone to rupture.

An aneurysm may not need treatment, but should be monitored. Emergency surgery is needed for a rupture, and surgery may be advised for a large aneurysm or one liable to rupture.

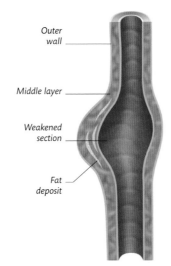

Common aneurysm
This type of aneurysm forms when the artery's middle layer is weakened, usually by fat deposits. Pressure causes the weakened area to bulge.

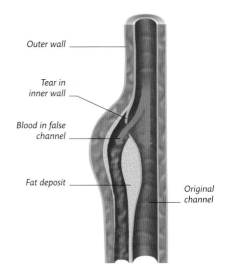

Dissecting aneurysm
In this type of aneurysm, blood is forced through a tear in the inner wall, creating a false channel between the layers of the wall.

RHEUMATIC FEVER

Rheumatic fever is a disease that causes inflammation throughout the body, especially in the joints, producing pain and swelling. It may also affect the heart, leading to heart valve problems (p.182); the skin, causing a rash; or sometimes the nervous system, causing uncontrollable jerking movements. Rheumatic fever develops after an infection, usually of the throat, caused by streptococcal bacteria. The disease is believed to be caused by the immune system attacking the body's tissues in response to the infection, rather than by the infection itself. Treatment is with medication and bed rest.

RAYNAUD'S DISEASE

In this condition, small blood vessels in the extremities suddenly narrow, restricting blood flow. In most cases, the underlying cause is not known and the condition is known as Raynaud's disease. If there is an identifiable cause, it is called Raynaud's phenomenon. Often the conditions are simply known collectively as Raynaud's. Possible causes of Raynaud's include rheumatoid arthritis, systemic lupus erythematosus (lupus), scleroderma (an immune disorder that affects the skin), taking certain medications, and hand–arm vibration syndrome.

Symptoms may be triggered by cold temperatures, stress, and smoking. The fingers, toes, ears, or nose whiten, cool, and turn blue as the blood vessels narrow. The vessels then widen again and blood flow increases, turning the tissues red. There may also be numbness, pain, and tingling. In severe cases, Raynaud's may lead to skin ulcers or gangrene (tissue death). Symptoms can be avoided by keeping the extremities warm, and also by not smoking. Medication may be prescribed in severe cases.

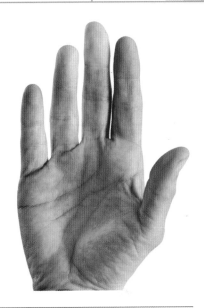

Raynaud's of the hand
An attack of Raynaud's in the hand restricts blood supply to the ends of the fingers, turning them pale. When the blood vessels widen again, pain and tingling often occur.

VARICOSE VEINS

Varicose veins are enlarged, distorted veins just under the skin, most commonly found in the legs. Normally, muscle contractions in the legs help to push blood through veins, and one-way valves in the veins prevent the blood from flowing backwards. Varicose veins develop when the valves fail to close properly, causing a backflow of blood; this increases pressure in the veins and makes them swell. Varicose veins are often caused by increased pressure from swelling of the abdomen during pregnancy or in obesity, or from prolonged standing. Rarely, they are due to the veins being abnormally stretchy or having too few valves.

In addition to their appearance, varicose veins may cause symptoms, such as aching, burning, or throbbing in the legs, swollen feet and ankles, and leg cramps. The skin over a varicose vein may also become dry and itchy, may bleed easily, and may become ulcerated.

Varicose veins usually do not require any treatment other than compression stockings and measures to prevent the condition from getting worse, such as weight loss, exercise, and avoiding prolonged standing. If necessary, varicose veins may be treated by sealing off the affected veins or by removing them completely.

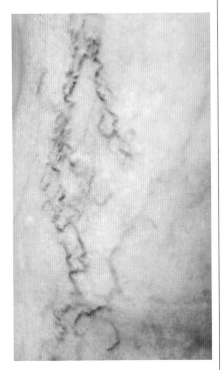

Varicose veins in the leg
Any vein can become varicose, but the most common site is the leg, where the swollen, distorted veins may become more prominent if the person stands for long periods of time.

HAND-ARM VIBRATION SYNDROME

In this condition, there is pain and numbness in the hands and arms due to prolonged use of vibrating tools causing repeated damage to blood vessels and nerves. Symptoms often also include blue or white coloration of the fingers, tingling in affected areas, and difficulty manipulating small objects. It may also cause Raynaud's. There is no specific treatment but avoiding the use of vibrating tools can help prevent the condition from worsening. Medication may also sometimes be prescribed.

KAWASAKI DISEASE

Kawasaki disease is an illness that most commonly affects children under five and causes a prolonged fever. The cause is not known. As well as a fever lasting one to two weeks, symptoms include sore eyes, cracked lips, and swelling and reddening of the hands and feet followed by peeling of the skin on the toes and fingers. Most children recover completely with treatment. Untreated, complications affecting the heart or blood vessels may develop, such as aneurysms (swellings in artery walls).

BLOOD, LYMPHATIC, AND IMMUNE DISORDERS

ANAEMIA

In anaemia, there is a reduction in the number of red blood cells in the body, or the haemoglobin in red blood cells is deficient or abnormal. Haemoglobin is the component of red blood cells that binds with oxygen in the lungs and carries it through the circulatory system to body tissues. If there are too few red blood cells or their haemoglobin is lacking or abnormal, the oxygen-carrying capacity of the blood is reduced and the body tissues may not receive enough oxygen.

Normally, stable haemoglobin levels in the blood are maintained by a balance between red-cell production in the bone marrow and red-cell destruction in the spleen. Anaemia may result if this balance is upset or if the haemoglobin is abnormal.

There are four main types of anaemia. The first is due to a deficiency of substances necessary for the formation of red blood cells. The most common form of this type is iron-deficiency anaemia. This is a result of low levels of iron in the body, and is most common in women who have heavy

menstrual bleeding. The second type of anaemia results from inherited disorders in which abnormal haemoglobin is produced, such as in sickle cell disease (see below). The third type of anaemia, known as haemolytic anaemia, occurs when red blood cells are broken down more rapidly than they can be replaced. This may be caused by the body's immune system

destroying red blood cells, by certain inherited disorders, or by infections, such as malaria. The fourth type of anaemia, called aplastic anaemia, is caused by failure of the bone marrow to produce enough red blood cells. The underlying cause is often unknown, but it may sometimes be due to toxins, radiation, or certain drugs.

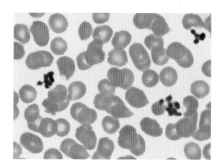

Normal blood cells
This colour-enhanced light micrograph view of human blood cells shows the characteristic appearance of healthy, normal red cells: round, bright red, and with a small pale area in the middle of the cells.

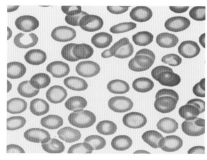

Iron-deficient red blood cells
This light micrograph shows iron-defecient red blood cells. In iron-deficiency anaemia, the red blood cells are slightly smaller than normal, generally paler overall, and have a larger pale area in their centres.

SICKLE CELL DISEASE

Sickle cell disease is an inherited disease in which red blood cells contain abnormal haemoglobin, (the substance that carries oxygen to body tissues). This makes the red cells fragile, rigid, and sickle shaped. The abnormal red cells may be destroyed prematurely, leading to anaemia (see above). They may also become lodged in small blood vessels, obstructing blood flow and depriving organs of oxygen. This may lead to episodes of severe pain (sickle cell crises) and eventual organ damage.

The condition is most common in people of African or Afro-Caribbean origin and is caused by an abnormal gene. If a child inherits two abnormal genes (one

from each parent), he or she will develop sickle cell disease. However, if a child inherits only one abnormal gene, a condition known as sickle cell trait results, which does not usually produce symptoms. Screening for sickle cell disease may be offered in pregnancy or shortly after birth. Treatment is aimed at preventing and treating the crises, with medication, rehydration, or blood transfusions. In some cases, a bone marrow transplant may be an option.

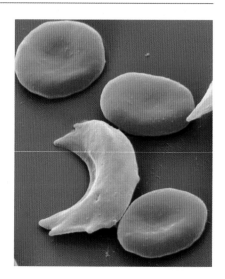

Sickle-cell diseased red blood cells
In sickle cell disease, some red blood cells are distorted into a sickle shape. These abnormal cells have a reduced lifespan, leading to anaemia.

LEUKAEMIA

Leukaemia is a group of cancers in which there is uncontrolled proliferation of abnormal white blood cells in the bone marrow and reduced production of normal blood cells. The cancerous white blood cells are unable to fight infection; lack of red blood cells leads to anaemia; and reduced levels of platelets lead to excessive bruising and bleeding. The cancerous white cells also spread to other organs. Leukaemia may develop rapidly (acute) or more slowly (chronic) and may be fatal without treatment, which may include anticancer drugs, blood transfusions, radiotherapy, or a bone marrow transplant.

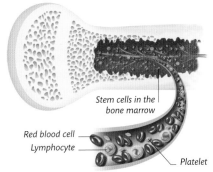

Blood cell production
All blood cells derive from stem cells found in the bone marrow. Red blood cells carry oxygen. Lymphocytes are a type of white blood cell that fights infection. Platelets help the blood to clot at injury sites, reducing blood loss.

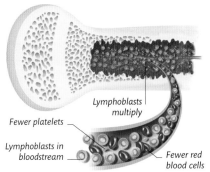

Acute lymphoblastic leukaemia
Lymphoblasts (immature malignant lymphocytes) proliferate rapidly in the bone marrow. As a result, the production of normal blood cells is disrupted. Lymphoblasts also spread via the bloodstream and carry the cancer to other tissues and organs in the body.

HYPERCALCAEMIA

An abnormally high level of calcium in the blood is called hypercalcaemia. It is commonly caused by overactivity of the parathyroid glands (small glands in the neck that help regulate the blood level of calcium). Cancer may also cause hypercalcaemia, either by spreading to bone or by producing abnormal hormones that cause bones to release calcium. Less commonly, the condition may result from too much vitamin D in the diet or from certain inflammatory conditions, such as sarcoidosis (thought to be due to overactivity of the immune system).

LYMPHANGITIS

This is an inflammation of lymphatic vessels due to the spread of bacteria from the site of an infection, usually an infected wound. The condition typically affects lymphatic vessels in an arm or leg. The infected vessels become tender and inflamed, and red streaks may appear on the overlying skin. Nearby lymph nodes may also become swollen, and sometimes ulcers form on the skin over the infected lymphatic vessels. If left untreated, the infection may spread into the blood and cause septicaemia (p.234), which may be life-threatening.

LYMPHADENOPATHY
Swollen lymph node

Lymphadenopathy is an enlargement of the lymph nodes (sometimes called glands), usually due to an infection or to the proliferation of white blood cells within the lymph nodes. A single node, a group of nodes, or sometimes all the lymph nodes may be affected.

Swelling of a single node or group of nodes is often due to a localized bacterial infection. For example, swollen lymph nodes in the neck are commonly due to a throat infection, and they usually subside when the infection clears up. Swollen nodes that are due to infection are often painful. Persistent swelling of many or all of the lymph nodes may be the result of some types of cancer, such as breast cancer, leukaemia, or lymphoma (lymphatic system cancer). Swollen nodes due to cancer are not normally painful. Persistent lymph node enlargement may also be caused by long-term infections, such as tuberculosis or HIV infection.

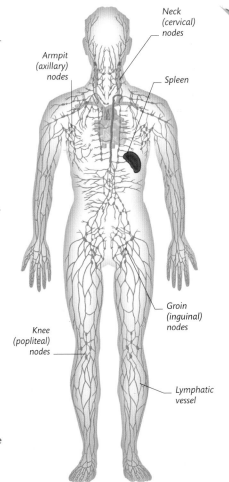

Lymphatic system
The lymphatic system consists of a network of lymph nodes connected by lymphatic vessels. The nodes generally occur in clusters, mainly in the neck, armpits, and groin. The lymphatic system also includes organs such as the spleen.

LYMPHOEDEMA

In lymphoedema, fluid accumulates in the lymphatic vessels, resulting in the painless swelling of a limb. There are various possible causes, including obstruction of the lymphatic vessels by cancer cells or parasitic worms. Surgical removal of lymph nodes or radiation therapy to an area containing lymph nodes may also result in lymphoedema. Rarely, it may be due to an inherited condition in which the lymphatic vessels fail to develop properly. In some cases, it occurs for no known reason. Lymphoedema is usually a lifelong condition and treatment is aimed at relieving symptoms.

LYMPHOMA

Lymphomas are cancers that develop when lymphocytes (a type of white blood cell) multiply and form tumours in the lymphatic system. They may also spread to other tissues. There are two main types, called Hodgkin's and non-Hodgkin's lymphoma. In Hodgkin's, a particular type of cancer cell is present. All the other types are classed as non-Hodgkin's. Hodgkin's most commonly affects those aged 15 to 35 or over 50. The other lymphomas mainly occur in people over 60. The cause is not known, but they may run in families. They are also more common in those with reduced immunity, and may be triggered by certain infections.

MESENTERIC ADENITIS

In mesenteric adenitis, the lymph nodes in the mesentery (the membrane that anchors organs to the abdominal wall) become inflamed. The condition most commonly affects children and is usually caused by a viral infection. The main symptoms are pain in the centre or lower right side of the abdomen, fever, nausea, and diarrhoea.

Usually, no treatment is needed other than painkillers, and the condition clears up by itself within a few days. However, a doctor should be consulted to rule out other possible causes of the symptoms, such as appendicitis (p.205).

HIV AND AIDS

HIV (human immunodeficiency virus) gradually destroys cells of the immune system and may eventually lead to AIDS (acquired immunodeficiency syndrome), a life-threatening condition. HIV is passed on by contact with infected body fluids, including blood, semen, vaginal fluids, and breast milk. It can also be passed from an infected woman to her fetus or to the baby at birth. Initially, there may be a short, flu-like illness, mouth ulcers, or rash, or no symptoms at all. The virus then multiplies over several years, damaging the immune system. The damage can be assessed by counting the number of immune system cells called CD4 lymphocytes. As the infection progresses, fever, night sweats, diarrhoea, weight loss, swollen lymph nodes, and recurrent infections may occur. In the late stage, known as AIDS, the CD4 count drops very low and various diseases develop, including infections that are not normally serious in otherwise healthy people (such as candidiasis, *Pneumocystis* pneumonia, and cytomegalovirus infection) but may be so in a person with AIDS. There is no vaccine or cure for HIV infection, but antiretroviral drugs can slow the damage to the immune system.

HIV budding from a lymphocyte
This micrograph shows clusters of virus particles (at the top) budding off from the surface of an infected lymphocyte (a type white blood cell).

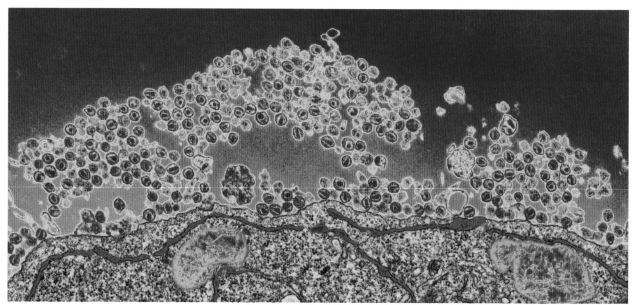

POLYMYALGIA RHEUMATICA

This condition is an inflammatory disorder that causes severe stiffness and pain in the muscles of the shoulders, neck, and hips. The stiffness and pain are worse in the morning after waking up, but improve with physical activity. There may also be other symptoms, such as tiredness, lack of energy, a general sense of feeling unwell, fever, night sweats, weight loss, and depression.

Polymyalgia rheumatica is most common in those over the age of about 60 and affects more women than men. The underlying cause is unknown, but the condition is thought to be due to a combination of genetic and environmental factors, although specific factors have not yet been identified. In some cases, polymyalgia rheumatica may occur together with giant cell arteritis (p.183), a more serious condition in which arteries in the head and scalp become inflamed. Polymyalgia rheumatica is usually treated with corticosteroid drugs.

FOOD ALLERGIES
Cow's milk allergy

A food allergy is an exaggerated reaction of the immune system to a specific food or food group, causing a range of symptoms, from a rash, to abdominal cramps, diarrhoea, and difficulty breathing or swallowing due to swelling of the lips, mouth, throat, and airways. In extreme cases, it may cause a life-threatening reaction called anaphylaxis, with sudden breathing difficulty and collapse.

Almost any food can cause an allergic reaction, although dairy products, nuts, eggs, seafood, and wheat are common triggers. A food allergy is different from a food intolerance, in which symptoms arise from food toxins, problems with digestive enzymes, or the direct action of chemicals in the food. The most effective treatment for allergy is to avoid the problem food. People with severe allergy may be advised to carry an epinephrine autoinjector for emergency treatment.

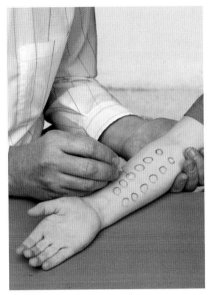

Skin prick testing for allergies
To test for food allergies, extracts of suspect foods are applied to the skin, which is then pricked with a needle. Any redness or swelling at the site of a prick is an indication of an allergy to that food.

LUPUS
Discoid lupus erythematosus (DLE) | Systemic lupus erythematosus (SLE)

Lupus is a type of autoimmune disease, one in which the immune system attacks the body's own tissues. In lupus, the immune system attacks the connective tissue. This is the material that supports, connects, or binds other tissues or organs and it occurs throughout the body – in the skin, joints, internal organs, and walls of blood vessels, for example.

The most common type of lupus is discoid lupus erythematosus (DLE), which affects only exposed areas of skin, such as the face, scalp, and behind the ears. A more serious form, systemic lupus erythematosus (SLE), can affect many tissues and organs, including the skin. In both types, symptoms subside and then recur with varying severity. In DLE, a red, itchy, scaly rash develops. Exposure to sunlight tends to trigger onset of the rash or make an existing rash worse. The rash may leave scars or, if it occurs on the scalp, bald patches. SLE can cause a wide variety of symptoms, depending on which parts of the body are affected. A common symptom is a butterfly-shaped rash on the face; other symptoms may include joint pain, fever, fatigue, weight loss, and mouth ulcers. There may also be other problems, such as anaemia, kidney failure, inflammation of the membranes around the lungs or the membrane around the heart, and if the nervous system is affected, headaches, blurred vision, and strokes. There is no cure for either type of lupus but medication can usually control symptoms.

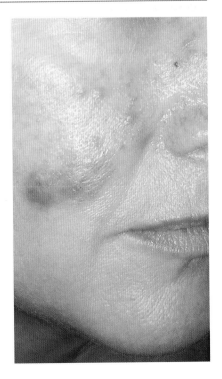

Butterfly rash
A common symptom of systemic lupus erythematosus is a red, raised rash across the nose and cheeks in a distinctive butterfly shape.

RESPIRATORY DISORDERS

NOSEBLEED

Nosebleeds often occur in dry or cold conditions, when the lining of the nose becomes dry and cracked, causing bleeding. They are also commonly caused by a blow to the nose, fragile blood vessels, or are a result of a common cold or other infection. Recurrent nosebleeds may sometimes occur as a side effect of certain drugs; rarely, they indicate an underlying disorder, such as high blood pressure, a bleeding disorder, or a tumour of the nasal passages.

The majority of nosebleeds can be treated with simple first aid and pressing both sides of the nose together for 15–20 minutes. However, a nosebleed that continues after first aid and lasts for more than 20 minutes requires medical attention.

NASAL POLYPS

Nasal polyps are growths in the lining of the nose, usually attached by a small stalk. Their cause is not known, although they are more common in people with asthma or rhinitis (inflammation of the lining of the nose). Small polyps may not cause symptoms, but if they are large or numerous, symptoms may include a stuffy or runny nose, reduced sense of smell, snoring, and post-nasal drip (mucus dripping from the back of the nose down the throat). They may also sometimes lead to recurrent sinusitis (inflammation of the sinuses).

Treatment is usually with medication (including nasal spray); large polyps may need to be removed by surgery.

DEVIATED NASAL SEPTUM

With a deviated nasal septum, the partition that separates the nostrils (which is called the nasal septum) is shifted to one side. A deviated septum may be present from birth or it may result from an injury to the nose.

A mildly deviated septum does not usually cause any problems. However, a severely deviated septum may impair breathing and cause snoring. It also increases the risk of developing sinusitis (inflammation of the sinuses).

Treatment for a deviated septum is usually not necessary. If the condition causes breathing difficulty or recurrent sinusitis, surgery to straighten the septum may be advised.

HAY FEVER
Allergic rhinitis |
Seasonal allergic rhinitis

In hay fever (also called seasonal allergic rhinitis), the lining of the nose becomes inflamed due to an allergic reaction to pollen. In other types of allergic rhinitis, the allergic reaction occurs in response to other normally harmless substances (allergens), such as house dust mites, flakes of skin shed from animals (such as cats or dogs), or feathers.

The allergic reaction is due to an exaggerated response of the immune system that, when exposed to the allergen, produces histamine and other chemicals that cause inflammation and fluid production in the nose and sinuses. This, in turn, produces symptoms such as a runny, stuffy, or itchy nose, sneezing, an itchy throat, and itchy, red, watery eyes.

Symptoms of hay fever and allergic rhinitis can be prevented by avoiding the allergen, if possible. Medication may be used relieve the symptoms of hay fever and allergic rhinitis. In severe cases, immunotherapy may be an option. This involves gradually introducing increasing amounts of the allergen into the body in order to desensitize the immune system.

Grass pollen grains
This micrograph shows a highly magnified view of grass pollen, a common cause of hay fever. The condition can also occur in response to tree, flower, or weed pollens, and spores from mould and fungi.

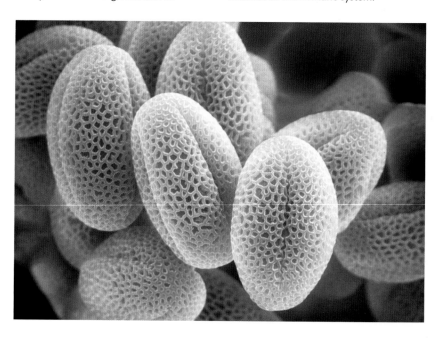

SINUSITIS

In sinusitis, the membrane that lines the sinuses becomes inflamed. It may be accompanied by inflammation of the nasal lining (rhinitis), in which case the condition is known as rhinosinusitis. The inflammation may be acute (developing and clearing up rapidly) or chronic (long-term). It is usually caused by a viral infection, such as the common cold. The blockage of the sinuses from a viral infection may lead to a build-up of mucus, which may then become infected with bacteria. Blockage is more likely in people with an abnormality of the nose, such as a deviated nasal septum or nasal polyps. Sinusitis is also more likely to develop in people with hay fever or another form of allergic rhinitis.

Symptoms typically include headache, a feeling of fullness around the sinuses, pain in the face that worsens when bending forward, a stuffy or runny nose, and sometimes fever. Sinusitis usually clears up without treatment, although medication may relieve symptoms. Surgery may be recommended for persistent sinusitis.

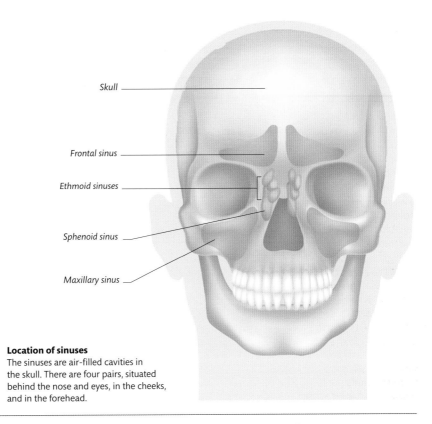

Skull

Frontal sinus

Ethmoid sinuses

Sphenoid sinus

Maxillary sinus

Location of sinuses
The sinuses are air-filled cavities in the skull. There are four pairs, situated behind the nose and eyes, in the cheeks, and in the forehead.

SLEEP APNOEA

In sleep apnoea, there are episodes of temporary breathing stoppage (lasting 10 seconds or longer) during sleep. Obstructive sleep apnoea is the most common type and most often affects men who are overweight. Causes include over-relaxation of muscles of the soft palate (at the roof of the mouth), or enlarged tonsils or adenoids. Central sleep apnoea occurs because of a problem with the nerves that control breathing, which may be due to various disorders, such as brain damage after a head injury or stroke.

As well as breathing stoppages, both types may cause loud snoring, disturbed sleep, daytime sleepiness, morning headaches, and poor concentration. Obstructive sleep apnoea may be treated by continuous positive airways pressure (CPAP), in which high-pressure air is breathed through a mask. Treatment of central sleep apnoea depends on the underlying cause.

EPIGLOTTITIS

Epiglottitis is a potentially life-threatening condition in which the epiglottis (the flap of tissue behind the tongue that prevents food from entering the airways) becomes inflamed, usually due to infection with *Haemophilus influenzae* type b (Hib) bacteria. Symptoms typically come on quickly and may include fever, a severely sore throat, difficulty swallowing, restlessness, and noisy, rapid, and laboured breathing. Without urgent medical treatment, the swollen epiglottis may completely obstruct breathing and cause suffocation.

Treatment for epiglottitis may include giving oxygen or possibly surgery, and medication. With prompt treatment, most people recover without any long-term problems. A vaccine against Hib is available to help prevent infection.

TONSIL STONE

Also known as tonsoliths, tonsil stones are accumulations of mucus, debris, and bacteria that form in the tonsils, forming white or yellow balls.

Tonsil stones do not always cause symptoms, but when symptoms do occur, they may include recurrent bad breath, a bad or metallic taste in the mouth, pain or difficulty when swallowing, swelling of the tonsils, and sometimes earache. The stones may also give off a putrid smell.

Tonsil stones that cause no symptoms do not usually need treatment. Large or troublesome tonsil stones may be removed by surgery.

PHARYNGITIS AND TONSILLITIS
Bacterial tonsillitis | Viral sore throat

Pharyngitis and tonsillitis are common disorders that are often described simply as a sore throat. The pharynx connects the back of the mouth and nose to the larynx (voice box) and oesophagus (gullet). The tonsils lie at the top of the pharynx. Tonsillitis (inflammation of the tonsils) is more common in children, because they have large tonsils, which shrink with age. Adults tend to get pharyngitis (inflammation of the pharynx). However, both conditions can occur together in adults and children.

Pharyngitis and tonsillitis are usually caused by a viral infection, such as the common cold (p.232) or infectious mononucleosis (glandular fever, p.235), but the conditions may sometimes be due to a bacterial or fungal infection. The symptoms of both conditions are similar and may include sore throat, difficulty swallowing, earache, and swollen lymph nodes in the neck. There may also be a fever. In severe cases, there may be breathing difficulty,

and occasionally an abscess forms near a tonsil, a condition called peritonsillar abscess or quinsy.

Treatment for pharyngitis and tonsillitis is usually with medication, although surgery may be needed for recurrent tonsillitis or a peritonsillar abscess.

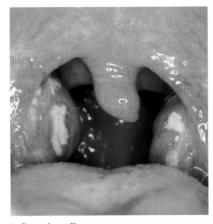

Inflamed tonsils
In tonsillitis, the tonsils at the back of the throat become inflamed. They may also have white, pus-filled spots on them, as shown above.

HERPANGINA

Herpangina is a throat infection caused by a specific group of viruses known as enteroviruses, most commonly by coxsackieviruses – a group of viruses that can cause a range of diseases, including hand, foot, and mouth disease (p.229), meningitis (inflammation of the membranes around the brain and spinal cord, p.168), and pneumonia (p194). The viruses are usually spread by infected droplets coughed or sneezed into the air, and the viruses can survive on surfaces for several days. Herpangina is most common in young children but can affect people of any age.

Symptoms of herpangina do not typically appear until two to seven days after infection, when there is a sudden onset of fever, sore throat, and sometimes also headache, abdominal discomfort, and muscle pain. Small blisters appear in the throat; they enlarge and then burst, forming ulcers.

The infection usually clears up within about a week without specific treatment, although symptoms of the infection may be relieved with medication.

CROUP

In croup (medically known as laryngotracheitis), the upper airways become inflamed and narrowed, producing hoarseness, a harsh, grating sound while breathing in (known as stridor), a distinctive barking cough, and sometimes breathing difficulty.

Croup is most common in infants and young children and is usually caused by a viral infection of the airways, although it may also occur as a result of an allergy, inhaling a small foreign body or an irritant chemical, or epiglottitis (inflammation of the epiglottis, which is the flap of tissue behind the tongue that stops food from entering the airways, p.191).

Mild cases of croup may be treated with medication. Severe cases with serious breathing difficulty need urgent medical treatment.

FUNCTIONAL DYSPHONIA
Voice overuse

Functional dysphonia is the medical term for abnormalities of the voice that are not due to any underlying disorder. Typical abnormalities may include a breathy, hoarse, or rough voice, changes in the pitch, loudness, or quality of the voice, a feeling of having to strain to speak, breaks in speaking when the sound cuts out briefly, and discomfort or pain when speaking.

The most common cause of the problem is overuse of the voice. Stress may also sometimes be a factor, and smoking may make symptoms worse.

Functional dysphonia usually clears up by itself from resting the voice. Speech therapy may be advised if the problem recurs repeatedly.

VOCAL CORD POLYPS AND NODULES

Vocal cord polyps and nodules are noncancerous growths on the vocal cords. A polyp is a small swelling that develops on the membrane covering the vocal cords. As it grows, the polyp may develop a small stalk. A nodule is a small, callus-like lump on the vocal cords.

Both polyps and nodules are usually caused by overuse of the voice and both produce similar symptoms. Symptoms include hoarseness, a harsh, breathy voice, and sometimes discomfort or pain when speaking.

Treatment for vocal cord polyps and nodules consists of resting the voice, although sometimes surgery to remove the growths may be advised. Tests to confirm that the growths are not cancerous may also be carried out.

LARYNGITIS

In laryngitis, the larynx (voice box) is inflamed, usually as a result of infection. The condition may be acute, lasting for only a few days, or chronic and persist for several months.

Acute laryngitis is usually caused by a viral infection, such as the common cold (p.232), but it may also occur after straining the voice. Chronic laryngitis is often caused by smoking or long-term overuse of the voice. Drinking alcohol may aggravate either type of laryngitis.

Symptoms of laryngitis may include hoarseness, gradual loss of the voice, and discomfort or pain in the throat, especially when speaking.

There is no specific treatment for this problem, other than resting the voice. Steam inhalations may help to relieve symptoms. If hoarseness lasts for more than about two weeks, medical advice should be sought to exclude the possibility of the symptoms being due to laryngeal cancer.

LARYNGEAL CANCER

In laryngeal cancer, a cancerous tumour develops on the vocal cords themselves or just above or below the cords. The exact cause is not known, but it is associated with smoking, high alcohol consumption, and exposure to certain substances, such as coal dust or asbestos.

The main symptom of lanryngeal cancer is hoarseness, especially when the tumour originates on the vocal cords. Other symptoms may include pain when swallowing or difficulty swallowing, a persistent sore throat, and a persistent cough. In advanced cases, there may also be difficulty breathing.

If the cancer has spread to nearby lymph nodes in the neck, the nodes become enlarged and cause swelling in the neck.

Treatment depends on how far advanced the cancer is but may include radiotherapy, surgery, chemotherapy, or a combination of these. In some cases, other medication may also be used.

ACUTE BRONCHITIS

Acute bronchitis is a short-term inflammation of the bronchi (the airways leading from the windpipe into the lungs). It is usually due to a viral infection, such as a common cold, that has spread from the nose, throat, or sinuses. Smokers, young children, older people, and those with an existing lung disease are particularly susceptible to bronchitis.

Symptoms of acute bronchitis typically develop over a day or two and include a hacking cough that may bring up phlegm, tightness of the chest, wheezing, headache, and mild fever. The cough may persist for several weeks after the other symptoms have disappeared.

In otherwise healthy people, acute bronchitis usually clears up by itself in a few days; over-the-counter painkillers may help to relieve symptoms. Medical advice should be sought if symptoms persist or worsen, if other symptoms develop, or if the person already has another health problem.

ASTHMA

Asthma is a lung disorder in which there is intermittent inflammation and narrowing of the airways in the lungs. People with asthma have recurrent attacks when the muscles in the walls of the airways contract, causing narrowing. This is usually in response to an allergen, such as pollen, house dust mites, or pet dander (minute scales from animal hair, feathers, and skin), but an attack may also be triggered by factors such as inhaled chemicals, irritants, or dusts, certain medications, stress, exercise, or respiratory infections.

An asthma attack causes the sudden onset of wheezing, shortness of breath, tightness of the chest, and coughing. In a severe attack, breathlessness may be so bad that speaking is impossible, the lips, fingers and toes may turn blue, and the person may become unconscious. Asthma is treated with medication to prevent or relieve attacks. A severe attack requires urgent medical help.

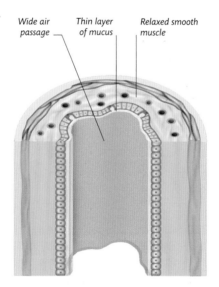

Healthy airway
In a healthy airway, the smooth muscle is relaxed and does not contract readily in response to triggers. There is a thin layer of mucus covering the lining of the airway and the air passage is wide.

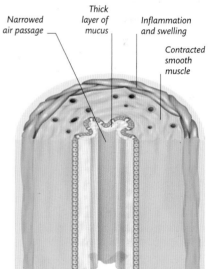

Airway in asthma
In asthma, the smooth muscle of the airway is contracted, the lining of the airway is inflamed, and the mucus layer is thickened. The air passage is narrowed, causing wheezing and breathlessness.

PNEUMONIA

Pneumonia is inflammation of the air sacs (alveoli) of the lungs, usually due to infection. Often, only part of one lung is affected, but in severe cases both lungs can be affected, which may be life-threatening.

Most cases are caused by infection with bacteria, including *Streptococcus pneumoniae* (also called pneumococcus), causing pneumococcal pneumonia; *Legionella pneumophila*, causing a form of pneumonia known as Legionnaires' disease; *Haemophilus influenzae*; and *Mycoplasma pneumoniae*. Viral causes of pneumonia include influenza and chickenpox. In some cases, pneumonia can be caused by fungi or protozoa. These infections may be serious in those with reduced immunity; for example, the protozoan *Pneumocystis jirovecii* may cause a severe type of pneumonia (*Pneumocystis* pneumonia) in people with AIDS. Pneumonia may also be caused by inhaling vomit, a form known as aspiration pneumonia.

Symptoms typically include fever, sharp chest pain, shortness of breath, and a cough that produces sputum, which may sometimes be bloody. Occasionally, the infection may spread from the lungs to the pleura (membranes around the lungs), causing pleurisy, or to the blood, causing blood poisoning (septicaemia, p.234).

Treatment depends on the cause and severity, but may include medication and, in severe cases, oxygen therapy. Vaccination against influenza and pneumococcus can help to prevent pneumonia.

Inflamed air sacs
The air sacs (alveoli) in the lungs become filled with white blood cells and fluid, which reduces the amount of oxygen passing from the lungs into the bloodstream.

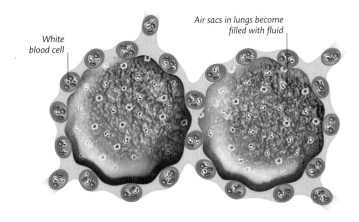

White blood cell

Air sacs in lungs become filled with fluid

CHRONIC OBSTRUCTIVE PULMONARY DISEASE

Chronic obstructive pulmonary disease (COPD), also called obstructive airways disease, refers to long-term damage to the airways, causing breathing difficulty. It consists primarily of chronic bronchitis (long-term inflammation of the airways) and emphysema (damage to the air sacs in the lungs). The most common cause is smoking, although COPD may also result from long-term exposure to harmful dusts or fumes, or from an inherited disorder that makes the lungs susceptible to damage. The main symptoms of COPD include: increasing breathlessness; a persistent cough that brings up phlegm; frequent chest infections; and persistent wheezing.

Without treatment, the symptoms gradually worsen. There is no cure for COPD. Stopping smoking is essential to prevent further lung damage from occuring. Other treatments may include medication and tailored physical exercises. Rarely, surgery or a lung transplant may be options.

PLEURISY

Pleurisy is inflammation of the pleura, the two-layered membrane that covers the outside of the lungs and lines the inside of the chest. Causes of the condition include a viral infection such as influenza; pneumonia; a pulmonary embolism (p.183), in which the blood supply to the lungs is blocked by a blood clot; or lung cancer. Occasionally, pleurisy may result from an autoimmune condition, such as rheumatoid arthritis or systemic lupus erythematosus, in which the immune system attacks the pleura.

Symptoms of pleurisy may come on suddenly or gradually, depending on the cause of the pleurisy. They may include a sharp chest pain that is worse when breathing in, shortness of breath, and coughing up phlegm or blood. Treatment is of the underlying cause, together with medication to relieve symptoms.

CYSTIC FIBROSIS

Cystic fibrosis (CF) is an inherited condition in which a faulty gene causes body secretions to be abnormal, especially in the lungs and digestive system, leading to progressive lung damage and difficulty absorbing nutrients from food. To be born with CF, a child must inherit two copies of the faulty gene. A person with only one copy does not have CF but is a carrier; each child of two carrier parents has a 25 per cent chance of having CF. Genetic tests are available to check if a person is a carrier. Newborn babies can also be tested for CF.

Symptoms tend to begin in early childhood and may include oily, foul-smelling faeces, failure to put on weight or grow at the normal rate, and recurrent respiratory infections. The sweat is also abnormally salty. Often, a constant cough develops. As the condition progresses, the lungs become damaged, and liver damage and diabetes may develop. Eventually, CF usually causes death from respiratory failure.

There is no cure, but treatment with medication, physiotherapy, and a special diet can help to control symptoms. A lung transplant may also sometimes be an option.

PNEUMOTHORAX

A pneumothorax occurs when air enters the pleural cavity – the space between the two layers of the pleural membrane surrounding the lungs – and causes a lung to collapse, leading to chest pain and shortness of breath. A pneumothorax may occur spontaneously – more commonly in tall, thin young men – or following a chest injury. A pneumothorax may also occur as a complication of conditions such as a chest infection, chronic obstructive pulmonary disease, cystic fibrosis, or lung cancer. A penetrating chest injury may cause a tension pneumothorax where, with each breath, more air is drawn into the pleural cavity. This prevents blood from returning to the heart from the lungs, causing fainting and shock; a tension pneumothorax can be life-threatening.

A small pneumothorax may clear up without treatment in a few days. A large pneumothorax or a tension pneumothorax may be treated by inserting a tube or hollow needle into the chest to allow the air to escape.

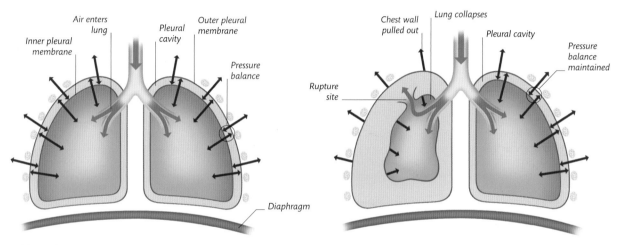

Normal breathing
When a person takes a breath in, the chest wall expands, lowering the pressure inside the pleural cavity. The lungs are pulled outwards by the pressure difference.

Collapsed lung
Air from the right lung leaks into the pleural cavity and the lung deflates; no longer acting as a sealed unit, the lung cannot be pulled outwards by the pressure difference.

LUNG CANCER

Malignant lung tumours are one of the common causes of cancer deaths worldwide. A tumour that originates in the lungs is known as primary lung cancer. A tumour that develops in the lungs as a result of the spread of cancer (metastasis) from elsewhere in the body is known as secondary lung cancer.

Smoking is the main cause of primary lung cancer, and passive smoking is a risk factor for nonsmokers. More rarely, primary lung cancer may be caused by toxic chemicals, radon (a radioactive gas), or mineral dusts, such as asbestos. Secondary lung cancer is a common feature of many other types of primary cancer, including breast, bowel, prostate, and kidney cancer.

The first and most common symptom of both types of lung cancer is usually a cough. Other symptoms may include coughing up blood, shortness of breath, and chest pain. A tumour may also cause pleurisy (inflammation of the membranes surrounding the lungs) or pneumonia. Primary cancer may also spread to other parts of the body, especially the liver, brain, or bones.

Treatment of primary lung cancer may involve surgery, radiotherapy, chemotherapy, or sometimes newer treatments, such as medications known as biological therapies or laser therapy. Treatment of secondary lung cancer is aimed at the underlying primary cancer.

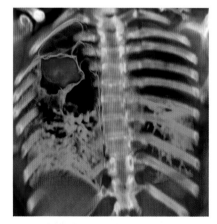

Tumour in the lung
In this colour-enhanced scan of the chest, a tumour in the right lung (on the left of the image) shows up as a red mass.

DIGESTIVE DISORDERS

CONSTIPATION

Constipation is infrequent bowel movements or the difficult passing of hard and dry faeces. In most cases, constipation is simply the result of insufficient fibre or fluids in the diet or lack of exercise. Other causes include difficult toilet-training in childhood, repeatedly ignoring the urge to move the bowels, prolonged immobility, pregnancy, or certain medications. Occasionally, constipation may be due to an underlying disorder, such as hypothyroidism (underactivity of the thyroid, p.220), haemorrhoids (p.207), irritable bowel syndrome (p.203), an anal fissure (p.207), diverticular disease (p.205), or bowel cancer (p.206).

Constipation usually clears up with self-help measures, such as increasing the amount of fibre and fluids in the diet and exercising more regularly. If constipation persists, medical advice should be sought.

DIARRHOEA
Bile acid diarrhoea | Overflow diarrhoea

Diarrhoea that comes on suddenly is often caused by an intestinal infection. Other causes include food allergy, stress, and certain medications. Long-term diarrhoea is often due to an intestinal disorder, such as irritable bowel syndrome (p.203), Crohn's disease (p.203), coeliac disease (p.204), ulcerative colitis (p.203), bowel cancer (p.206), or a condition called bile acid diarrhoea (in which diarrhoea results from digestive juices called bile acids

remaining in the intestine instead of being reabsorbed). Long-term constipation can sometimes cause overflow diarrhoea, in which a solid faecal mass in the rectum leads to leakage of watery faeces.

Diarrhoea often clears up by itself in a day or two. To prevent dehydration, plenty of fluids should be drunk. Medical advice should be sought if diarrhoea persists. If a baby or elderly person shows signs of dehydration, prompt medical attention is necessary.

TODDLER'S DIARRHOEA

Toddler's diarrhoea is a common, harmless condition that affects some children for a period after the introduction of an adult diet. As well as frequent bowel movements, there are often recognizable pieces of food

in the faeces. The cause of toddler's diarrhoea is not known. It does not cause any lasting adverse effects and does not need medical treatment, although a doctor should be consulted as a precaution to exclude other possible causes of diarrhoea.

GASTROENTERITIS
Infective gastroenteritis | Norovirus

Gastroenteritis is inflammation of the stomach and intestines, typically causing the sudden onset of nausea, vomiting, diarrhoea, and stomach cramps. It is most commonly due to infection (infective gastroenteritis) with viruses, bacteria, or parasites such as protozoa. Viruses that can cause gastroenteritis include norovirus and rotaviruses. Bacterial causes for gastroenteritis include *Salmonella*, *Campylobacter*, and *Escherichia coli*. Parasitic causes for gastroenteritis include the protozoa that cause amoebiasis (*Entamoeba histolytica*, p.237) and giardiasis (*Giardia lamblia*, p.237). The infection is usually acquired from contaminated food or water or from close contact with infected people. Less commonly, gastroenteritis may have a non-infectious cause, such as Crohn's disease (p.203), food intolerance, or certain medications.

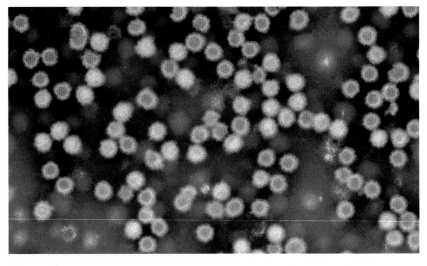

A mild attack of gastroenteritis usually clears up by itself. Drinking plenty of fluids and taking paracetamol for any pain can relieve symptoms. If symptoms are severe or prolonged, seek medical advice.

Norovirus
This coloured micrograph shows particles of norovirus, a common cause of gastroenteritis worldwide. The virus can be spread by direct contact with infected people or objects. It may also be caught from contaminated oysters.

FOOD POISONING

Food poisoning is sudden illness caused by consuming food or drink contaminated with an infectious organism or toxin. Bacteria that can cause food poisoning include *Salmonella*, *Campylobacter*, *Escherichia coli*, *Staphylococcus*, *Listeria*, *Clostridium difficile*, and *Clostridium botulinum* (which causes botulism). Viral causes include norovirus, rotaviruses, and some adenoviruses. Protozoal infections include cryptosporidiosis (p.237), amoebiasis (p.237), and giardiasis (p.237). Food poisoning can be caused by eating poisonous mushrooms or food contaminated with high doses of pesticides.

The main symptoms include nausea, vomiting, diarrhoea, and abdominal cramps. Some food poisoning may cause more widespread symptoms; for example, botulism may cause muscle weakness and paralysis.

In most cases, symptoms clear up by themselves within a few days. They can be relieved by self-help measures, such as drinking plenty of fluids and eating a bland diet. If symptoms are severe or prolonged, or if other, unusual symptoms develop (muscle weakness or paralysis, for example), medical advice should be sought.

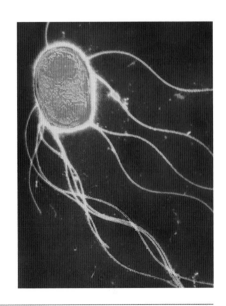

Salmonella enteritidis bacterium
The *Salmonella enteritidis* bacterium is one of the causes of bacterial food poisoning. Infection typically occurs by eating contaminated and undercooked chicken eggs or meat.

UNDERNUTRITION

Undernutrition – not getting enough nutrients – may simply be the result of an inadequate diet or may be due to any of a wide range of disorders. For example, it may result from diseases in which the absorption of nutrients is impaired, such as cystic fibrosis (p.194), coeliac disease (p.204), Crohn's disease (p.203), ulcerative colitis (p.203), and giardiasis (p.237) or similar parasitic intestinal infections. Various long-term problems that cause nausea, vomiting, loss of appetite, or diarrhoea may also lead to undernutrition. These include some types of cancer, liver disease, and some respiratory disorders. Undernutrition may also be a feature of various mental health problems or nervous system disorders, such as anorexia (p.243), depression (p.242), dementia (p.170), and alcohol misuse (p.243).

General symptoms include tiredness, weakness, weight loss, poor concentration, low mood, frequent illnesses, and a slow recovery time from illness. In children, undernutrition may cause slower than normal growth.

Treatment of undernutrition depends on the underlying cause and the degree of deficiency, but it may involve dietary changes or nutrient supplements.

DENTAL ABSCESS

A dental abscess is a pus-filled sac that develops in or around the root of a tooth. It may occur when bacteria invades a tooth as a result of tooth decay, a tooth fracture, or gum disease. Symptoms include severe pain on touching the affected tooth and when eating; loosening of the tooth; and a red, painful swelling of the gum over the root of the tooth.

Treatment may involve drilling the tooth to drain the abscess, followed by root-canal treatment (removing the tooth's inner tissues and then sealing the tooth). In some cases, it may be necessary to extract the affected tooth. An abscess around the root of a tooth may be treated by scraping away the affected material. Antibiotics may also be prescribed.

TOOTH DECAY

Also known as dental caries, tooth decay is the gradual erosion of the outer enamel of a tooth and sometimes also the inner dentine. Initial decay usually occurs on the grinding surfaces of the back teeth and areas around the gum line. The main cause of decay is the acid produced by bacteria in plaque (a sticky deposit of food particles, dead cells, saliva, and bacteria on the surface of teeth). Early-stage decay often causes no symptoms. Later, there may be toothache, sensitivity of the tooth to heat, cold, or sugary foods, and bad breath.

Superficial decay may be treated by applying fluoride to the decayed area. More advanced decay may need a filling or root canal treatment (removing the tooth's inner tissues then sealing the tooth). With very advanced decay, the tooth may need to be extracted.

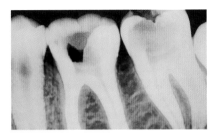

Tooth decay
In this coloured X-ray, the gum is red and healthy teeth are yellow. One of the teeth has some decay (black area) due to acid produced by bacteria in dental plaque.

GINGIVITIS

Gingivitis is inflammation of the gums, usually due to the build-up of plaque (a deposit of food particles, dead cells, saliva, and bacteria) as a result of poor oral hygiene. Symptoms of gingivitis include soft, red, swollen gums that bleed easily when brushing.

Untreated, the gums may recede and the teeth may become loose or even fall out. Mild gingivitis can often be reversed by good oral hygiene – brushing at least twice a day for about two minutes each time and flossing regularly. In more advanced cases, a dentist may have to remove hardened plaque deposits. An antiseptic mouthwash may help to prevent plaque from building up.

MOUTH ULCER

Also known as aphthous ulcers or canker sores, mouth ulcers are painful open sores inside the mouth. The exact cause of mouth ulcers is unknown, though a combination of factors may contribute, including minor mouth injuries, vitamin deficiencies, and stress. The ulcer forms a small, pale pit, and the area around it may become swollen.

Most ulcers clear up by themselves within about three weeks. Symptoms may be relieved by over-the-counter antiseptic mouthwashes, painkillers, corticosteroid lozenges, or anaesthetic gels. A doctor or dentist should be consulted if an ulcer lasts for more than about three weeks or becomes more painful or red, or if ulcers keep recurring.

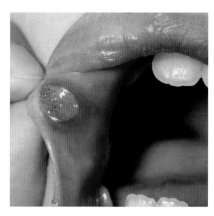

Ulcer inside lip
Mouth ulcers are open sores on the inside of the mouth. They usually occur on the inside of the lips (as shown here) or inside of the cheeks, but they may also sometimes affect the tongue.

LEUKOPLAKIA

In leukoplakia, there are small, thickened, white patches in the mouth, usually on the lining of the mouth or tongue, but sometimes on the gums or floor of the mouth. The main feature of the patches is that they cannot be scraped off.

Leukoplakia is linked to irritation from substances such as tobacco, alcohol, and betel leaves or nuts, or from the tongue or cheek rubbing on a rough tooth or denture. A type of leukoplakia called hairy leukoplakia affects people with reduced immunity. In this type, the patches have a rough surface. Leukoplakia is associated with an increased risk of mouth cancer, but hairy leukoplakia is not.

Stopping smoking and reducing alcohol consumption may cause the patches to shrink or disappear. The patches are usually harmless, but medical advice should be sought if they haven't cleared up after two weeks to check whether the leukoplakia is likely to become cancerous. If so, surgical removal may be advised.

ORAL CANCER

Also known as mouth cancer, oral cancer is a cancerous tumour of the lip, tongue, lining of the mouth, or gums. Lip cancer and tongue cancer are the most common types of oral cancer.

Risk factors for developing oral cancer include smoking or chewing tobacco, excessive alcohol use; chewing betel leaves or nuts, infection with human papillomavirus (HPV), and leukoplakia. Repeated exposure to sunlight increases the risk of lip cancer. Other factors that may increase the risk include a poor diet and reduced immunity.

Symptoms may include an ulcer or sore that does not heal; a white or red patch in the mouth that does not clear up; persistent pain in the mouth; a swelling that develops anywhere inside the mouth or on the lips; and pain when swallowing. Untreated, oral cancer may spread to other parts of the body.

Treatment for oral cancer is usually by surgical removal of the tumour, often followed by radiotherapy. Cosmetic surgery may also be offered after removal of the tumour to restore a more normal facial appearance. If the cancer has spread, treatment is usually with chemotherapy and radiotherapy.

SALIVARY GLAND PROBLEMS
Parotid tumour | Parotitis | Salivary gland stone

A stone can form in a salivary gland, such as a parotid gland, causing a visible swelling on the outside of the mouth or the sensation of a lump inside the mouth. There may also be pain while eating. It is often possible to remove a salivary gland stone by surgery, although in some cases the entire gland may need to be removed.

The salivary glands can also become infected and inflamed. For example, the parotid glands can become inflamed (parotitis) due to infection with the mumps virus. The inflammation subsides when the underlying infection clears up. Occasionally, a bacterial infection may lead to an abscess, which may need to be treated with antibiotics or drained.

Tumours of the salivary glands (such as parotid tumours) are rare. They cause a lump that may be felt protruding inside the mouth or on the face. Cancerous tumours usually grow quickly, feel hard, and are sometimes painful. Noncancerous tumours are usually painless and rubbery in consistency. Treatment is with surgery to remove the tumour or, sometimes, all of the affected salivary gland. After surgery, radiotherapy may also be given for cancerous tumours.

GEOGRAPHIC TONGUE

In geographic tongue, there are irregular, raw, red patches with white borders on the tongue. The cause is not known.

This condition usually causes no symptoms, although occasionally there may be discomfort when eating spicy or acidic foods. The condition is harmless and usually clears up on its own. A doctor or dentist should be consulted if any unusual patch in the mouth persists for more than a few weeks, to exclude the possibility of a more serious condition.

OESOPHAGEAL CANCER

Malignant tumours of the oesophagus, which carries food from the throat to the stomach, tend to develop slowly and often cause no symptoms in the early stage. Later, symptoms may include difficulty swallowing, regurgitation of food, coughing, persistent indigestion, loss of appetite, and weight loss. The cause of is not known, but risk factors include smoking, prolonged excessive alcohol consumption, being overweight, an unhealthy diet low in fruit and vegetables, and persistent gastro-oesophageal reflux disease.

Treatment is usually with surgery to remove the cancer and a tube (stent) may be inserted to keep the oesophagus open and allow swallowing.

OESOPHAGITIS

Oesophagitis is inflammation of the lining of the oesophagus. There are two main types: reflux and corrosive. Reflux oesophagitis is due to leaking of stomach acid into the oesophagus (gastro-oesophageal reflux disease); the acid inflames the oesophageal lining, causing heartburn. Treatment may include lifestyle changes, such as avoiding heavy meals, medication to reduce stomach acidity, or sometimes surgery. Corrosive oesophagitis is due to swallowing caustic chemicals. Treatment consists of reducing pain and nursing care until the oesophagus heals.

GASTRO-OESOPHAGEAL REFLUX DISEASE

Commonly known as acid reflux or dyspepsia, gastro-oesophageal reflux disease (GORD) is regurgitation of stomach acid into the oesophagus, causing pain in the upper abdomen and chest. It is usually due to poor functioning of the sphincter muscle in the oesophagus, which normally prevents regurgitation of the stomach contents. Factors that may result in GORD include poor muscle tone in the sphincter, pressure in the abdomen due to pregnancy or obesity, or a hiatus hernia (p.204). Symptoms include heartburn, an acid taste in the mouth, a persistent cough, belching, and in severe cases, blood in the vomit or faeces.

GORD can often be treated with self-help measures, such as eating smaller meals, losing any excess weight, and using over-the-counter heartburn remedies. If such measures are ineffective, a doctor may prescribe medication to reduce stomach acidity. Severe, persistent GORD may be treated with surgery.

GASTRITIS
Helicobacter pylori infection

Inflammation of the stomach lining (gastritis) may occur as due to infection or irritation. It may develop suddenly (acute) or be long-term (chronic). Acute gastritis is commonly caused by excessive alcohol consumption or the use of nonsteroidal anti-inflammatory drugs. Chronic gastritis is usually due to infection with *Helicobacter pylori* bacteria. Symptoms include upper abdominal pain and nausea. Some people have no symptoms. Mild gastritis can often be relieved by self-help measures, such as using over-the-counter medications to reduce stomach acidity. If symptoms are severe or persist for more than a week, a doctor should be consulted to investigate the cause. If *H. pylori* is identified as the cause, antibiotics and medication to reduce stomach acid usually clear up the gastritis.

Bacterium

Stomach lining

Bacteria in the stomach
More than 50 per cent of people carry *H. pylori* bacteria, but often it does not cause any problems. However, in some people it may cause chronic gastritis, stomach ulcers, or stomach cancer.

STOMACH ULCER
Peptic ulcer | Perforated ulcer

Also known as peptic ulcers, stomach ulcers are eroded areas in the lining of the stomach or duodenum. Most ulcers result from infection with *Helicobacter pylori* bacteria (p.199) or from long-term use of nonsteroidal anti-inflammatory drugs. Other contributory factors include smoking, consuming alcohol, and a family history of the condition. Symptoms include upper abdominal pain, loss of appetite, weight loss, nausea, and sometimes vomiting. Bleeding ulcers may also cause vomiting of blood or black, tarry faeces. Rarely, a perforated ulcer may form, creating a perforation (hole) in the wall of the stomach or duodenum, which may lead to peritonitis (p.205).

Most ulcers can be treated with medication to eliminate the *H. pylori* bacteria and reduce stomach acid production. A bleeding or perforated ulcer requires emergency treatment, which may involve surgery.

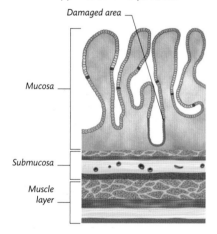

Damaged area

Mucosa

Submucosa

Muscle layer

Early ulcer
The lining of the stomach is normally protected by a layer of mucus. If this layer is breached, stomach acid can attack and damage mucosal cells.

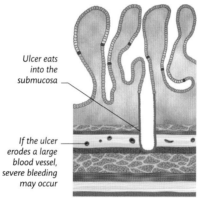

Ulcer eats into the submucosa

If the ulcer erodes a large blood vessel, severe bleeding may occur

Progressive ulceration
If an ulcer erodes the deeper layers of the stomach, it may damage blood vessels or it may even break through (perforate) the wall of the stomach or duodenum.

STOMACH CANCER

Stomach cancer is a malignant tumour that develops in the lining of the stomach wall. The cause of the condition is unknown, but factors that increase the risk of developing stomach cancer include infection with *H. pylori* bacteria (p.199); smoking; high alcohol consumption; a family history of the condition; certain disorders, such as pernicious anaemia (a type of anaemia caused by failure to absorb vitamin B12); and previous stomach surgery. A diet high in salted, pickled, or smoked foods and low in fruit and vegetables may also increase the risk.

Early symptoms are often mild and vague. They may include heartburn and stomach pain after eating, feeling full very quickly, loss of appetite, weight loss, nausea, and vomiting. In the later stages, there may be jaundice and bleeding from the stomach, which may result in vomiting up blood; black, tarry faeces; and symptoms of anaemia, such as breathlessness, tiredness, and pale skin.

Treatment is with surgery to remove part or all of the stomach, together with chemotherapy and sometimes radiotherapy. Medication to relieve symptoms may also be given. The outlook depends on factors such as the person's age and general health and how advanced the cancer is when it is treated.

HEPATITIS

Hepatitis is inflammation of the liver. Acute (short-term) hepatitis is usually due to infection with one of the hepatitis viruses, although it may also be due to other infections, such as cytomegalovirus, or to non-infectious factors, such as excessive alcohol intake or an overdose of paracetamol. Chronic (long-lasting) hepatitis is commonly a result of a hepatitis virus infection or long-term alcohol abuse. Other causes include certain medications or diseases, such as haemochromatosis (in which iron builds up in the body).

Symptoms include tiredness, fever, loss of appetite, nausea, vomiting, pain in the upper right side of the abdomen, and jaundice. Chronic hepatitis may also cause abdominal swelling due to fluid build-up; vomiting of blood; and black, tarry faeces. Severe hepatitis may lead to liver failure.

Acute hepatitis is usually treated with rest and medication to relieve symptoms. Most people recover, although in some cases the condition becomes chronic. Severe cases require hospital treatment and sometimes a liver transplant. Chronic hepatitis due to a viral infection is usually treated with medication. In other cases, treatment depends on the cause. In all cases, alcohol should be avoided. Vaccines against some of the hepatitis viruses are available to help prevent infection.

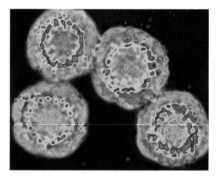

Hepatitis B virus
The hepatitis B virus is a common cause of hepatitis worldwide. It can be transmitted in blood, blood products, or other body fluids, by sexual contact, and from a mother to her baby during childbirth.

JAUNDICE

Jaundice is yellow discolouration of the whites of the eyes and skin, and is the chief sign of many disorders of the liver and biliary system. It is caused by the build-up of a substance called bilirubin, which is produced when red blood cells die. It is broken down by the liver and excreted in bile, which normally eventually passes out of the body in the urine and faeces.

In haemolytic jaundice, too many red blood cells are broken down, leading to excessive amounts of bilirubin. In obstructive jaundice, a blockage prevents bilirubin from leaving the liver. In hepatic jaundice, the liver cannot break down and excrete bilirubin normally. Jaundice requires medical investigation, because the underlying cause may be serious.

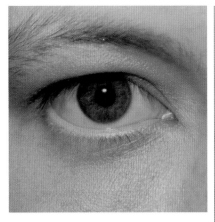

Yellowing of the eye
In jaundice, the white of the eye (sclera) appears yellow because of a build-up of bilirubin in the overlying, usually clear conjunctiva of the eye.

CIRRHOSIS

Cirrhosis is scarring of the liver arising from long-term damage to its cells. As a result, liver function becomes impaired, which may eventually lead to liver failure. The most common causes of cirrhosis are long-term, excessive alcohol consumption and long-term infection with a hepatitis virus. Other causes include non-alcoholic fatty liver disease (NAFLD), disorders of the bile ducts (the tubes that carry bile from the liver to the gallbladder and intestines), certain inherited disorders of body chemistry, cystic fibrosis, heart failure, and certain poisons or medications.

Cirrhosis often produces no symptoms in the early stages. As the condition progresses, there may be tiredness, nausea, loss of appetite, weight loss, jaundice, swelling of the legs or abdomen due to the build-up of fluid, vomiting of blood, a tendency to bleed or bruise easily, itchy skin, and black, tarry faeces. Cirrhosis may also cause toxins to build up in the brain, producing symptoms such as confusion, difficulty concentrating, and changes in personality; eventually, it may even lead to coma.

Liver damage due to cirrhosis is usually irreversible. Treatment is directed towards relieving symptoms and slowing the rate of liver damage, if possible, by treating the underlying cause. It is also important to avoid alcohol. In some cases, however, liver failure develops and a liver transplant is the only treatment option.

CHOLANGITIS
Primary biliary cholangitis

Cholangitis is inflammation of the bile ducts, the tubes that carry bile from the liver to the gallbladder and intestines. It is usually caused by bacterial infection, often as a result of blockage of a bile duct, and typically causes upper abdominal pain, fever, chills, nausea, vomiting, and jaundice. Treatment is with antibiotics and, if necessary, surgery to clear any blockage. Primary biliary cholangitis is a long-term condition in which the bile ducts become damaged. It is thought to be due to the immune system mistakenly attacking the ducts. Symptoms include tiredness, itchy skin, and bloating.

Treatment may include medication to minimize liver damage and relieve symptoms. In severe cases, a liver transplant may be needed.

LIVER CANCER

Most cancerous liver tumours are due to a cancer having spread from another part of the body (metastases), most commonly from a cancer in the colon (bowel), stomach, breast, ovary, lung, kidney, or, in men, prostate gland. Cancer that originates within the liver (primary liver cancer) may result from chronic viral hepatitis, cirrhosis from long-term alcohol abuse, exposure to toxins, or, mainly in parts of Asia, infection with a type of liver fluke (p.238). People with the inherited disorder haemochromatosis (in which iron builds up in the body) are also at risk of developing liver cancer.

Symptoms, which typically do not appear until the cancer is advanced, may include weight loss, fever, pain in the upper right side of the abdomen, jaundice, and abdominal swelling due to fluid build-up.

Treatment may involve surgery to remove part of the liver, microwave or radio-wave therapy to destroy the cancerous cells, a liver transplant, or chemotherapy.

LIVER FAILURE

In liver failure, normal functioning of the liver is severely impaired. It may occur suddenly (acute liver failure), for example, as a result of acute hepatitis or toxins, or gradually (chronic liver failure), which is commonly due to chronic hepatitis or cirrhosis from long-term alcohol abuse. Symptoms of acute failure develop rapidly and may include confusion, drowsiness, unconsciousness, and death. Chronic failure develops more slowly and may produce jaundice, itching, abdominal swelling due to fluid build-up, and, in men, enlarged breasts and shrunken testes.

Acute liver failure requires immediate hospital treatment; it is often ultimately fatal without a liver transplant. Chronic liver failure is treated with medication to relieve symptoms, and lifestyle measures, such as a diet low in salt and protein and stopping drinking alcohol.

PANCREATIC CANCER

Pancreatic cancer is relatively rare overall but is a common cause of cancer deaths, because it is often not diagnosed until it has reached an advanced stage. The cause of the cancer is unknown, but risk factors include smoking, being overweight, high alcohol consumption, diabetes, chronic pancreatitis, and a family history of pancreatic cancer.

Symptoms usually do not appear until late in the disease and often develop gradually. They may include pain in the upper abdomen that spreads out to the back, loss of appetite, weight loss, jaundice, and itching. There may also sometimes be indigestion, tiredness, nausea, vomiting, and diarrhoea.

Treatment depends on the individual case but typically includes surgery, radiotherapy, chemotherapy, and medication. The aim of treatment is to eradicate the cancer, but often this is not possible, and treatment is focused on relieving symptoms and limiting the spread of the cancer.

PANCREATITIS

Pancreatitis is inflammation of the pancreas. Acute (sudden-onset) pancreatitis may be caused by gallstones, alcohol abuse, an abdominal injury, a viral infection, or certain medications. Chronic (long-term) pancreatitis is commonly due to long-term alcohol abuse; other causes include cystic fibrosis (p.194) and hyperlipidaemia (high levels of fat in the blood).

Symptoms of both forms include severe upper abdominal pain that may spread to the back; nausea, vomiting, and fever. In severe acute pancreatitis, the abdominal lining may become inflamed (peritonitis, p.205). Chronic pancreatitis may lead to malabsorption or diabetes (p.219).

Acute pancreatitis usually requires monitoring and treatment in hospital until the inflammation clears up. Chronic pancreatitis is treated with painkillers, pancreatic hormones, insulin, and sometimes surgery.

GALLSTONES

Gallstones are hard masses formed from bile (a digestive juice produced by the liver) that occur in the gallbladder or bile ducts (tubes that carry bile from the liver to the gallbladder and intestines). Gallstones are more common in women, those who are overweight, people who eat a high-fat diet, those over about the age of 40, and people with certain disorders, such as cirrhosis (p.201) or Crohn's disease.

Gallstones take years to form and often cause no symptoms unless they become lodged in the cystic or common bile duct. If this happens, it can cause an attack of biliary colic: sudden, severe upper abdominal pain, often with nausea and vomiting. Less commonly, there may be also be fever, persistent pain, jaundice (p.201), and diarrhoea. Occasionally, a gallstone may lead to infection and inflammation of the gallbladder (cholecystitis).

Gallstones that cause no symptoms do not usually need treatment. Those that cause only mild or infrequent symptoms may be treated with painkillers and a diet that is low in fat. If symptoms are severe or occur frequently, surgical removal of the gallbladder is usually recommended.

CHOLECYSTITIS

Cholecystitis is inflammation of the gallbladder. It most commonly comes on suddenly (acute cholecystitis), due to a gallstone blocking the outflow of bile along the main duct leading out of the gallbladder. The trapped bile causes irritation of the gallbladder, which may become infected. Rarely, acute cholecystitis may be due to other causes, such as a serious injury.

The main symptom of acute cholecystitis is severe, persistent pain in the upper right abdomen that spreads to the right shoulder. Other symptoms may include fever, nausea, vomiting, loss of appetite, and a bulge in the abdomen. Treatment is usually with painkillers, antibiotics, and surgery to remove the gallbladder.

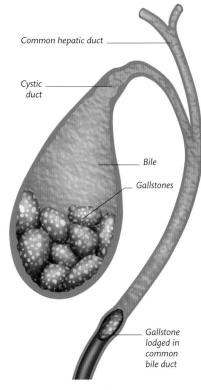

Common hepatic duct

Cystic duct

Bile

Gallstones

Gallstone lodged in common bile duct

Gallstone in common bile duct
A stone can block the flow of bile into the first part of the small intestine, leading to jaundice. Stagnant bile behind the stone may become infected, leading to inflammation of the bile duct (cholangitis, p.201).

MALABSORPTION

Malabsorption is a general term for impaired absorption of nutrients by the small intestine. It may be caused by many conditions, including cystic fibrosis (p.194), coeliac disease (p.204), Crohn's disease, pancreatitis, parasitic diseases (such as giardiasis, p.237), and intestinal damage. Certain medications and surgery on the intestine or stomach may also be causes. Common symptoms of malabsorption are weight loss, diarrhoea, bloating, wind, abdominal pain, tiredness, and weakness. In severe cases, there may also be malnutrition, vitamin or mineral deficiencies, or anaemia.

Treatment is of the underlying cause, if possible. Dietary modification or supplements may also be needed.

IRRITABLE BOWEL SYNDROME

Irritable bowel syndrome (IBS) is a long-term condition in which there is intermittent abdominal pain and constipation, diarrhoea, or bouts of each in the absence of any diagnosed disease. The cause is unknown, but it may result from abnormal contractions of the intestines. An increased sensitivity to certain foods may also contribute. In some cases, IBS may be triggered by an episode of gastroenteritis (p.196). Stress and anxiety tend to worsen the condition.

Symptoms tend to come and go, but attacks often recur for years. They vary widely among individuals and with each episode. Symptoms may include bloating and excessive wind; abdominal pain that may be relieved by defecation or passing wind; diarrhoea, constipation, or both; and passing mucus during defecation.

IBS can often be controlled by self-help measures, such as a change in diet, exercising regularly, and relaxation techniques to reduce stress. In some cases, medication may be prescribed to relieve specific symptoms.

LACTOSE INTOLERANCE

In lactose intolerance, the body cannot digest lactose, a natural sugar in milk and dairy products. The condition usually appears in adolescence or adulthood and is more common in those of African, Native American, Asian, or Jewish origin. The cause is lack of the enzyme lactase, which breaks down lactose. High levels of the enzyme are present at birth but in many ethnic groups levels naturally drop with age, eventually resulting in lactose intolerance.

Symptoms usually appear within a few hours of consuming products containing milk. They typically include wind, abdominal bloating and cramping, diarrhoea, and vomiting.

The condition is usually lifelong, but symptoms can be avoided by following a lactose-free diet. In addition, a doctor may suggest supplements to improve digestion of lactose.

INFLAMMATORY BOWEL DISEASE

Inflammatory bowel disease (IBD) is a collective term for persistent disorders that affect the small intestine or large intestine, or both. It causes symptoms such as recurrent or bloody diarrhoea, abdominal pain, abdominal swelling, weight loss, and tiredness.

The most common types of IBD are Crohn's disease (which can affect any part of the digestive tract but most commonly occurs in the last part of the small intestine or in the colon) and ulcerative colitis (which affects the colon and rectum).

CROHN'S DISEASE

Crohn's disease is a long-term condition in which there is inflammation of the intestine, most commonly the last part of the small intestine (ileum) or colon. The cause is unknown, but it is thought to be due to an immune system problem.

Symptoms tend to occur intermittently. During an attack, they may include diarrhoea, abdominal pain, fever, and weight loss; there may also sometimes be bloody diarrhoea; bleeding from the rectum; joint pain, inflamed eyes, and a rash. Possible complications include intestinal obstruction and malabsorption.

Treatment is usually with medication to reduce inflammation and alleviate symptoms. In some cases, surgery to remove affected parts of the intestine may be needed.

ULCERATIVE COLITIS

Ulcerative colitis is a long-term condition in which the colon and rectum become inflamed and ulcerated. The cause is unknown, but it is thought to be an autoimmune disorder.

Symptoms are often intermittent, with months or even years when there are few or no symptoms. Symptoms may include recurrent diarrhoea, sometimes containing blood, mucus, or pus; abdominal cramps; tiredness; loss of appetite; weight loss; and sometimes fever and abdominal swelling.

Treatment with medication, such as corticosteroids and immunosuppressants, can often relieve symptoms and prevent problems from developing. In severe cases, treatment is with surgery to remove the diseased part of the intestine.

MECKEL'S DIVERTICULUM

Meckel's diverticulum is a small, hollow, wide-mouthed pouch that protrudes from the last part of the small intestine. The pouch is present at birth. It often causes no problems and does not need treatment.

Symptoms only occur if the pouch becomes obstructed, inflamed, or twisted. The most common symptom is painless bleeding from the rectum. This bleeding may be sudden and severe; it requires treatment with an immediate blood transfusion. Inflammation may cause pain in the lower abdomen. Occasionally, the diverticulum results in telescoping (intussusception) or twisting (volvulus, p.204) of the small intestine.

Inflammation, intussusception, and volvulus are treated by surgical removal of the affected part of the intestine.

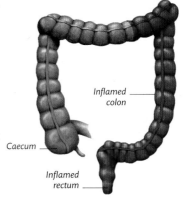

Inflamed colon

Caecum

Inflamed rectum

Inflammation and ulceration
In ulcerative colitis, the inflammation is usually continuous, extending from the rectum up to the colon to a varying extent. It sometimes reaches all the way to the caecum, a condition called pancolitis.

COELIAC DISEASE

In coeliac disease, the lining of the small intestine is damaged due to an adverse reaction to gluten, a protein that is found in wheat, barley, and rye. The condition is thought to be due to an abnormal immune response to gluten. Coeliac disease tends to run in families. Symptoms vary widely but may include diarrhoea, with bulky, foul-smelling faeces; abdominal pain and swelling; wind; weight loss; and sometimes a persistent rash. The disease may also lead to malabsorption and malnutrition, and sometimes anaemia.

Treatment is to follow a gluten-free diet, which usually clears up the symptoms rapidly (normally within a few weeks). The diet needs to be followed for life to avoid symptoms recurring.

VOLVULUS

Volvulus is a twisting of a loop of intestine or, rarely, of the stomach. It is a serious condition that causes obstruction of the passage of intestinal contents. Volvulus also carries the risk of strangulation, in which the blood supply to the affected area of the gastrointestinal tract is cut off. This blockage may lead to gangrene (death of tissues) in that area, which is potentially fatal. Volvulus may be present at birth or may result from adhesions (areas of scar tissue) binding together loops of intestine or portions of the stomach.

The main symptoms of volvulus are severe episodes of painful abdominal cramps followed by vomiting. The abdomen is tense (hard) and often bloated, and there is frequently constipation. Volvulus usually requires emergency surgical treatment to untwist the intestine.

HERNIA
Femoral hernia | Hiatus hernia | Inguinal hernia | Strangulated femoral hernia

A hernia is protrusion of part of an organ, usually the intestine, through a tear or weak area of muscle or surrounding tissue.

In an inguinal hernia, part of the intestine protrudes into the groin; this type mainly affects men and is visible as a bulge in the groin or scrotum.

A femoral hernia also occurs when the intestine protrudes into the groin. This type of hernia mainly affects women and is visible as a bulge at the top front of the thigh.

In a hiatus hernia, part of the stomach protrudes into the chest through an opening in the diaphragm called the hiatus. This type of hernia often causes no symptoms, although it may sometimes lead to gastro-oesophageal reflux disease (p.199), with symptoms such as heartburn and swallowing difficulties.

If left untreated, a hernia may cause intestinal obstruction, or the blood supply to the herniated tissue may become cut off (a strangulated hernia) and gangrene (tissue death) may develop in that area. Most hernias can be successfully treated by surgery.

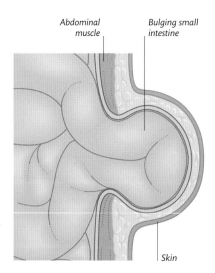

Abdominal muscle   *Bulging small intestine*

Skin

How a hernia develops
Part of the small intestine pushes through a weak area of muscle in the abdominal wall, which may cause a noticeable bulge to appear on the surface of the body.

POLYP

Also called bowel polyps or colorectal polyps, these are growths that project out from the lining of the colon or rectum. In most cases, the cause is unknown.

Polyps usually produce no symptoms and are discovered only during medical investigations for other reasons, such as during screening for bowel cancer. If symptoms do occur, they may include diarrhoea or constipation, blood in the faeces, or bleeding from the rectum. Polyps themselves are not cancerous, but some may develop into cancer, so if they are discovered, they need to be removed, usually by minimally invasive surgery. Rarely, it may be necessary to remove part of the colon.

Multiple polyps may occasionally be due to a rare inherited condition called familial adenomatous polyposis, in which hundreds of polyps grow in the lining of the colon and there is a high risk of bowel cancer. For this reason, people with familial adenomatous polyposis may be advised to have the colon completely removed.

INTESTINAL OBSTRUCTION
Bowel obstruction

Partial or complete blockage of the small intestine can have numerous possible causes. The causes include obstruction by a tumour, a strangulated hernia, or scar tissue; volvulus (twisting of the intestine); intussusception (telescoping of the intestine inside itself); and diseases that affect the intestinal wall, such as Crohn's disease (p.203) or paralysis of muscles in the intestinal wall. Less commonly, intestinal obstruction may be due to impacted food or faeces, gallstones (p.202), or a swallowed object.

Symptoms of intestinal obstruction may include abdominal pain and swelling, vomiting, and failure to pass wind or faeces. Treatment often involves surgery to relieve the obstruction.

DIVERTICULAR DISEASE
Diverticulitis

Diverticular disease is the presence of small pouches (diverticula) in the wall of the intestines, and the symptoms or complications caused by them. The term diverticulosis signifies the presence of the pouches; if the pouches become infected and inflamed, the condition is known as diverticulitis. Risk factors for diverticular disease include smoking, being overweight, a history of constipation, a family history of diverticular disease, and use of nonsteroidal anti-inflammatory drugs (such as ibuprofen).

Diverticulosis often causes no symptoms. If symptoms do occur, they may include episodes of abdominal pain that are relieved by defecation or passing wind; intermittent diarrhoea or constipation; and sometimes bleeding from the rectum.

If diverticulitis develops, the symptoms worsen and may be accompanied by severe, left-sided lower abdominal pain, fever, nausea, and vomiting.

Diverticulosis can, if necessary, be treated with a high-fibre diet and paracetamol. Diverticulitis can usually be successfully treated with antibiotics, although severe cases may need surgery to remove the affected area of bowel.

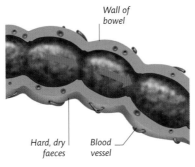

Wall of bowel

Hard, dry faeces *Blood vessel*

Hard faeces
If faeces are small, hard, and dry, the muscles in the bowel wall must contract harder to push them along than if they are large and soft.

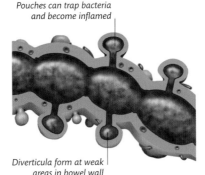

Pouches can trap bacteria and become inflamed

Diverticula form at weak areas in bowel wall

Pouches form
Pressure from pushing can cause diverticula to form at weak areas in the bowel wall. The pouches may become infected and inflamed.

PERITONITIS

Peritonitis is inflammation of the peritoneum, the membrane surrounding the abdominal organs and lining the abdominal wall. It is caused by infection, usually occurring as a complication of another disorder, such as appendicitis, a ruptured stomach ulcer, or diverticular disease.

Symptoms usually develop rapidly and may include severe, constant abdominal pain, fever, abdominal swelling, nausea, and vomiting. It is potentially life-threatening and needs urgent treatment. This usually involves medications to eliminate the infection, and sometimes surgery to treat the underlying cause.

HIRSCHSPRUNG'S DISEASE

In Hirschsprung's disease, nerves that control muscle contractions of the bowel to push faeces along are missing from the end of the bowel. As a result, faeces build up and block the bowel. The condition is present from birth. Symptoms, which are usually apparent within weeks of birth, include constipation, bloating, vomiting, poor feeding, and failure to gain weight. Treatment is with surgery to remove the affected part of the bowel and then later to rejoin healthy sections.

APPENDICITIS

Appendicitis is inflammation of the appendix, leading to severe abdominal pain. Blockage and infection in the appendix can cause it to fill with pus and swell. As the swelling worsens, the appendix starts to die. Eventually, it bursts and infected material leaks out, which may then lead to peritonitis.

The first symptom of appendicitis is usually vague discomfort around the navel. Within hours, this develops into severe pain in the lower right side of the abdomen. There may also be nausea, vomiting, fever, and diarrhoea. Treatment is by prompt surgical removal of the appendix.

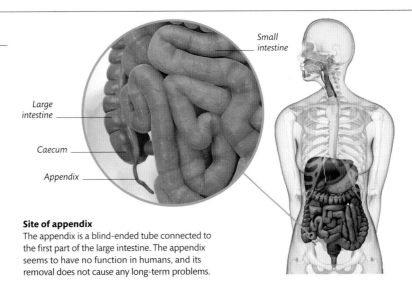

Small intestine

Large intestine

Caecum

Appendix

Site of appendix
The appendix is a blind-ended tube connected to the first part of the large intestine. The appendix seems to have no function in humans, and its removal does not cause any long-term problems.

PROCTITIS

Proctitis is inflammation of the rectum. It commonly occurs as a feature of diseases such as ulcerative colitis (p.203), Crohn's disease (p.203), amoebiasis (p.237), schistosomiasis (fluke infestations, p.238), sexually transmitted infections, and tuberculosis (p.236). Other possible causes include radiotherapy to the lower abdomen and injury from a foreign object inserted into the rectum.

Symptoms may include blood, mucus, or pus in the faeces; pain the rectum that is more severe with a bowel movement; diarrhoea or constipation; and an increased urge to defecate. Proctitis due to a sexually transmitted infection may also cause fever and pelvic pain. Treatment depends on the underlying cause.

PROCTALGIA FUGAX

Proctalgia fugax is severe, cramping pain in the rectum that is not due to any disease. The cause is not understood, but it may be due to spasms in the muscles of the anus. In some cases, the pain may be triggered by sexual intercourse, defecation, a bout of constipation, stress, or a menstrual period.

The pain typically comes on suddenly and lasts only a few seconds or minutes. In many cases, attacks occur in clusters, with no pain between episodes. The clusters tend to occur infrequently.

Usually, no treatment is needed, although a doctor should be consulted to rule out more serious conditions. If the condition is troublesome, medication to relieve the pain may be prescribed.

ANORECTAL ABSCESS

An anorectal abscess is an infected, pus-filled cavity in the anal or rectal area that develops when bacteria infect a mucus-secreting gland in the anus or rectum. The abscess may occur deep inside the rectum or close to the anus. Anorectal abscesses are associated with inflammatory bowel disorders, such as Crohn's disease (p.203) or ulcerative colitis (p.203), and anal sex.

Symptoms may include swelling and redness in the anal area; throbbing pain in the anal area that worsens with defecation; a discharge of pus from the rectum; and sometimes fever. Treatment usually involves surgery to drain the abscess, antibiotics to eliminate infection, and medication to relieve pain.

BOWEL CANCER
Rectal cancer

Also known as colorectal cancer, bowel cancer is a malignant tumour of the rectum or colon. Rectal cancer affects the last part of the bowel. The cause of bowel cancer is usually unknown, but risk factors include a diet high in red or processed meat and low in fibre; being overweight; lack of exercise; smoking; excessive alcohol consumption; a family history of bowel cancer; and a personal medical history of certain long-standing inflammatory bowel disorders, such as ulcerative colitis or Crohn's disease. Rarely, bowel cancer is due to the inherited disorder familial adenomatous polyposis, in which numerous polyps (p.204) grow in the bowel.

Symptoms include changes in the frequency of bowel movements or in the general consistency of the faeces; persistent blood in the faeces; persistent lower abdominal pain, bloating, or discomfort; a sensation of incomplete emptying of the bowel after defecation; and loss of appetite.

Treatment depends on the location and stage of the cancer. In most cases, treatment involves surgery to remove the affected section of bowel, sometimes combined with chemotherapy, radiotherapy, or biological treatments (medications that shrink the tumour). Some countries have screening programmes to detect the disease early.

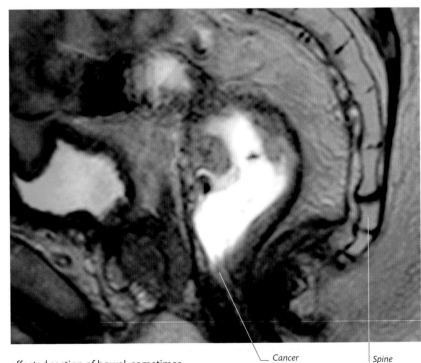

Cancer | _Spine_

Bowel cancer
This magnetic resonance imaging (MRI) scan shows cancer in the rectum (the last part of the bowel). The image has been artificially coloured to highlight the cancer, which is shown in purple.

RECTAL PROLAPSE

In a rectal prolapse, the lining of the rectum protrudes outside the anus. It is often a result of increased pressure in the abdomen, due, for example, to constipation, pregnancy, or persistent coughing. The condition is more common in women and older people, and may be a recurrent problem in those who have weak pelvic floor muscles. Rectal prolapse also sometimes occurs temporarily in young children during toilet training.

The main symptom is a lump protruding out of the anus. Initially, this may appear only when straining to defecate and then it disappears when standing up, but later it may be present all the time. Other symptoms may include discomfort or pain when defecating, and bleeding and a discharge of mucus from the anus. If the prolapse is large, there may also be faecal incontinence.

In many cases, the prolapse can be treated by pushing it back, followed by treatment to relieve the cause, such as a high-fibre diet for constipation. Sometimes, however, surgery is needed to fix the rectum in position permanently.

HAEMORRHOIDS

Commonly known as piles, haemorrhoids are swollen veins inside the rectum or around the anus. They result from increased pressure inside the abdomen, commonly due to straining to defecate because of constipation or diarrhoea, excess body weight, or pregnancy.

Haemorrhoids that occur inside the rectum may bleed, showing as bright red blood on the faeces, toilet paper, or in the toilet bowl. Larger internal haemorrhoids may protrude out of the anus, typically after defecation, but often go back in by themselves or can be pushed back by hand. External haemorrhoids develop outside the anus. Both types can form itchy, tender, painful lumps.

Small haemorrhoids do not usually need treatment, and those due to pregnancy usually disappear after the birth. Lifestyle measures, such as a high-fibre diet, can prevent constipation, and over-the-counter haemorrhoid preparations can relieve symptoms. More severe haemorrhoids may be treated by placing a tight band around the haemorrhoid, causing it to fall off, or by surgery.

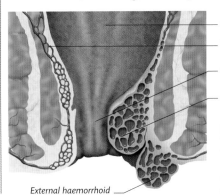

Rectum

Vein network

Anal canal

Internal haemorrhoid

External haemorrhoid

Haemorrhoids
The veins on the left are normal. Those on the right have become swollen, protruding into the anal canal at the end of the rectum (internal haemorrhoids) or outside the anus (external haemorrhoids).

ANAL FISSURE

An anal fissure is a tear or ulcer in the lining of the anal canal. It is most commonly caused by damage from passing hard, dry faeces due to constipation. It is also common during pregnancy and after delivery. Less common causes include an inflammatory bowel disease, such as Crohn's disease (p.203) or ulcerative colitis (p.203), or having unusually tight anal sphincter muscles.

The main symptoms are severe pain when defecating and bleeding when defecating (often visible as bright red blood on the faeces, toilet paper, or in the toilet bowl). Most fissures heal by themselves within a few weeks. Measures such as a high-fibre diet to prevent constipation and painkillers can relieve symptoms and help the healing process. If such treatments are ineffective, surgery may be recommended.

ANAL FISTULA

An anal fistula is an abnormal channel connecting the inside of the anal canal with the skin around the anus. In most cases, it is the result of an abscess that develops for unknown reasons in the wall of the anus and does not heal properly. An anal fistula may also sometimes develop as a result of an intestinal disorder such as Crohn's disease (p.203), ulcerative colitis (p.203), or bowel cancer.

Symptoms of an anal fistula may include a discharge of pus onto the skin around the anus; passing blood or pus in the faeces; irritation, swelling, redness, and constant, throbbing pain around the anus; and, in some cases, fever and faecal incontinence.

A fistula rarely heals by itself and usually requires treatment with surgery.

ANAL CANCER

Cancer of the anus or anal canal is rare and its cause is not known, although it may be linked with infection with human papillomaviruses (HPV), which cause genital warts (p.218) and are also associated with cervical cancer (p.215).

Symptoms of anal cancer usually develop gradually. They may include bleeding from the anus, itching and pain around the anus, a frequent need to defecate or faecal incontinence, a discharge of mucus from the anus, and a lump in or near the anus.

The usual treatment is chemotherapy combined with radiotherapy. In many cases, this causes the tumour to shrink so that surgery is not needed. However, if this treatment is ineffective, surgery to remove the anus and part of the rectum is necessary.

URINARY AND REPRODUCTIVE DISORDERS

KIDNEY STONES

Also known as renal calculi, kidney stones may be associated with dehydration; a high-protein, low-fibre diet; certain medications; or various disorders, such as gout, hyperparathyroidism (overactivity of the parathyroid glands), kidney disease, or a urinary tract infection.

Small stones may pass out of the body unnoticed in the urine. Larger stones or stone fragments that pass into the ureter (the tube from the kidney to the bladder) may cause severe back pain; nausea; vomiting; and frequent, painful urination, sometimes with blood in the urine.

Small stones may be treated with medication to relieve symptoms, and plenty of fluids to flush out the stones. A larger stone may be treated with shock waves to break it up so that it can pass out in the urine. Alternatively, surgery may be used to remove or break up the stone.

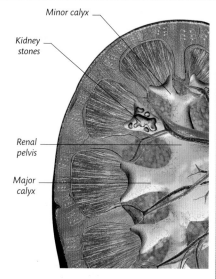

Minor calyx

Kidney stones

Renal pelvis

Major calyx

Growth of kidney stones
Kidney stones can occur in any urine-collecting part of the kidney. Larger stones form in the calyces and renal pelvis. Stones usually grow slowly, sometimes taking years to form.

KIDNEY INFECTION

The kidney may become infected as a result of bacterial infection entering the urinary tract through the urethra (the tube that carries urine out of the body) and travelling up through the bladder and ureters (the tubes between the bladder and kidneys) to the kidney. This causes inflammation of the kidney (pyelonephritis).

Symptoms typically appear suddenly and may include intense pain in the lower back (usually only on one side), fever, nausea, vomiting, and frequent, painful urination; the urine may be cloudy, bloodstained, or foul-smelling.

Untreated, pyelonephritis may cause complications such as septicaemia (p.234) or kidney damage. Treatment is with paracetamol to relieve pain and antibiotics to destroy the bacteria causing the infection. With prompt treatment, most people recover within about two weeks.

KIDNEY CYSTS

Simple kidney cysts are fluid-filled sacs that develop in the outer layer of the kidney. They can occur singly or multiply, and one or both kidneys may be affected. They are very common, especially in people over about 50, but their cause is not known. The cysts are not cancerous and do not usually cause symptoms. Rarely, there may be blood in the urine or a cyst may become large enough to press on surrounding tissues, causing back pain.

Treatment is not usually necessary, although a cyst that is causing pain may be drained or removed surgically.

KIDNEY FAILURE

In kidney failure, the kidneys do not function normally and there is a build-up of waste products and water in the body, disrupting the body's chemical balance. Kidney failure may occur suddenly (which is referred to as acute kidney injury) or more gradually (called chronic kidney disease).

Acute kidney damage may occur as a result of conditions such as infection, dehydration, very low blood pressure, a heart disorder such as heart failure (p.181), the effects of certain medications or poisons, or an underlying problem with the urinary system. Symptoms may include nausea, vomiting, a greatly reduced amount of urine, back pain, build-up of fluid in the body, drowsiness, and confusion.

Untreated, acute kidney injury may be life-threatening. Treatment depends on the underlying cause, but may include rehydration with intravenous fluids, and in severe cases, kidney dialysis.

CHRONIC KIDNEY DISEASE

In chronic kidney disease, there is a gradual and progressive loss of function affecting both kidneys. It is usually caused by a long-term condition, such as high blood pressure, diabetes (p.219), kidney infection, or longstanding obstruction to urine flow – for example, due to an enlarged prostate gland (p.212). It may also occur with prolonged use of some medications and the inherited disorder polycystic kidney disease. Chronic kidney disease typically produces few symptoms until it is advanced, when tiredness, weakness, nausea, itching, blood in the urine, and swelling of the ankles, feet, or hands may occur. Treatment is directed at the underlying cause. In severe cases, dialysis or a kidney transplant may be needed.

KIDNEY CANCER

Most kidney cancers originate within the kidney itself; only rarely are they due to the spread of cancer from elsewhere in the body. There are often no symptoms in the early stages. Later symptoms may include blood in the urine; pain in the back or sides; frequent, painful urination; and weight loss. Kidney cancer may also spread to other organs, such as the bones or lungs.

The main treatment is surgery to remove all or part of the affected kidney and sometimes also the ureter and part of the bladder. Other treatments may include radiotherapy, embolization (cutting off the blood supply to the cancer), destroying the cancer with heat or cold, or biological therapies (medications that help prevent the cancer from growing or spreading).

BLADDER INFECTION
Interstitial cystitis (painful bladder syndrome)

This condition, also called cystitis, is the inflammation of the bladder lining. More common in women, it is usually due to a bacterial infection. In men, it is usually due to a urinary tract disorder. There is also a type called interstitial cystitis (painful bladder syndrome), which has no known cause.

All types of cystitis produce similar symptoms, including painful urination, a frequent and urgent need to urinate, and a feeling of incomplete emptying of the bladder. In interstitial cystitis there may also be intense pain below the belly button and blood in the urine. Cystitis due to infection may also cause fever, and pain in the lower abdomen or lower back.

Symptoms may be relieved by drinking plenty of fluids, such as unsweetened cranberry juice or water. A bacterial infection is usually treated with antibiotics. Treatment for interstitial cystitis depends on the specific cause. Various treatments may be tried, including medication, physiotherapy, and bladder training (techniques to delay urination), In some cases, surgery may be recommended.

URINARY TRACT INFECTION

Urinary tract infection (UTI) is a general term for infection anywhere in the urinary tract – the kidneys, bladder, ureters (the tubes from the kidneys to the bladder), or urethra (the tube from the bladder to outside the body).

Infection of the kidney (pyelonephritis) and bladder (cystitis) is usually due to bacteria. Infection of the urethra (urethritis) is often due to a sexually transmitted infection, such as gonorrhoea (p.218), but may also have other causes. Various factors increase the risk of developing a urinary tract infection, including kidney or bladder stones (p.210), diabetes (p.219), reduced immunity, difficulty emptying the bladder fully, and, in men, an enlarged prostate gland (p.212).

Treatment is usually with antibiotics. Painkillers and drinking plenty of fluids may relieve symptoms.

URINARY INCONTINENCE
Overactive bladder | Stress incontinence | Total incontinence | Urge incontinence

There are various types of urinary incontinence, which is the involuntary passing of urine. The main ones are: stress incontinence, in which urine leaks when the bladder is under pressure (for example, while coughing or sneezing); urge incontinence, when urine leaks immediately after a sudden urge to urinate; overactive bladder, in which there is a frequent, urgent need to urinate; nocturia, with frequent waking at night in order to urinate; and total incontinence, when there is no bladder control at all.

There are many possible causes for incontinence, including weakness, damage, or overactivity of the muscles that control urine flow; various diseases, such as urinary tract infections, nervous system disorders, bladder stones, or, in men, an enlarged prostate gland; the effects of certain medication; or simply drinking too much caffeine or alcohol.

Treatment of incontinence depends on the type and cause. It may involve lifestyle changes; pelvic floor exercises to strengthen muscles involved in urinating; bladder training (techniques to delay urination); medication; or, occasionally, surgery.

Stress incontinence
This type of incontinence results from weakness of the urethral sphincter and pelvic floor muscles. When pressure in the bladder increases, the muscles are not strong enough to retain the urine.

Urine in bladder

NORMAL BLADDER   *Urethra*   *Pelvic floor muscle*

Pressure on bladder increases

INCONTINENT BLADDER   *Leaking urine*   *Weakened pelvic floor muscle*

URINARY RETENTION
Overflow incontinence

Urinary retention is the inability to empty the bladder completely or at all. It may occur suddenly (acute retention) or develop gradually (chronic retention). In chronic retention, there may be constant dribbling of urine, a condition known as overflow incontinence.

In men, causes of retention include an enlarged prostate (p.212), phimosis (tight foreskin), or a narrowed urethra (the tube from the bladder to outside the body). In women, causes include fibroids (noncancerous growths, p.215) in the uterus, and, in pregnancy, pressure on the urethra from the growing fetus. In both sexes, retention may result from constipation (p.196), bladder stones, or bladder tumours. Other causes include spinal injury, multiple sclerosis (p.171), or diabetes (p.219). It may also occur after surgery or as a side effect of some medications.

Treatment depends on the underlying cause, although acute retention requires urgent medical treatment to drain the accumulated urine.

BLADDER CANCER

Most cancerous growths in the bladder arise in the lining of the bladder wall, but they can also develop in muscle and other cells in the bladder. Bladder tumours are more common in men and in people whose jobs involve exposure to carcinogens in the rubber, textile, and printing industries; in smokers; and in those with persistent irritation of the bladder from bladder stones or the worm infestation schistosomiasis.

Initially, there may be no symptoms, but over time there may be blood in the urine, difficulty passing urine, and weight loss. A large tumour may cause urinary retention.

Untreated, the cancer may spread to other parts of the body. Treatment may include surgery, chemotherapy, radiotherapy, or a combination of these.

BLADDER STONE

Bladder stones are hard lumps of minerals that gradually form inside the bladder, usually as a result of incomplete emptying of the bladder (urinary retention). They are also more likely to develop in people who have recurrent cystitis (inflammation of the bladder) or certain disorders of body chemistry, such as gout (p.159). A small stone may not cause any symptoms and may be passed out naturally in the urine. A large stone may cause pain and difficulty passing urine, a frequent and sometimes urgent need to pass urine, and blood in the urine. Treatment is usually with surgery.

EPIDIDYMO-ORCHITIS
Epididymitis | Orchitis

In epididymo-orchitis, the epididymis (the coiled tube that runs along the back of the testis and stores sperm, which then pass to the vas deferens) and testis become inflamed, causing pain and swelling at the back of the testis and, in severe cases, swelling, redness, and extreme pain in the scrotum. It is usually one-sided. An inflammation that only affects the epididymis is called epididymitis. Inflammation of the testis is called orchitis. Orchitis may cause swelling and pain in one or both testes, fever, nausea, and vomiting.

Epididymo-orchitis, epididymitis, and orchitis are usually caused by a sexually transmitted infection, such as chlamydia (p.218) or nongonococcal urethritis (p.218), or a urinary tract infection (p.209); rarely, it is due to an infection carried through the bloodstream from elsewhere in the body, such as tuberculosis (p.236). Treatment is with medication.

TORSION OF TESTIS

Each testis is suspended in the scrotum on a spermatic cord, which contains blood vessels and the vas deferens (the tube that carries sperm from each testis). In torsion of the testis, the testis rotates, causing the spermatic cord to become twisted. This restricts the blood supply to the testis and causes pain. The condition usually affects only one testis and sometimes occurs after strenuous activity, but may develop for no apparent reason.

Symptoms usually appear suddenly and, as well as pain in the scrotum, may include swelling of the testis, redness of the scrotum, nausea, and vomiting. This is a medical emergency and without prompt treatment, the testis may be permanently damaged. Treatment is with surgery.

EPIDIDYMAL CYST

An epididymal cyst is a harmless, fluid-filled sac that forms in the epididymis (the coiled tube that runs along the back of the testis and stores sperm from the testis). Epididymal cysts often occur in both testes and are most common in middle-aged and older men. The cysts are usually painless and need no treatment.

Occasionally, an epididymal cyst may become large and cause discomfort, or, very rarely, may become twisted and painful (a condition called torsion of an epididymal cyst), which is a medical emergency and requires surgery.

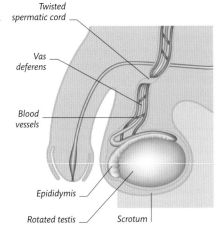

Torsion of the testis
In addition to twisting of the spermatic cord, the testis lies in a different position in the scrotum, which may distort the scrotum's usual shape.

TESTICULAR CANCER

A cancerous tumour of the testis (testicle) is one of the most common cancers in young to middle-aged men, although it is relatively rare overall. Risk factors for testicular cancer include having an undescended testis or a family history of testicular cancer.

Testicular cancer usually affects only one testis. Symptoms include a hard, painless lump in the affected testis, a change in the usual size and texture of the testis, a dull ache in the scrotum, and a feeling of heaviness in the scrotum. Sometimes there may be a sharp pain in the affected testis, or fluid may accumulate in the scrotum, causing visible swelling. In advanced cases, the cancer may spread to other parts of the body, such as the lymph nodes or lungs.

Treatment is usually with surgery to remove the affected testis. This may be combined with chemotherapy or radiotherapy. If the cancer has spread, additional treatment may be needed to treat the secondary cancer.

HYDROCELE

A hydrocele is a soft, painless swelling in the scrotum that is due to a build-up of fluid in the double-layered membrane that partially surrounds each testis.

The condition is most common in infants and older men. In most cases, there is no apparent cause, although occasionally a hydrocele may be associated with infection, inflammation, or injury of the testis or, rarely, it may be associated with testicular cancer.

A hydrocele in an infant usually clears up by itself. In older children and adults, treatment to drain the fluid may be advised if a hydrocele is large or troublesome. Treatment may also be needed for any underlying cause that is identified.

Swollen scrotum
The fluid of a hydrocele is contained within the double-layered membrane that partially surrounds each testis. The accumulated fluid causes swelling of the scrotum but is not usually painful.

Prostate gland

Urethra

Epididymis

Testis

Scrotum

Accumulated fluid in hydrocele

VARICOCELE

A varicocele is a collection of swollen, enlarged veins – varicose veins – in the scrotum. The condition is caused by leaking valves in the veins that carry blood away from the testes, although there is usually no identifiable reason for the leakage. Varicoceles most commonly occur on the left side of the scrotum.

There may be no obvious symptoms, or they may include a swelling that is described as "feeling like a bag of worms", and an aching pain in the scrotum. The affected side of the scrotum may also hang lower than normal. A varicocele may also reduce fertility.

Small, painless varicoceles often disappear by themselves. Larger ones, those causing discomfort, or varicoceles that affect fertility may be treated by surgery to tie off swollen veins.

ERECTILE DYSFUNCTION

Also known as impotence, erectile dysfunction is the inability to get or keep an erection. Psychological causes include stress, fatigue, depression, and relationship problems. Possible physical causes include atherosclerosis (narrowing of the blood vessels), diabetes (p.219), or nervous system problems, such as multiple sclerosis (p.171) or spinal cord damage. Some medications also cause erection difficulties as a side effect, as can drinking too much alcohol. Erectile dysfunction can also result if nerves supplying the penis are damaged during surgery – for example, in operations on the prostate gland.

Treatment of erectile dysfunction depends on the cause, but may include counselling or psychological therapy, lifestyle changes, medication, devices to help with erections, or, rarely, surgery.

PROSTATITIS

Prostatitis is inflammation of the prostate gland. It may develop suddenly and cause severe symptoms (acute prostatitis) or more gradually (chronic prostatitis). Acute prostatitis is due to an infection, usually a bacterial one, whereas the cause of chronic prostatitis is usually unknown. It is more common in men between 30 and 50.

Symptoms of acute prostatitis include fever and chills; pain around the base of the penis and in the lower back; pain during bowel movements; and frequent, urgent, and painful urination. Chronic prostatitis may cause pain and tenderness at the base of the penis, and in the testes, groin, pelvis, or back; pain when ejaculating; blood in the semen, and frequent, painful urination.

Both types of prostatitis are treated with medication The condition may be slow to clear up and tends to recur.

ENLARGED PROSTATE

Prostate enlargement may be due to inflammation (prostatitis, p.211), prostate cancer, or benign prostatic hyperplasia (BPH). Symptoms of BPH may include frequent urination, delay in starting to pass urine, a weak urine flow, dribbling after urinating, and a feeling that the bladder has not emptied completely. Occasionally, urine flow may be completely blocked, causing rapidly increasing pain. This requires urgent treatment to drain accumulated urine.

Mild BPH can often be controlled by lifestyle changes, such as reducing caffeine and alcohol intake, limiting evening beverages, eating a healthy diet, staying active, urinating when you first feel an urge, and urinating regularly every four to six hours during the day. More severe cases may be treated with medication to shrink the prostate or improve urine flow. If these treatments are ineffective, surgery may be recommended.

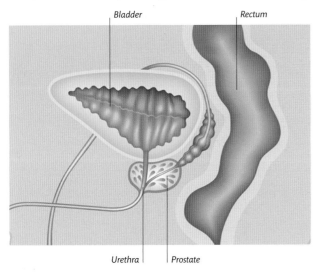

Bladder   *Rectum*

Urethra | *Prostate*

Normal prostate
The prostate gland surrounds the urethra at the point where it exits the bladder. The prostate secretes prostatic fluid, which forms part of the seminal fluid during ejaculation.

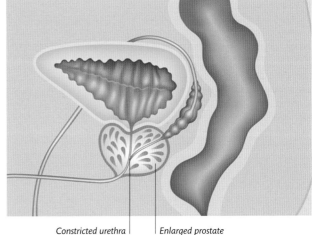

Constricted urethra | *Enlarged prostate*

Enlarged prostate
As the prostate enlarges, it constricts the urethra and impedes the flow of urine, leading to symptoms such as poor, dribbling urine flow, and a frequent need to pass urine.

PROSTATE CANCER

Cancer of the prostate gland is a slow-growing cancer that mainly affects older men. It is often not fatal. The cause is unknown, although it is more common in men with a family history of the disease and in those of Afro-Caribbean or African descent. Symptoms do not usually develop until the cancer constricts the urethra, causing problems such as frequent urination, weak flow, and a feeling that the bladder has not emptied completely.

Treatment depends on the stage of the cancer and the age, health, and wishes of the man. In some cases, the cancer may only need to be monitored. If treatment is necessary, options include surgery, radiotherapy, chemotherapy, and hormone therapy to limit growth of the cancer.

GYNAECOMASTIA

Gynaecomastia is a noncancerous enlargement of one or both breasts in men or boys. It is often due to an excess of the female hormone oestrogen (which is also produced naturally in males, but normally only in small amounts). Mild, temporary gynaecomastia can occur at birth as a result of maternal hormones, and is also common at puberty. Gynaecomastia in later life may be a result of being overweight, due to increased oestrogen produced by fat cells. Adult gynaecomastia may also be due to some medications, long-term liver disease, or a hormone-secreting testicular or pituitary tumour.

Treatment depends on the cause. If there is no underlying disorder, the excess breast tissue may be removed surgically.

PREMENSTRUAL SYNDROME

Also known as premenstrual tension, premenstrual syndrome (PMS) is the combination of physical and psychological symptoms that many women experience in the week or so before menstruation. The cause is unknown, but it is thought to be linked to changing levels of hormones.

Symptoms can vary from woman to woman, and also from month to month, and may be severe enough to disrupt normal everyday activities.

No single treatment has proved consistently successful. Treatments that may be suggested include lifestyle changes, relaxation techniques, medication to relieve symptoms, psychological therapy, and hormone treatment, such as the combined oral contraceptive pill.

OVARIAN CYSTS

Ovarian cysts are fluid-filled sacs in an ovary. There are several types of cyst. The most common are ones that develop in the follicles (cavities where eggs develop) or corpus luteum (the empty follicle remaining after an egg is released). Other types include dermoid cysts and cystadenomas, which can grow very large. Multiple ovarian cysts, together with other characteristic features, occur in polycystic ovary syndrome.

Most cysts cause no symptoms. When symptoms do occur, they may include abdominal discomfort, pain during sex, and menstrual irregularities. Occasionally, a cyst may rupture or become twisted, causing symptoms such as severe abdominal pain, nausea, and fever. Rarely, a cyst may become cancerous.

In most cases, cysts disappear naturally without treatment. A large cyst, one that has ruptured or twisted, or one that may become cancerous is treated by surgical removal.

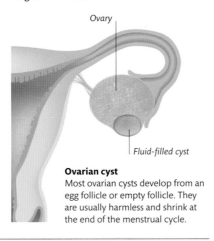

Ovary

Fluid-filled cyst

Ovarian cyst
Most ovarian cysts develop from an egg follicle or empty follicle. They are usually harmless and shrink at the end of the menstrual cycle.

OVARIAN CANCER

Cancer of the ovary mainly affects women after menopause. The cause is not known, although it sometimes develops from an ovarian cyst. Risk factors include never having had children and a family history of ovarian or breast cancer.

Often, the cancer causes no symptoms until it is advanced. Then, symptoms may include swelling and discomfort in the abdomen, frequent urination, and, rarely, abnormal vaginal bleeding. Untreated, it may spread to other organs, such as the liver or lungs.

The main treatments are surgery to remove the cancer and chemotherapy. However, often the cancer is not diagnosed until it is advanced, and a complete cure is not possible.

POLYCYSTIC OVARY SYNDROME

Polycystic ovary syndrome is characterized by multiple ovarian cysts, high levels of male sex hormones (which are produced naturally in women, but usually only in small amounts), and certain other features, such as excessive hair, menstrual irregularities, and reduced fertility. The cause of polycystic ovary syndrome is unknown.

Symptoms of polycystic ovary syndrome may include irregular or absent periods;

excessive hair growth, usually on the face, chest, back, or buttocks; thinning of the hair on the head; acne; and weight gain. Polycystic ovary syndrome also increases the risk of developing diabetes, high blood pressure, heart disease, and uterine cancer (p.214).

Treatment for polycystic ovary syndrome includes medications to treat symptoms such as excessive hair, irregular periods, and fertility problems. If a woman wants to conceive and medications are ineffective, surgery may be an option.

MITTELSCHMERZ

Mittelschmerz is pain in the lower abdomen that some women have at the time of ovulation. The pain usually occurs on one side of the abdomen and lasts only a few minutes or hours, although it may sometimes continue for a day or two. Occasionally, there may also be slight vaginal bleeding. Symptoms can usually be relieved with over-the-counter painkillers. In severe cases, oral contraceptives may be recommended to suppress ovulation and eliminate the pain.

PELVIC INFLAMMATORY DISEASE

Pelvic inflammatory disease (PID) is inflammation of the upper part of the female reproductive organs, including the ovaries, fallopian tubes, uterus, and cervix. This disorder is usually due to a sexually transmitted infection, however, it may also sometimes occur after a miscarriage, abortion, or childbirth. The insertion of an intrauterine contraceptive device (IUD, commonly known as a coil) may also sometimes lead to PID.

Sometimes there may be no symptoms. If symptoms do occur, they may include lower abdominal pain; fever; an abnormal vaginal discharge; heavy, painful, or prolonged periods; and pain during sex. PID that develops suddenly may cause severe pain, nausea, and vomiting, and it requires urgent medical treatment. PID may cause infertility or increase the risk of ectopic pregnancy (p.217).

Treatment is usually with antibiotics, and painkillers to relieve symptoms. Sex should be avoided until recovery is complete. Recent sexual partners should also be checked for infection.

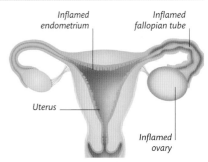

Inflamed endometrium

Inflamed fallopian tube

Uterus

Inflamed ovary

Possible areas of inflammation
Pelvic inflammatory disease can affect various parts of the reproductive tract, including the ovaries, fallopian tubes, and endometrium (lining of the uterus).

ENDOMETRIOSIS

In endometriosis, tissue that normally lines the uterus is found in other parts of the body, such as the ovaries, fallopian tubes, vagina, cervix, bladder, or intestines. The cause is not known. Sometimes there are no symptoms. If symptoms do occur, they may include heavy, painful periods, abdominal or lower back pain, and pain when having a bowel movement.

Treatment may include medication to relieve symptoms, such as painkillers; hormone therapy; or surgery to remove the tissue or part or all of the organs affected.

UTERINE CANCER

Most uterine cancers originate in the endometrium (lining of the uterus). The cause is unknown, but risk factors include obesity; taking oestrogen-only hormone replacement therapy; not having had children; and certain disorders, such as diabetes and polycystic ovary syndrome.

Symptoms in premenopausal women may include periods that are heavier than normal, and vaginal bleeding between periods or after sex. In postmenopausal women, the main symptom is vaginal bleeding (from spotting to heavier bleeding).

The main treatment is surgery to remove the uterus (hysterectomy). Radiotherapy or chemotherapy may also be used.

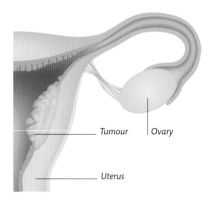

Uterine tumour
In most cases of uterine cancer, the endometrial cells, which line the inside of the uterus, develop into a tumour that grows into the uterus.

PROLAPSE OF UTERUS AND VAGINA

A prolapse of the uterus or vagina is when one or both of these organs is displaced due to weakening or stretching of their supporting tissues (which might happen during childbirth). In a uterine prolapse, the uterus moves down into the vagina. In the type of vaginal prolapse called a cystocele, the bladder presses inwards against the front vaginal wall. In the other main type of vaginal prolapse, a rectocele, the rectum bulges against the back vaginal wall.

Symptoms may include a feeling of fullness in the vagina; a bulge protruding into or out of the vagina; difficulty passing urine or faeces; frequent urination; and discomfort during sex. Mild cases often require only measures such as pelvic floor exercises to prevent the condition from worsening. Other treatments include a vaginal pessary to keep the prolapsed organ in place or, occasionally, surgery.

Types of prolapse
A uterine prolapse may be associated with a vaginal prolapse involving the rectum or bladder. Any of these types of prolapse can occur together or alone.

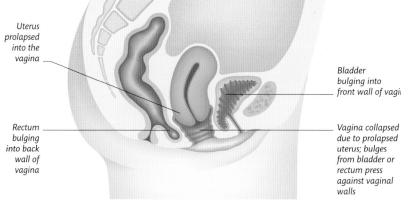

Uterus prolapsed into the vagina

Rectum bulging into back wall of vagina

Bladder bulging into front wall of vagina

Vagina collapsed due to prolapsed uterus; bulges from bladder or rectum press against vaginal walls

DYSMENORRHOEA

Dysmenorrhoea, commonly known as period pain, is cramp-like lower abdominal pain just before or during a menstrual period, sometimes accompanied by lower back pain. There are two types: primary and secondary. Primary dysmenorrhoea has no obvious cause. It typically begins two to three years after menstruation starts and often disappears by about the age of 30. Secondary dysmenorrhoea most commonly affects women aged 30 to 45 and is due to an underlying disorder, such as endometriosis or fibroids.

Primary dysmenorrhea can often be relieved by painkillers. In severe cases, hormonal treatments may relieve symptoms. Treatment of secondary dysmenorrhoea depends on the cause.

CERVICAL ECTROPION

Also sometimes called cervical ectopy or cervical erosion, cervical ectropion is a condition in which cells that are normally found in the inner lining of the cervix also appear on its outer surface. In many cases, there is no obvious cause for the condition, but it may sometimes be present from birth or may be associated with long-term use of oral contraceptives or pregnancy.

Most women have few or no symptoms, and the condition disappears by itself without treatment. However, some women experience vaginal bleeding at unexpected times or have a vaginal discharge. In such cases, medical advice should be sought. Treatments to destroy abnormally located tissue may be offered.

CERVICAL CANCER

Cervical cancer is most commonly associated with infection with certain strains of human papillomavirus (HPV), which is spread by intimate skin-to-skin sexual contact, including vaginal, anal, and oral sex. The cancer typically develops slowly and often causes no symptoms in its early stages. Later, symptoms may include vaginal bleeding, a watery, bloodstained, and foul-smelling vaginal discharge, and pelvic pain. Untreated, the cancer may spread to the uterus and other organs.

Cervical cancer can be detected early by cervical screening. Treatment is usually with surgery. Advanced cancer is usually treated with radiotherapy, chemotherapy, or both, although surgery may also be used. An HPV vaccine is available to protect against strains of HPV associated with cervical cancer.

VAGINISMUS

Vaginismus is spasm of the muscles around the entrance to the vagina, making sexual intercourse painful and difficult, or sometimes even impossible. The cause is usually psychological, although it may also sometimes result from certain physical disorders, such as inflammation of the vagina due to infection.

If vaginismus is due to a physical cause, treatment is of that cause. Vaginismus due to a psychological problem is treated with psychotherapy or sex therapy.

UTERINE POLYPS

Uterine polyp are painless growths attached to the inside of the uterus. They may occur singly or in groups, and typically produce bleeding between periods or after menopause, bleeding after intercourse, and heavy periods. Polyps are usually harmless, but they may occasionally become cancerous.

They may be removed by a minor surgical procedure called a hysteroscopy. Polyps may sometimes recur after treatment, and then further surgery may be required.

FIBROIDS

Fibroids are slow-growing, noncancerous growths in the uterus that consist of muscle and fibrous tissue. Their cause is unknown, although they are thought to be linked to the hormone oestrogen, because they develop mainly during the reproductive years and shrink after menopause.

Small fibroids often do not cause symptoms. However, fibroids may grow very large and cause symptoms such as painful, heavy periods, abdominal pain, lower back pain, and frequent urination. Untreated, they may lead to infertility or cause problems during childbirth.

Small, symptomless fibroids may not need treatment. Larger fibroids may be treated with medication to shrink them. If medication proves ineffective, surgery may be recommended.

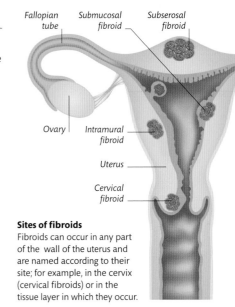

Fallopian tube   Submucosal fibroid   Subserosal fibroid

Ovary   Intramural fibroid

Uterus

Cervical fibroid

Sites of fibroids
Fibroids can occur in any part of the wall of the uterus and are named according to their site; for example, in the cervix (cervical fibroids) or in the tissue layer in which they occur.

VULVODYNIA

Vulvodynia is the medical term for persistent pain in the vulva that has no apparent cause. The pain may be a stinging, burning, or sore sensation, and may be triggered by touch. It may affect all or part of the vulva, and may sometimes spread to the inner thighs or buttocks. This condition is more common in young women.

There is no one treatment that works for everybody. Treatments that may be tried include avoiding scented soaps and personal hygiene products, and using an anaesthetic gel or vaginal lubricant. Over-the-counter painkillers are usually ineffective, although a doctor may prescribe other medications to relieve the symptoms or may advise other treatments, such as physiotherapy or cognitive-behavioural therapy.

Persistent vulval pain may be due to a condition other than vulvodynia, so medical advice should be sought.

BACTERIAL VAGINOSIS

In bacterial vaginosis, there is excessive growth of some of the types of bacteria that normally live in the vagina. The cause is not known, but bacterial vaginosis is more common in women who are sexually active. Bacterial vaginosis often causes no symptoms. However, some women have a greyish-white vaginal discharge with a fishy or musty smell and itching of the vagina or vulva. Seek medical advice if the condition persists or if it occurs during pregnancy.

Treatment with antibiotics usually clears up the problem, although it often recurs.

ATROPHIC VAGINITIS

In atrophic vaginitis, the lining of the vagina becomes thin, fragile, and prone to inflammation due to reduced levels of oestrogen hormones after the menopause. As a result, the vagina may be dry and itchy, and there may be pain, discomfort, or bleeding during sex. Other symptoms of atrophic vaginitis may include the need to pass urine more frequently, and painful urination. It is common after menopause.

The condition may be treated with hormone replacement therapy (HRT) or oestrogen-containing creams, pessaries, or vaginal tablets.

BREAST CANCER

Worldwide, breast cancer is the most common cancer in women. It can also occur in men but it is very rare. The causes of the cancer are not fully understood, but various risk factors have been identified. The principal one is age: the risk of developing it increases with age, and most cases occur in women over 50. Other risk factors include: a family history of the disease; having started periods at an early age or having a late menopause; not having had children or having them late in life; being overweight; moderate to heavy alcohol intake; using the combined oral contraceptive pill; and hormone replacement therapy. In some cases, breast cancer may be linked to inherited genes, including the genes known as BRCA1 and BRCA2.

The first noticeable symptom of breast cancer is often a painless lump. Other symptoms include a change in breast size or shape; a lump or swelling in the armpit; dimpling of the skin over the breast lump; a rash around the nipple; a change in the appearance of the nipple, such as becoming inverted (retracted inwards); and an unusual nipple discharge, which may contain blood. The cancer may spread to other parts of the body, such as the lungs.

Possible treatments include surgery, chemotherapy, and radiotherapy. In some cases, hormone therapy or biological therapy medication may also be used. Mammography screening to detect breast cancer early is available in some countries.

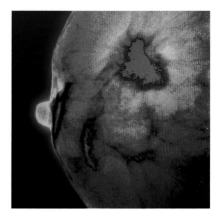

Breast tumour
A mammogram is an X-ray of the breast that is used to screen for breast cancer. This coloured mammogram shows a lump of dense green, which is a cancerous tumour.

BREAST PAIN

Known medically as mastalgia, breast pain is a common problem. It is often due to hormonal changes during the menstrual cycle (cyclical breast pain). This pain tends to affect both breasts, is most severe before periods, and may be aggravated by stress, caffeine, and smoking. Breast pain not related to menstruation (noncyclical breast pain) may have various causes, including muscle strain, a breast cyst (a fluid-filled sac in the breast), inflammation of the breast (mastitis), a breast abscess, or engorgement of the breast with milk after childbirth. Sore, tender breasts may also be an early sign of pregnancy. Only very rarely is breast pain by itself a sign of cancer.

Mild cyclical breast pain does not normally need treatment. Severe cases may be treated with medication. A supportive bra may also help to relieve the pain. For noncyclical breast pain, treatment depends on the cause.

FAT NECROSIS

Fat necrosis is a noncancerous lump that forms in an area of fatty breast tissue. The lump forms in response to damage to the tissue – for example, following an injury, breast surgery, a breast biopsy (taking a sample of tissue for analysis), or radiotherapy. The lump is usually firm and painless, and the surrounding area may look red or sometimes dimpled; occasionally, the nipple may be inverted (retracted inwards).

Fat necrosis often clears up by itself, although surgery may be advised if it persists or gets larger. A biopsy may also be advised to exclude the possibility of breast cancer.

MASTITIS

Mastitis is inflammation of the breast tissue. It is usually due to bacteria entering the nipple during breast-feeding, but it may also be caused by changes in levels of sex hormones – for example the changes that occur at the start of puberty.

Typical symptoms include breast pain, tenderness, and swelling in one or both breasts. Bacterial mastitis during breast-feeding may also cause redness and engorgement, and may result in a breast abscess (collection of pus).

Mastitis due to infection may be treated with medication. Mastitis caused by hormonal changes usually clears up in a few weeks without treatment

NIPPLE PROBLEMS

There are three main types of problems that may affect the nipple: retraction into the breast tissue (nipple inversion), disorders affecting the skin on or around the nipple, and discharge of fluid.

Inversion may occur during puberty if the breasts do not develop properly. This is usually harmless, although it may later make breast-feeding difficult. Inversion may also develop in older women due to ageing. Cracked nipples are common during breast-feeding and may lead to mastitis (inflammation of the breasts). Dry, flaky skin on or around the nipples is often due to eczema (p.222) but may occasionally be due to a type of cancer called Paget's disease of the nipple. Discharge from the nipple may occur naturally in early pregnancy, and a milky discharge may persist once breast-feeding is over. A discharge in a woman who is not pregnant or breast-feeding may be due to a hormone imbalance or, rarely, a cyst under the areola. A discharge containing pus indicates a breast abscess. A bloodstained discharge may be due to either a noncancerous breast disorder or a cancerous tumour.

Medical advice should be sought for any nipple problem to get an accurate diagnosis and, if necessary, appropriate treatment.

BREAST CYST

A breast cyst is a round, fluid-filled lump that forms within the milk-producing tissue of the breast. They are usually not cancerous. Breast cysts can occur in women of any age, but they most commonly affect women between the ages of 35 and 50, especially those approaching menopause. Postmenopausal women taking hormone replacement therapy can also develop breast cysts. Cysts may occur singly, but typically multiple cysts develop and both breasts may be affected. The cysts do not usually cause pain.

Medical advice should be obtained to check for the possibility of breast cancer. Treatment is usually by draining the cysts.

FIBROADENOMA

Fibroadenomas are noncancerous growths in the breast tissue. They occur most often in women under 30 and may develop in one or both breasts. Their cause is not fully understood but they are thought to be linked to sensitivity of breast tissue to female sex hormones. The lumps are painless, round, firm, and movable. They do not usually require treatment, although large lumps that cause discomfort may be removed by surgery. Medical advice should be sought to exclude the possibility of breast cancer.

FIBROCYSTIC BREAST DISEASE

Fibrocystic breast disease is the term used to describe the general lumpiness that is a normal feature of some women's breasts. It is also called fibroadenosis. Cyclical changes in hormone levels often lead to lumpiness, which is more obvious before a menstrual period.

Fibrocystic breast disease does not increase the risk of developing breast cancer and does not usually need treatment. However, a new solitary, discrete breast lump should be assessed by a doctor to rule out the possibility of breast cancer.

ECTOPIC PREGNANCY

In an ectopic pregnancy, a fertilized egg implants itself outside the uterus, usually in a fallopian tube. Symptoms include severe pain in the lower abdomen and vaginal bleeding. If the pregnancy continues, the tube may rupture, causing internal bleeding and shock; this may be life-threatening and requires emergency medical help. Most ectopic pregnancies are discovered early. In such cases, treatment may involve monitoring, as the egg may die naturally, or, if that does not occur, treatment is with medication to end the pregnancy or surgery to remove the fertilized egg.

PLACENTAL ABRUPTION

In a placental abruption, the placenta separates from the wall of the uterus before the baby is born. The cause is usually not known, but abruption is more common in women with long-term high blood pressure, those who have had an abruption previously, and women who have had several pregnancies. Smoking, high alcohol consumption, and drug abuse also increase the risk.

Symptoms usually occur suddenly and may include vaginal bleeding, cramps in the abdomen or severe, constant abdominal pain, backache, and reduced fetal movements. A small abruption is usually treated with bed rest. In severe cases, it may be necessary to induce labour or carry out an emergency caesarean operation. With treatment, the mother is not usually in danger, but there is a risk of the baby having health problems or dying.

MISCARRIAGE

Miscarriage is natural loss of a baby during the first 23 weeks of pregnancy. The majority of miscarriages occur in the first 12 weeks of pregnancy and may be mistaken for a late menstrual period. In many cases, there is no obvious cause. The main symptoms of a miscarriage are heavy bleeding and cramping and pain in the lower abdomen.

PREMATURE LABOUR

Also known as pre-term labour, premature labour is birth of a baby before the 37th week of pregnancy. If labour occurs very early, the baby may have health problems or even die. Because of the risks to the baby, who may be born before his or her internal organs (especially the lungs) are mature, medication may be used to delay labour long enough for corticosteroid drugs to be given to help the baby's lungs mature. After birth, premature infants are usually nursed in a special baby unit.

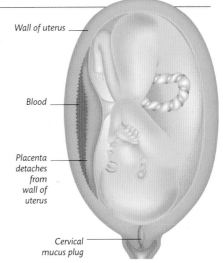

Wall of uterus

Blood

Placenta detaches from wall of uterus

Cervical mucus plug

Placental detachment
In most cases, the placenta becomes partly detached and blood either passes out through the vagina or collects between the placenta and wall of the uterus (as shown here). Rarely, the entire placenta may become detached.

After a miscarriage, an examination is carried out to check that all of the contents of the uterus have been expelled. If so, no further treatment is usually needed. If some contents remain, medication may be given to cause the remaining tissue to pass out or the tissue may be removed surgically.

CHLAMYDIA INFECTION

Chlamydia is a sexually transmitted infection caused by the bacterium *Chlamydia trachomatis*. The infection can also be transmitted from a mother to her baby during birth.

Chlamydia often does not cause symptoms. If symptoms do occur, they may include painful urination and abnormal discharge from the vagina, rectum, or penis. In women, there may also be abdominal pain and bleeding between periods or during sex. Men may also have pain and swelling in the testes.

Untreated, chlamydia may lead to pelvic inflammatory disease (p.213) in women; or to epididymo-orchitis (p.210) in men. In developing countries, chlamydia is a cause of the eye disease trachoma (p.177).

Treatment with antibiotics usually clears up the infection. Sexual partners should be tested for the infection and, if necessary, offered treatment.

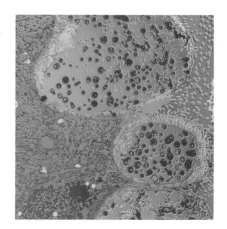

Tissue infected with Chlamydia
In this coloured micrograph of a tissue sample from the fallopian tube, numerous *Chlamydia trachomatis* bacteria can be seen as small red areas within the larger blue regions.

GONORRHOEA

Gonorrhoea is a sexually transmitted infection caused by the bacterium *Neisseria gonorrhoeae*. It can also be transmitted from a mother to her baby during birth.

Gonorrhoea often produces no symptoms. If symptoms do occur, in men they may include a discharge of pus from the penis and painful urination. In women, there may be a yellowish-green discharge of pus from the vagina, painful urination, and irregular vaginal bleeding. Gonorrhoea may lead to pelvic inflammatory disease (p.213) in women or inflammation of the prostate (p.211) or bladder in men. Treatment with antibiotics usually clears up the infection.

GENITAL WARTS

Genital warts are small, fleshy growths on or around the genitals or anal area caused by infection with certain strains of human papillomavirus (HPV). The virus can be spread by genital contact of any sort. It may also be spread from a mother to her baby during birth. The warts may take weeks or even years to develop after infection. Most eventually disappear, although this may take a long time. Infection is most likely to be passed on when warts are present.

Treatment may involve destroying the warts by freezing, heating, or applying medication, or surgery to remove them.

GENITAL HERPES

Genital herpes is caused by infection with the herpes simplex virus. The virus is spread by close contact with the skin or moist membranes. A mother may also transmit the virus to her baby during birth. Neonatal herpes may result in encephalitis (p.168), which can lead to permanent neurological damage or death of an infant.

Symptoms may include painful, fluid filled blisters, sores, or ulcers on or around the genitals, swollen lymph nodes in the groin, headache, fever, painful urination, and, in women, a vaginal discharge. Symptoms usually disappear within a few weeks but the virus remains dormant and may reactivate, causing another attack. The person is not highly infectious during the dormant period.

Attacks of genital herpes may be treated with antiviral medication. This reduces the severity of the symptoms but does not eliminate the virus.

NONGONOCOCCAL URETHRITIS

Nongonococcal urethritis (NGU) is inflammation of the urethra (the tube that carries urine out of the body) due to a cause other than gonorrhoea. It may be caused by sexually transmitted infections, including chlamydia, trichomoniasis, or genital warts, as well as other infections, such as thrush (p.238). Occasionally, NGU may occur without infection, for example, due to sensitivity to soap or spermicides.

NGU typically does not cause symptoms in women. In men, it may cause a discharge from the penis, painful urination, and soreness at the opening of the urethra.

NGU due to infection is usually treated with medication to kill the microorganism that caused it. Sexual partners should also be treated. Treatment of non-infective NGU depends on the cause.

TRICHOMONIASIS

Trichomoniasis is a sexually transmitted infection caused by the protozoan *Trichomonas vaginalis*. Rarely, the infection may also be passed from a pregnant woman to her baby.

Often, there are no symptoms. If symptoms do occur, in women they may include a profuse, yellowish-green, foul-smelling vaginal discharge, painful inflammation of the vagina (vaginitis, p.215), and painful urination; some women may also develop cystitis (inflammation of the bladder, p.209). In men, symptoms may include a white discharge from the penis and painful urination; some men also develop nongonococcal urethritis.

Treatment with antibiotics usually clears up the infection. Sexual partners should also be offered treatment to prevent reinfection.

ENDOCRINE AND METABOLIC DISORDERS

DIABETES
Hypoglycaemia

In diabetes, the level of glucose (sugar) in the blood is too high (hyperglycaemia) because the body produces too little or no insulin (a hormone that regulates blood glucose levels) or because body cells do not respond adequately to the hormone. The body takes in glucose from food, and body cells use it to produce energy. Insulin is produced by the pancreas and maintains a steady blood glucose level by helping body cells to absorb glucose.

There are two main types of diabetes: type 1 and type 2. Type 1 is an autoimmune disorder in which the immune system destroys insulin-producing cells in the pancreas. The underlying cause is unknown but it may be triggered by a viral infection and some people may also have a genetic predisposition to developing it. In type 2 diabetes, the pancreas produces too little insulin or the body cells are resistant to it. This type is strongly linked to obesity; genetics may also play a role. Another type of diabetes sometimes develops in pregnancy due to hormonal changes. Known as gestational diabetes, it usually disappears after delivery but may recur in future pregnancies; it also increases the risk of developing diabetes later in life.

Diabetes can be controlled with medication, dietary measures, or insulin injections. Untreated or poorly controlled diabetes may lead to various complications, including a potentially fatal metabolic disturbance called ketoacidosis, or disorders of the nerves, vision, heart and circulation, and kidneys. Another potential problem in people with diabetes is hypoglycaemia, an extremely low level of blood glucose that may lead to unconsciousness. It mainly affects people who take too much insulin, miss a meal, or exercise too hard. It can usually be corrected by eating something sugary. In severe cases, medication may be given.

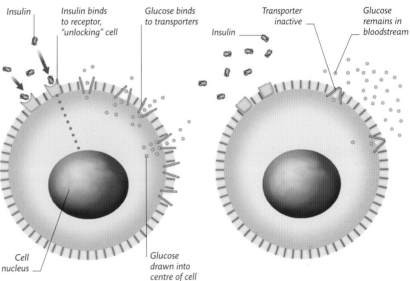

Glucose intake in a normal cell
Insulin binds with receptors on a cell to allow glucose to enter the cell. This triggers transporters within the cell membrane to draw glucose inside.

Insulin resistance in type 2 diabetes
In type 2 diabetes, the cell membrane receptors are resistant to insulin attachment and therefore take in too little glucose from the blood.

DIABETIC FOOT
Diabetic foot ulcer

Diabetic foot is the term used to describe a group of conditions that can affect the feet of people with diabetes due to nerve damage, poor blood supply, and infection. Diabetes may affect the blood vessels, leading to poor circulation in the legs and feet. It may also result in nerve damage (called diabetic neuropathy), which can lead to a gradual loss of sensation in the feet. The loss of sensation can mean that small injuries go unnoticed and this, together with poor circulation, may lead to a foot ulcer. Furthermore, an ulcer may become infected, and gangrene (death of tissue) may develop, which in severe cases may ultimately mean that the amputation of the foot becomes necessary.

The risk of developing diabetic foot can be minimized by ensuring that blood glucose levels are well controlled, and by paying particular attention to foot care: wearing well-fitting shoes, checking the feet every day, and ensuring that any wounds or infections are treated promptly.

DIABETIC NEUROPATHY

A potential complication of diabetes is nerve damage (neuropathy). The most common type affects sensory nerves, leading to tingling or numbness in the extremities, particularly the feet. The motor nerves (which help to control movement) may also be affected, leading to deformity (most often of the feet) or muscle wasting. In some cases, nerves that regulate automatic body functions may be affected, leading to symptoms such as low blood pressure on standing, diarrhoea, or erectile dysfunction.

DIABETIC RETINOPATHY

In diabetic retinopathy, the small blood vessels in the retina (the light-sensitive layer of the eye) become damaged as a result of high blood glucose (sugar) levels. Initially, the vessels develop bulges and leak small amounts of fluid and blood. Later, more severe bleeding occurs, and scar tissue and fragile new blood vessels develop on the retina. The condition usually affects both eyes. Initially, it may not affect vision, but it can progress quickly and lead to loss of vision. The longer a person has had diabetes and the less well it is controlled, the greater the risk of developing the condition. Treatment can usually halt progress of the condition, but not restore any vision already lost.

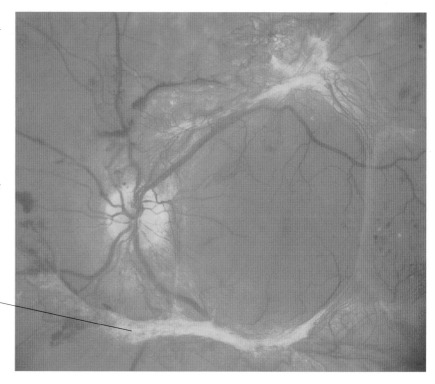

Scar tissue

Retinal damage
In diabetes, the retina can be damaged by the growth of fragile, new blood vessels, scarring, and bleeding.

HYPERTHYROIDISM

In hyperthyroidism, the thyroid gland overproduces thyroid hormones. These hormones regulate the body's metabolism (the chemical reactions that keep the body functioning), and excessive amounts cause body processes to speed up. Hyperthyroidism is most commonly caused by Graves' disease, an autoimmune disorder in which the immune system attacks the thyroid, stimulating it to produce more hormones. Other causes include benign tumours called thyroid nodules and the side effects of certain medications.

Symptoms tend to develop slowly and include weight loss, rapid heartbeat, restlessness, anxiety, insomnia, twitching or trembling, increased sweating, and, in severe cases, enlargement of the thyroid (goitre). In Graves' disease, the eyes may also bulge out. Untreated, hyperthyroidism may lead to complications such as heart problems and osteoporosis (thinning of

the bones, p.154). Treatment may be with medication, radioactive iodine to destroy excess thyroid tissue, or surgery to remove part of the thyroid gland.

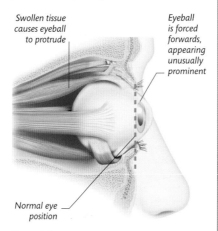

Swollen tissue causes eyeball to protrude

Eyeball is forced forwards, appearing unusually prominent

Normal eye position

Graves' disease
The autoimmune reaction in Graves' disease causes inflammation and abnormal deposits in the muscles and tissue behind the eyes, causing the eyes to protrude and affecting their function.

HYPOTHYROIDISM

In hypothyroidism, the thyroid gland does not produce enough thyroid hormones. These hormones regulate metabolism (chemical reactions that keep the body functioning) and insufficient amounts cause body processes to slow down. This produces a range of symptoms, including fatigue, weight gain, dry skin, mental slowness, and sometimes enlargement of the thyroid (goitre). Babies with hypothyriodism may have feeding difficulties and jaundice (yellowing of the skin and whites of the eyes, p.201).

Hypothyroidism is most common in adults and is usually due to an autoimmune disorder in which the immune system attacks thyroid tissue, although it may also be caused by the removal of thyroid tissue to treat hyperthyroidism (overactivity of the thyroid, see left). Rarely, babies are born with an underactive thyroid. Treatment is with replacement thyroid hormone.

HYPERCHOLESTEROLAEMIA

In this condition, the blood contains high levels of cholesterol, which does not usually cause symptoms itself but increases the risk of heart and circulation disorders, such as heart attack and stroke. Many people have a high cholesterol level, due to an unhealthy lifestyle, but some have an inherited disorder called familial hypercholesterolaemia that is associated with extremely high cholesterol levels. Treatment is with lifestyle measures and medication to reduce blood cholesterol.

GOITRE

Goitre is a condition in which the thyroid gland becomes enlarged. The thyroid may enlarge naturally at certain times, such as during puberty and pregnancy. Abnormal enlargement may be due to a thyroid disorder, such as hyperthyroidism (overactivity of the thyroid gland), hypothyroidism (underactivity of the thyroid gland), or a thyroid tumour; as a side effect of certain medications; or from lack of iodine (needed for proper thyroid function) in the diet.

Most goitres do not cause symptoms, but a large one may make swallowing or breathing difficult. Treatment may involve medication, radioactive iodine to shrink the thyroid, iodine supplements, or sometimes surgery.

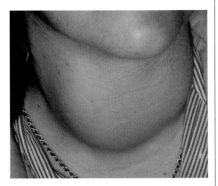

Enlarged thyroid gland
This swelling in the neck is due to enlargement of the thyroid (goitre). Most goitres do not cause pain or other symptoms.

ADDISON'S DISEASE

In this disorder, the adrenal glands do not produce enough corticosteroid hormones, which help the body respond to stress, help regulate metabolism (chemical reactions that keep the body functioning), control blood pressure, and balance the body's salt and water levels. Addison's disease is usually caused by an autoimmune reaction in which the immune system attacks the adrenal glands. Other causes include infections such as tuberculosis (TB) or HIV, certain medications, and suddenly stopping corticosteroid treatment.

Symptoms of Addison's disease include fatigue, muscle weakness, weight loss, depression, and abnormal skin

Adrenal gland structure
The adrenal glands sit on the kidneys. The cortex produces corticosteroid and other hormones; the medulla produces adrenaline and noradrenaline.

colouring. In addition, a sudden illness, injury, or other stress may cause an Addisonian crisis, in which there is a potentially fatal circulatory collapse that requires urgent medical attention.

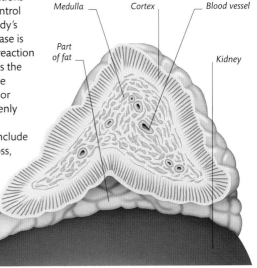

Medulla Cortex Blood vessel
Part of fat Kidney

CUSHING'S SYNDROME

In Cushing's syndrome, the body's adrenal glands produce too much cortisol. This is a corticosteroid that regulates the body's use of fats, helps the body cope with stress, and reduces inflammation. The condition is often caused by prolonged treatment with corticosteroid medication. Other causes include a tumour of the adrenal gland, or a pituitary tumour that causes overproduction of a pituitary hormone that stimulates the adrenal glands. Symptoms of Cushing's syndrome include weight gain, excess fat deposits (especially on the face and shoulders), reddish-purple stretch marks on the body or limbs, excessive hair growth, depression, weakness, reduced sex drive, and irregular or absent menstrual periods. If it remains untreated, osteoporosis (thinning of the bones), high blood pressure, diabetes, and kidney stones may develop. Treatment depends on the underlying cause.

PARATHYROID DISORDERS

The four parathyroid glands produce a hormone that regulates levels of calcium in the blood. Underactivity of the glands (hypoparathyroidism) causes low blood calcium, producing symptoms such as tingling, muscle spasms, and sometimes seizures (fits). Hypoparathyroidism may be due to accidental damage during surgery or the immune system mistakenly attacking parathyroid tissue. Treatment is with calcium and vitamin D supplements. Overactivity of the parathyroids (hyperparathyroidism) causes high blood calcium. Symptoms may include depression, tiredness, excessive urination, weakness, confusion and, in severe cases, unconsciousness. The high calcium levels may also cause kidney stones. Hyperparathyroidism may be caused by a benign tumour in one of the glands or may be due to another disorder, such as kidney disease. Treatment is with surgery or medication, or of the underlying cause.

SKIN, HAIR, AND NAIL DISORDERS

PSORIASIS

Psoriasis is a long-term disorder in which skin cells reproduce too rapidly, causing red, thickened patches. Psoriasis tends to recur in attacks, which may be triggered by factors such as infection, injury, stress, or certain medications. In the most common type, called plaque psoriasis, red, flaky patches

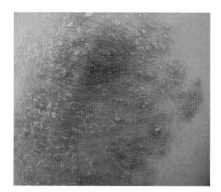

(plaques) covered in silver scales appear, usually on the elbows, knees, and scalp, which are itchy and sore. In guttate psoriasis, small, scaly, red patches occur all over the body. In flexural psoriasis, large, smooth, red patches develop in skin folds. Psoriasis may also affect the nails, which become pitted, discoloured, and loose. Psoriasis may also cause psoriatic arthritis (p.157).

Psoriasis can often be improved by topical treatments with corticosteroids, emollients, vitamin D analogues (forms of vitamin D), coal-tar preparations, or dithranol preparations. Ultraviolet light therapy may also help. If such treatments are ineffective, tablets or injected medication may be used.

Psoriasis on the elbow
Psoriasis can occur on skin anywhere on the body, typically causing thickened red patches that may be covered by silvery scales. Common sites are the elbow (as shown here), knee, and scalp.

LICHEN PLANUS
Oral lichen planus

Lichen planus is an itchy rash of small pink or purple spots that most commonly affects the arms, legs, lower back, or scalp. It may also affect the nails or the inside of the mouth (oral lichen planus).

If lichen planus affects the nails, they typically become ridged and loose. Oral lichen planus produces a lacy network of white spots on the inside of the cheeks.

Treatment of skin lichen planus may include over-the-counter antihistamines to relieve itching. A doctor may also prescribe topical corticosteroids or, if the scalp or nails are affected, corticosteroid tablets. Oral lichen planus may be treated with antiseptic or corticosteroid mouthwashes or corticosteroid tablets.

ECZEMA AND DERMATITIS
Contact dermatitis | Pompholyx (dyshidrotic eczema) | Seborrhoeic dermatitis

Both eczema and dermatitis are terms that refer to an inflammation of the skin, which causes patches of red, dry, itchy, and sometimes blistered skin.

Atopic eczema is the most common type of eczema and often appears in infancy. The cause is unknown, but people with an inherited tendency to allergies are more susceptible. The main symptom of atopic eczema is an intensely itchy rash, which often becomes scaly.

Contact dermatitis is due to direct contact with an irritant substance or an allergen. It can occur at any age and typically causes patches of red, itchy, flaky skin that may develop into raw patches or oozing blisters. Contact dermatitis usually affects

only the area of skin that has been in direct contact with the irritant or allergen.

Seborrhoeic dermatitis can occur at any age and causes a red, scaly, itchy rash on the face, scalp, chest, or back. The cause is unknown, but the rash often develops during times of stress and is sometimes associated with excessive growth of a yeast that is normally present on the skin.

Pompholyx, also called dyshidrotic eczema, causes small, itchy blisters on areas where the skin is thickest, such as the fingers, palms, and soles. The cause of pompholyx is unknown.

Symptoms of eczema may be relieved by measures such as avoiding irritant substances and known allergens; using hypoallergenic moisturizers on the skin; and covering the affected area with a dressing to prevent scratching. A doctor may also recommend more specific treatment, depending on the type and severity of the eczema.

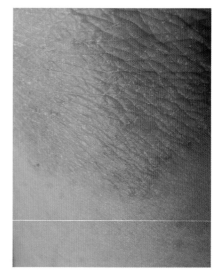

Contact dermatitis
Contact with an irritant substance can cause a localized area of red, itchy skin, as shown here. Common irritants include detergents, nickel, latex, certain plants, and cosmetics.

PITYRIASIS ROSEA

Pityriasis rosea is a mild skin condition in which a rash of scaly-edged pink spots or patches appears on the body and upper arms. It mainly affects children and young adults. The cause of pityriasis rosea is unknown.

The first sign of this condition is a large, round spot, called a herald patch, on the body. The rash typically appears a week later and may cause itching. The rash usually lasts for four to eight weeks and clears up without treatment, although moisturizers, or prescribed topical corticosteroids or antihistamines may relieve symptoms.

URTICARIA

Also called hives or nettle rash, urticaria is an itchy, raised rash that may affect the whole body or just a small area of skin. It usually lasts for only a few hours (acute urticaria) but may persist for months (chronic urticaria). Urticaria is usually due to an allergic reaction; sometimes it may be triggered by an infection, stress, or exposure to heat or cold.

Acute urticaria usually clears up without treatment. Chronic urticaria may be treated with antihistamines to relieve itching. In severe cases, corticosteroid tablets may be prescribed. Avoiding known triggers can help to prevent recurrences.

PHOTOSENSITIVITY

Photosensitivity is an abnormal reaction of the skin to any ultraviolet light. Exposed areas typically develop a red, often painful rash, small, itchy blisters, and scaly skin. It may be present at birth but more commonly develops later in life, sometimes as a result of using certain medications or cosmetics. It may also be a feature of systemic lupus erythematosus (p.189).

Treatment includes avoiding ultraviolet light, using sunblocks and covering the skin when outdoors, and avoiding substances that may cause photosensitivity. A doctor may also prescribe corticosteroids or antihistamines to relieve symptoms.

ACNE VULGARIS

In acne, the sebaceous glands become blocked and inflamed, leading to spots on the face, back, and chest. Acne most commonly affects teenagers but can occur at any age. Teenage acne is thought to be due to changes in sex-hormone levels that occur around puberty. In adults, acne mainly affects women and tends to occur just before menstrual periods or during pregnancy. Certain medications may also cause acne.

Various types of spot may develop, including blackheads, whiteheads, papules (small red lumps), and pustules (small, pus-filled lumps). In severe cases, there may be nodules (large, hard lumps) and cysts (large, pus-filled lumps that look like boils). These may scar when they rupture.

Mild acne can often be treated with lotions containing benzoyl peroxide. For more severe cases, prescribed medications may be used, including antibiotics, azelaic acid, and retinoids. In women, hormone medication therapy or the combined contraceptive pill may also be effective. It may take several months before there is any visible improvement.

Bacteria build up

Plug blocking sebaceous gland

Sebaceous gland

Excess sebum

Hair follicle

Inflamed hair follicle
Blockage of a sebaceous gland leads to a build-up of an oily substance (sebum). Bacteria that normally live harmlessly on the skin multiply in the sebum, causing inflammation and leading to spots.

ROSACEA

Rosacea is a long-term skin condition that primarily affects the face of fair-skinned people, causing episodes of flushing. Various things may trigger an episode, including sunlight, caffeine, alcohol, spicy foods, and stress. Eventually, there may be persistent facial redness, visible blood vessels in the skin (telangiectasia, p.224), spots and pustules, thickening of the skin, and the nose may become bulbous (rhinophyma).

Treatment includes avoiding triggers, and antibiotics or other prescribed medications to clear up severe spots. Telangiectasia may be treated with laser therapy.

RHINOPHYMA

Rhinophyma is a bulbous deformity and redness of the nose that occurs almost exclusively in older men. It is a complication of severe rosacea. In rhinophyma, the tissue of the nose thickens, small blood vessels in the nose enlarge and become prominent, and the sebaceous glands become overactive, making the nose excessively greasy.

Various medications used for rosacea may be tried for rhinophyma, but they are rarely effective and in most cases surgery to remove the thickened skin and reshape the nose is the recommended treatment.

LUPUS PERNIO

In lupus pernio, purple swellings resembling chilblains develop on the ears, nose, or cheeks. However, unlike chilblains, the swellings do not itch or cause pain.

Lupus pernio is a characteristic feature of sarcoidosis, a disorder in which areas of inflamed tissue (called granulomas) develop in one or more parts of the body, most often the lungs, lymph nodes, skin, and eyes. The cause of sarcoidosis is unknown, but it is thought to be an exaggerated response of the immune system, possibly to an infection.

Lupus pernio is usually treated with corticosteroids, which usually improve appearance, although the facial swellings may not disappear completely.

CHLOASMA

Also known as melasma, chloasma is a skin condition is which dark patches appear on the face, mainly on the forehead, nose, and cheeks. Exposure to sunlight makes the condition worse. The cause of chloasma is unknown, but it sometimes develops during pregnancy or is associated with the menopause or use of oral contraceptives.

The patches usually fade by themselves within a few months. Avoiding triggers, such as sunlight, can help. The patches can be hidden with special camouflage creams. In severe cases, a doctor may recommend a skin-lightening cream, laser treatment, or chemical peels to remove the outer layer of skin.

VITILIGO

In vitiligo, patches of skin lose their colour. This occurs most commonly on the face, hands, armpits, and groin. It is thought to be an autoimmune disorder in which the immune system attacks skin cells that make the pigment melanin. The condition usually develops in early adulthood.

There is no cure for vitiligo, but a combination of light therapy and medication may help to repigment the areas. Camouflage cosmetics can be used to disguise smaller areas. Other possible treatments include topical corticosteroids, topical immunomodulators (drugs that act on the immune system), and the vitamin D derivative calipotriol. Despite treatment, the patches often continue to enlarge slowly.

HAEMANGIOMA

A haemangioma is a birthmark caused by abnormal blood vessels under the skin. Types of haemangioma include stork marks (small, flat, pink or red patches); strawberry marks (raised, bright red marks); and port-wine stains (flat, red or purple patches). Stork marks and strawberry marks usually disappear by themselves. Port-wine stains are usually permanent.

Haemangiomas do not usually need any treatment. However, one that is very large, bleeds persistently, is near the eye and causing vision problems, or is unsightly may be treated with medication to shrink it or with surgery (such as laser treatment) to remove it.

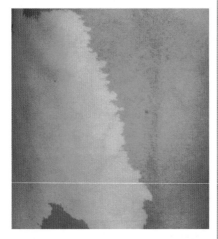

Vitiligo
In vitiligo, pale skin patches develop due to loss of the pigment melanin. Usually, the patches enlarge slowly despite treatment, although some people regain their natural skin colour spontaneously.

TELANGIECTASIA

In telangiectasia, the small blood vessels just beneath the skin become enlarged, causing redness and a "broken veins" appearance. It most commonly occurs on the nose and cheeks. Telangiectasia may be due to a skin disorder, such as rosacea (p.223), overexposure to the sun, or long-term excessive alcohol consumption. Often, there is no obvious cause.

Telangiectasia is not a cause for concern, but if it is unsightly the veins may be removed by laser treatment.

LIVEDO RETICULARIS

Livedo reticularis is a net-like, purple or blue mottling of the skin. It most commonly occurs on the lower legs and is due to enlargement of the blood vessels under the skin. The condition is more common in people with vasculitis (inflammation of the blood vessels), antiphospholipid syndrome (a disorder in which blood clots more readily than normal), and in those who have an extreme sensitivity to cold.

Livedo reticularis itself is harmless and does not need treatment, although any associated disorder may need medical attention.

INTERTRIGO

Intertrigo is inflammation of the skin due to two surfaces rubbing together. It often affects skin under the breasts, between the thighs, in the armpits, or between the buttocks. It is more common in people who are overweight. The affected skin is red and moist, may have an unpleasant odour, is often accompanied by a fungal infection, and may develop scales or blisters. Sweating makes symptoms worse.

Treatment consists of losing weight, if necessary, and keeping the affected area clean and dry. Topical antifungal and corticosteroid medication may be used to treat any infection and reduce inflammation.

BRUISE

A bruise is a discoloured area under the skin that is caused by bleeding from small blood vessels in the underlying tissues. Over a few days, the bruise gradually changes colour as the haemoglobin pigment in the leaked blood breaks down, and eventually the bruise fades completely. Applying an ice-pack can help to limit bleeding.

If a bruise does not disappear by itself within about two weeks or if bruising occurs unusually easily or for no obvious reason, a doctor should be consulted, because unusual bruising may be a sign of a blood clotting problem.

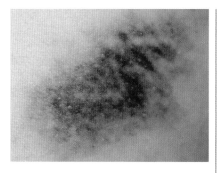

Bruise
Bruises change colour due to haemoglobin from red blood cells being broken down to form chemicals of various colours, including green, yellow, and light brown. The discolouration usually fades in about a week or two.

CHILBLAINS

Also called pernio, chilblains are itchy, painful swellings on the fingers or toes that occur as a result of the excessive narrowing of small blood vessels under the skin in cold weather. The swellings are typically painful when exposed to cold but become intensely itchy when the skin warms again.

Chilblains usually clear up by themselves within a few weeks but may recur. They can usually be prevented by keeping warm and exercising to encourage good blood flow to the hands and feet. Severe, recurrent chilblains may be treated with medication to widen blood vessels.

BLISTERS
Callus

Blisters are fluid-filled swellings in the skin. They may be a symptom of a wide variety of disorders, in which case they are usually accompanied by other symptoms.

Blisters by themselves are commonly due to friction from poorly fitting footwear, or from a burn. Regular or prolonged friction or pressure may also cause a patch of thickened skin, called a callus. A blister caused by minor damage usually heals by itself. It should be left intact and may be protected with a dry, sterile dressing. If a blister fills with pus or there is spreading redness around it, it may be infected and a doctor should be consulted. A serious burn also requires medical attention.

PRESSURE SORE

Also known as a bedsore or decubitus ulcer, a pressure sore is an ulcer that develops in pressure spots on the skin of people whose mobility is impaired. Pressure sores start as red, painful areas that become purple before the skin breaks down. Common sites for pressure sores are the hips, base of the spine, buttocks, shoulders, heels, and ankles.

Pressure sores may be treated with dressings and medication to speed up healing. In some cases, antibiotics and plastic surgery may be needed.

Pressure sores can usually be prevented by good nursing care, including regularly changing the person's position and protecting vulnerable areas with special cushions and mattresses.

VENOUS ULCER

A venous ulcer is a painful open sore, usually on the lower leg or ankle. Venous ulcers usually develop as a result of poor circulation and are common in people with varicose veins (p.185). They may occur spontaneously or after a minor injury. Venous ulcers typically appear as a shallow, pink area of broken skin; sometimes the skin surrounding the ulcer is swollen too.

Treatment usually involves cleaning and dressing the ulcer regularly and using compression bandages or support stockings to improve circulation. If the ulcer has become infected, antibiotics may be prescribed. With treatment, most ulcers heal within a few months.

SEBACEOUS CYST

Also called skin cyst or an epidermoid cyst, a sebaceous cyst is a smooth lump that forms under the skin due to inflammation of a hair follicle. The cyst contains a yellow, cheesy material composed of dead skin cells and sebum. Sebaceous cysts most commonly occur on the scalp, face, neck, body, and genitals. Although harmless, the cysts occasionally become very large and unsightly. If a cyst becomes infected, it may become painful and may eventually burst.

A cyst that is not causing problems does not need treatment. A large, painful, or infected cyst may be surgically removed. Antibiotics may also be prescribed for an infected cyst.

Sebaceous cyst on the neck
Sebaceous cysts are usually round and dome-shaped. They are harmless and can safely be left untreated, although they can be removed if they are troublesome or become infected. However, removal may leave a scar.

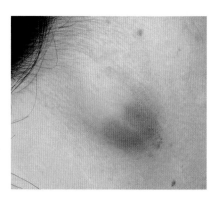

SKIN TAG

A skin tag is a small, soft, painless, noncancerous growth attached to the skin by a stalk. Tags usually occur spontaneously and may grow on any part of the body; common sites are the neck, armpits, around the groin, and under the breasts. Tags usually cause no problems, although they may bleed or become sore if rubbed by clothing. They are harmless and do not need treatment, although troublesome ones can be removed by a doctor by burning, freezing, or cutting them off.

LIPOMA

A lipoma is a noncancerous lump under the skin caused by excessive growth of fat cells. Lipomas may develop anywhere on the body but most commonly occur on the shoulders, neck, chest, back, buttocks, or thighs. They feel soft, smooth, and rubbery. When pressed, they may move about under the skin. Lipomas grow very slowly, are painless, and do not usually cause any problems. They are harmless and do not need treatment, although they can be surgically removed for cosmetic reasons.

SYRINGOMA

A syringoma is a noncancerous tumour of the sweat ducts. Syringomas are most commonly found in clusters on the eyelids, but they may also occur elsewhere on the face, or on the scalp, neck, chest, abdomen, armpits, or groin. They are yellow or skin-coloured, small, firm, rounded lumps, and rarely cause any other symptoms, although occasionally they may be itchy. They are harmless and do not need treatment. They may be removed by heat or laser treatment, but this can leave scars.

SOLAR KERATOSIS

Also known an actinic keratosis, a solar keratosis is a scaly skin growth caused by prolonged exposure to sunlight. The growths typically appear on the face, ears, hands, and bald parts of the scalp. They have a rough texture and may be sore or itchy. Sometimes, a solar keratosis may develop into squamous cell carcinoma, a type of skin cancer.

Some keratoses may simply need to be monitored and any changes should be checked by a doctor. However, if they are troublesome or may become cancerous, they may be removed by freezing or scraping them off; by using a special cream or gel; or by using a type of light treatment called photodynamic therapy.

BASAL CELL CARCINOMA

Basal cell carcinoma (BCC) is a type of skin cancer that arises from the basal (innermost) layer of skin. It is usually caused by excessive exposure to ultraviolet light (in sunlight, for example) and most commonly develops on the face. Typically, the growth appears as a small, painless lump with a smooth surface and a pearl-like border. The lump grows slowly and may become ulcerated. Untreated, it may destroy surrounding tissue, but it rarely spreads to other parts of the body.

Treatment is by surgical removal, freezing, radiotherapy, anticancer creams, or light treatment. With treatment, most people are cured, although occasionally the cancer may recur.

SQUAMOUS CELL CARCINOMA

Squamous cell carcinoma (SCC) is a type of skin cancer that arises from the outer skin layer. It may be caused by prolonged exposure to ultraviolet light (in sunlight, for example), chemical carcinogens, or develop from solar keratoses. SCC commonly affects exposed areas of skin but may also affect the genitals. It starts as an area of thickened skin and enlarges into a hard, painless lump resembling a wart. Untreated, SCC may spread and be fatal.

If detected early, SCC can often be treated with surgery to remove the cancer, or sometimes with radiotherapy. In advanced cases, chemotherapy may also be necessary. With early treatment, most people are cured.

MALIGNANT MELANOMA

Malignant melanoma is a type of skin cancer that arises from pigmented skin cells called melanocytes. It is caused by excessive exposure to ultraviolet light (for example, in sunlight). Sunburn, in particular, significantly increases the risk.

The most common symptom is the appearance of a new mole or a change in an existing one. Some melanomas appear as fast-growing dark lumps; others as irregular, flat, pigmented patches. Rarely, a melanoma has little or no colour (known as amelanotic melanoma). Untreated, melanoma can spread rapidly.

Treatment depends on the site of the melanoma and how far it has spread. The main treatment is surgery to remove the cancer, and maybe the surrounding lymph nodes. Additional treatments may include radiotherapy, chemotherapy, and sometimes other medications to destroy cancer cells or inhibit their growth. With early treatment, most cases can be cured. Melanomas that have spread widely are often fatal.

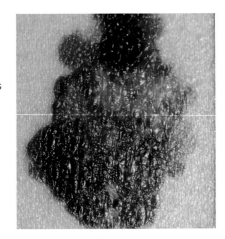

Melanoma
Most melanomas have an irregular edge and are unevenly coloured. Some take the form of flat patches (as here), whereas others are raised and lumpy.

MOLES

Moles are small, coloured skin growths caused by overproduction of pigmented skin cells called melanocytes. They are typically flat or raised, may vary in colour from light to dark brown, may be rough or smooth, and may be hairless or hairy. Less commonly, a mole may be a bluish-black colour, may be surrounded by a ring of paler skin, or may be larger than normal and unevenly coloured.

Moles may be present at birth, but most appear later; and almost all adults have several moles. Most moles are noncancerous, but occasionally they may develop into malignant melanoma. Warning signs in an existing mole include a change in shape or size; a change in colour or uneven colouring; crustiness; itching; inflammation; ulceration; bleeding; and

an irregular edge. The sudden appearance of a new mole may also indicate melanoma. Any such changes should be reported to a doctor promptly.

Most moles are harmless and do not need treatment, although they can be surgically removed for cosmetic reasons.

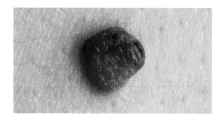

Mole
Overproduction and build-up of melanoctyes leads to a (sometimes raised) pigmented area. As the cells are not cancerous, they do not invade underlying tissue.

BOILS

A boil is an inflamed, painful, pus-filled swelling under the skin. It is caused by a bacterial infection of a hair follicle. Clusters of boils may interconnect to form a carbuncle. Common sites of boils are moist areas of skin, such as the groin, or areas where friction occurs, such as the neck. Recurrent boils may occur in people with diabetes (p.219) or those whose resistance to infection is lowered.

Boils often clear up without treatment. They may burst, release pus, and then heal, or may just gradually disappear. A large, persistent, or very painful boil may need to be drained by a doctor. Antibiotics may also be prescribed.

LICHEN SCLEROSUS

Lichen sclerosus is a long-term condition that affects skin in the genital or anal area. In females, it usually affects the vulva and skin around the anus. The affected skin develops small white patches that enlarge and may become cracked and sore. The patches are often itchy. Eventually, the vulva may scar and shrink.

In males, sore, white, sometimes itchy patches develop on the tip of the penis, and skin there becomes firm and white. There may also be difficulty retracting the foreskin.

Treatment for lichen sclerosus is with topical corticosteroids, although surgery to widen the vaginal opening or remove the foreskin may be recommended in severe cases.

KELOID

A keloid is a firm, itchy, irregularly shaped overgrowth of scar tissue that forms on the surface of a wound. Keloids are the result of overproduction of the skin protein collagen during the healing process. They are more common in dark-skinned people, and susceptibility to them may run in families. They usually develop after skin damage – even minor damage from, say, a small cut may cause a keloid – but they can also sometimes occur without any apparent cause.

Keloids are harmless and do not require treatment. Possible treatments include corticosteroids, silicone preparations, pressure dressings, freezing, or certain chemotherapy or wart medications. However, treatment is not always successful.

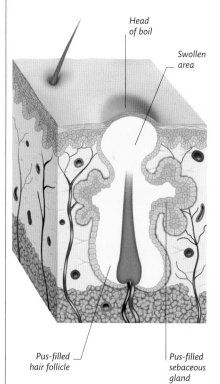

Head of boil

Swollen area

Pus-filled hair follicle

Pus-filled sebaceous gland

Boil
Often caused by infection with *Staphylococcus* bacteria, a boil is a collection of pus in a hair follicle and sometimes also in the associated sebaceous gland. Most boils burst and heal by themselves within about two weeks.

PUSTULE

A pustule is a small, pus-filled spot. Pustules usually appear as pale or red lumps with a white centre. The skin around them may be inflamed and sometimes itchy or painful. Pustules are a feature of a large number of conditions, probably

the most common of which is acne vulgaris (p.223), although sometimes an isolated pustule appears without any apparent cause and then disappears spontaneously.

A sudden outbreak of a large number of pustules may indicate an underlying disorder and should be seen by a doctor.

SEBORRHOEIC KERATOSIS

Also called seborrhoeic warts, seborrhoeic keratoses are harmless, wart-like growths that most commonly occur on the trunk but may also affect the head, neck, forearms, or backs of the hands. Typically, they appear as crusty or greasy spots, usually brown or black in colour. They are painless but may be itchy.

The growths do not need treatment, although a doctor should be consulted to check that the growth is not a type of skin cancer. If a seborrhoeic keratosis is troublesome, it may be removed by scraping it off or by freezing.

MOLLUSCUM CONTAGIOSUM

Molluscum contagiosum is a viral infection that produces shiny, pearly white or flesh coloured pimples on the skin. The pimples are dome-shaped and have a depression in their centre. They may be itchy and may spread to form small clusters. Molluscum contagiosum is harmless but contagious; it can be spread by close skin contact, sexual intercourse, or contact with contaminated objects.

Children are not usually treated because treatment may be painful and leave scars. It usually clears up by itself within about 12 months. In adults, the pimples may be removed for cosmetic reasons, by scraping them off, freezing or burning, laser therapy, or by using various topical medications.

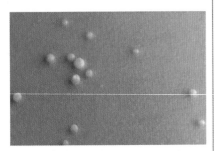

Molluscum contagiosum
Most common in children, molluscum contagiosum produces small, raised pimples on the skin. The condition is contagious until all of the pimples have disappeared.

IMPETIGO

Impetigo is a bacterial skin infection, common in children, that usually occurs around the chin, mouth, and nose. The condition is highly contagious and is spread by direct physical contact. It causes reddening of the skin, followed by the appearance of tiny, fluid-filled blisters. The blisters then burst, leaving weeping areas that dry to give yellowish crusts. There may also be fever and swelling of the lymph nodes in the neck or face.

Impetigo is treated with topical or oral antibiotics. With treatment, the infection usually clears up in a few days. To prevent the spread of the infection, bed and bath linen should not be shared, and those who are infected should stay at home.

ERYSIPELAS

Erysipelas is a bacterial infection of the upper layers of the skin, usually as a result of bacteria entering through a break in the skin – for example, from a cut or ulcer or from a skin condition such as athlete's foot or eczema (p.222).

The condition typically occurs on the face or legs, although any area of skin may be affected. The infected area of skin becomes warm, swollen, and inflamed, and blisters may form. There may also be fever, tiredness, and swelling of nearby lymph nodes.

Erysipelas is treated with antibiotics, which usually clears up the infection within about two weeks. Painkillers, such as paracetamol, may help to relieve symptoms.

SKIN ABSCESS

A skin abscess is a collection of pus under the skin, which is usually caused by a bacterial infection. A skin abscess typically appears as a smooth, firm swelling that may be tender or painful. The swelling and the immediately surrounding area may be warm and inflamed, and there may be a visible accumulation of pus under the swelling. In some cases, there may also be a fever and chills.

A small skin abscess may not require treatment and will disappear by itself. A large or persistent skin abscess will probably need to be drained by a doctor, who may also prescribe antibiotics to clear up the infection.

ANGULAR STOMATITIS

Also called angular cheilitis, angular stomatitis is the inflammation of the corners of the mouth, usually due to a bacterial or fungal infection. It typically causes redness, soreness, cracking, crusting, and sometimes bleeding at the corners of the mouth. The condition is most likely to develop in those with poorly fitting dentures; people whose diet is low in vitamin B12, folic acid, or iron; those with certain long-term bowel problems; and people who salivate excessively.

Angular stomatitis is treated with antifungal or antibiotic medication and, if necessary, the treatment of any associated condition, such as a dietary deficiency. Good oral hygiene can help to prevent a recurrence.

CELLULITIS

Cellulitis is a bacterial infection of the deeper layers of the skin and the underlying tissue. It usually affects the lower legs but may occur anywhere, including the face around the eyes. It is most commonly caused by bacteria entering the skin through a wound.

Symptoms usually appear within a few hours of infection and include redness, swelling, heat, and pain in the affected area, and sometimes fever and chills. Untreated, the infection may spread rapidly through the body and may be life-threatening.

Treatment is with antibiotics. In severe cases, these may need to be given intravenously at a hospital. With prompt treatment, most make a full recovery.

WARTS
Verrucas

Warts are small, firm growths on the skin caused by a viral infection. Verrucas, also called plantar warts, are warts on the sole of the foot that have been flattened by the body's weight. Most warts occur on the hands or feet, but they may also affect the genitals (genital warts, p.218).

Warts are usually round and firm, have a rough, raised surface, and may be dotted with tiny dark spots. Verrucas are flattened, firm, have a thickened surface, and are often painful to walk on.

Most warts eventually disappear by themselves, although this may take months or years. Various over-the-counter wart treatments are available, or a wart may be removed by a doctor by freezing, scraping, or burning it off. Genital warts should always be treated by a doctor.

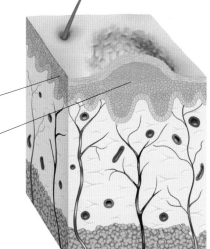

Epidermis (outer layer of skin)

Overgrowth of cells in the skin's outer layer

Wart formation
A wart is an overgrowth of skin cells caused by infection with a human papillomavirus. Warts can be passed on by direct physical contact or by contact with contaminated objects or surfaces.

SCABIES

Scabies is a skin infestation caused by a mite that burrows into the skin. It is contagious and can be passed on by close physical contact. Symptoms include intense itching; a widespread rash of raised, pinkish-red spots, and short lines on the skin caused by the mite's burrows. The itching may persist for up to three weeks after the rash has disappeared.

Treatment is with an antiparasitic lotion or cream. A topical corticosteroid may be prescribed to relieve itching. To prevent reinfection, all family members should be treated. Nightwear and bed and bath linen should be washed at a high temperature.

HAND, FOOT, AND MOUTH DISEASE

Hand, foot, and mouth disease is an infectious disease (caused by a virus) that mainly affects young children. Symptoms usually develop three to five days after infection. They may include blisters inside the mouth that may develop into painful ulcers, blisters on the hands and feet, a sore throat, and fever.

Hand, foot, and mouth disease usually clears up by itself within about seven to ten days. Self-help measures, such as avoiding hot or irritating foods and drinks and taking paracetamol or ibuprofen, can help to relieve the symptoms.

ATHLETE'S FOOT

Also called tinea pedis, athlete's foot is a ringworm (fungal) infection of the skin of the feet that can be picked up by contact with infected skin or with contaminated surfaces or objects. The infection usually affects skin between the toes or on the soles of the feet. The affected skin becomes cracked, sore, itchy, and soggy. Sometimes, the infection spreads to the toenails, which may become yellow, thickened, and brittle. Athlete's foot is unlikely to clear up by itself, but it can usually be treated with over-the-counter antifungal medications. If this treatment is ineffective, a doctor may prescribe a stronger antifungal drug.

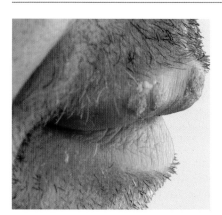

COLD SORE

Cold sores are small blisters that form around the mouth or on the lips. They are caused by the herpes simplex virus. The first attack of the virus may cause a flu-like illness. The virus then lies dormant, but it may be reactivated and cause cold sores.

Cold sore blisters
Cold sores first appear as tiny, fluid-filled spots but soon develop into larger, crusty blisters. New skin starts to form under the blisters, which gradually shrink then disappear entirely.

In many cases, an outbreak of cold sores is preceded by a tingling sensation on the lips. This is followed by the appearance of small blisters that enlarge and become painful and itchy. The blisters then burst and become crusty, before gradually disappearing.

Cold sores usually clear up by themselves within about seven to ten days. Treatment with an over-the-counter antiviral cream may prevent individual outbreaks if used at the first sign of tingling. However, it does not eliminate the virus or prevent further attacks.

ALOPECIA
Alopecia areata | Diffuse alopecia | Traction alopecia

Alopecia is the medical term for hair loss. The most common type is male-pattern baldness, in which hair is lost from the temples and crown. In female-pattern baldness, hair is usually lost from only the top of the head. Generalized hair loss may occur temporarily after pregnancy or as a result of chemotherapy; other causes include stress, malnutrition, acute illness, and telogen effluvium. Alopecia areata, caused by the immune system attacking hair follicles, usually causes patchy hair loss. Other causes of patchy hair loss include ringworm, lichen planus (p.222), thyroid problems, and trichotillomania.

Treatment depends on the underlying cause. Medications such as corticosteroids may stimulate hair regrowth. Other options include a hair transplant or wearing a wig.

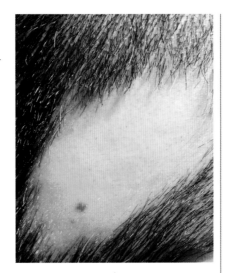

Hair loss
Alopecia areata most commonly affects teenagers and young adults. It typically causes patchy hair loss but may rarely lead to loss of all hair on the head and body.

RINGWORM
Jock itch | Tinea cruris infection | Tinea capitis infection

Ringworm is the commonly used term for various fungal infections of the skin, scalp, and nails. The infections may be acquired by physical contact with infected people or animals, or from contaminated objects or surfaces.

The most common type of ringworm is probably athlete's foot (p.229). Body ringworm (tinea corporis) produces an itchy, red or silvery ring on the skin of the body. Groin ringworm (tinea cruris, commonly called jock itch) produces a reddened, itchy, flaky patch that spreads from the genitals over the inside of the thighs. Scalp ringworm (tinea capitis) produces round, itchy, scaly patches of hair loss on the scalp. In all these types of ringworm, blisters or sores may form around the edge of the affected area. Ringworm of the nails typically causes thick, discoloured nails.

Treatment is usually with topical antifungals, although antifungal tablets may be needed for widespread infections or those affecting the scalp or nails.

DANDRUFF

Dandruff is a harmless condition in which dead skin is shed from the scalp, accumulating in the hair and sometimes causing itching. It is commonly due to seborrhoeic dermatitis (p.222), which is associated with overgrowth of a yeast that normally lives on the skin. Other causes include eczema (p.222), psoriasis (p.222), and scalp ringworm (tinea capitis).

Dandruff usually clears up with regular use of an antidandruff shampoo. If it persists despite such treatment or is accompanied by other symptoms, a doctor should be consulted to investigate possible causes or prescribe a stronger treatment.

TRICHOTILLOMANIA

Trichotillomania is an impulse-control disorder in which a person compulsively and repeatedly pulls out his or her own hair. The person typically pulls or twists off hair from the scalp, often leaving visible bald patches. They may also sometimes pull out eyelashes, eyebrows, or pubic hair. The cause of the condition is unknown but it can be associated with severe learning difficulties or with psychological problems, such as obsessive-compulsive disorder.

Treatment usually involves psychotherapy, such as cognitive-behavioural therapy, although medications (antidepressants) may also be recommended.

TELOGEN EFFLUVIUM

In telogen effluvium, there is widespread thinning of the hair on the scalp. Often, the cause of the condition is unknown, but telogen effluvium may sometimes be triggered by factors such as childbirth, a severe illness, stress, or extreme dieting and weight loss.

Usually, the only symptom is increased hair loss - noticeable, for example, as more than normal amounts of hair shed when brushing, combing, or washing the hair - although sometimes the scalp may be more sensitive than normal.

Telogen effluvium does not need treatment, because the hair grows back once the trigger has disappeared.

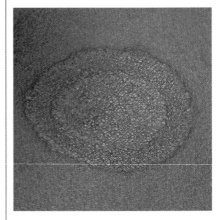

Body ringworm
A raised red ring with healthy looking skin in the centre is characteristic of tinea corporis (body ringworm). In severe cases, pus-filled blisters may develop around the ring.

PILONIDAL SINUS

A pilonidal sinus is a pit in the skin, often containing hairs, in the upper part of the cleft between the buttocks. The cause is probably a broken hair fragment growing inwards into the skin.

A pilonidal sinus is usually harmless, does not cause symptoms, and does not need treatment. However, it may become infected, which may result in a painful, swollen, pus-filled abscess (called a pilonidal cyst) that does need treatment. Treatment is usually with antibiotics and surgery to drain the pus. If there are repeated infections, the sinus may be surgically removed.

HEAD LICE

Head lice are tiny insects that live in hair and lay eggs (nits) on the base of hairs. Head lice are harmless, but their bite causes intense itching. They can be transmitted by close personal contact or by sharing items such as combs and hats.

Lice can be treated using over-the-counter insecticide medications. These are not suitable for everybody, so a pharmacist should be consulted first. Alternatively, lice can be removed by repeatedly combing the hair with a special comb. All family members should be treated to prevent reinfestation.

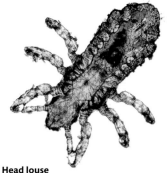

Head louse
The adult head louse is a tiny, greyish-brown insect, about the size of a sesame seed, that most commonly lives on scalp hair but can also sometimes infest the eyelashes or eyebrows.

CLUBBING

In clubbing, the fingertips and ends of the toes become broader, thicker, and bulbous, and there is increased curvature of the nails so that they look like upside-down spoons. Clubbing can sometimes occur without any apparent cause, and rarely the condition runs in families and is harmless. More commonly, however, it is a sign of an underlying disorder, such as lung cancer (p.195), bronchiectasis (abnormal widening of the bronchi, the large airways in the lungs), cystic fibrosis (p.194), heart disease, liver disease, thyroid disease, stomach cancer (p.200), bowel cancer (p.206), or inflammatory bowel disease (p.203).

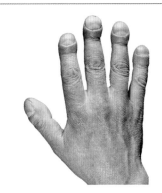

Clubbing of the fingers
The broadening and thickening of the ends of the fingers usually indicates an underlying health problem, often a disorder of the heart or lungs, but it could be caused by a wide range of conditions.

PARONYCHIA

Paronychia is infection of the fold of skin surrounding a nail (the nail fold). It may develop suddenly (acute paronychia), due to a bacterial infection, or gradually (chronic paronychia), usually due to a yeast infection. Acute paronychia causes pain and swelling on the side of the nail fold and a build-up of pus around the nail. Chronic paronychia causes similar symptoms but does not usually produce a build-up of pus.

Treatment is with antibiotics or antifungal medications. With acute paronychia, it may also be necessary to drain a build-up of pus.

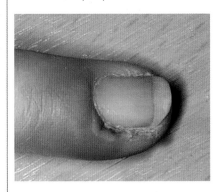

Acute paronychia
Acute paronychia is usually the result of a bacterial infection entering the nail fold through a minor cut or break in the skin. It causes rapid inflammation and a build up of pus.

FUNGAL NAIL INFECTION

Known medically as onychomycosis, fungal nail infections cause the nails to become discoloured, thickened, distorted, and brittle. Affected nails may also cause pain when under pressure – from shoes, for example. The toenails are affected more often than the fingernails. Most fungal nail infections result from the spread of fungi that cause athlete's foot (p.229).

Treatment is with antifungal tablets, topical antifungal drugs, or by softening the nail and scraping away the infected areas. In severe cases, removal of the nail may be recommended.

INGROWN TOENAIL

An ingrown toenail occurs when one or both edges of the nail curl round and grow into the adjacent skin. This often causes the skin to become inflamed and painful. It may also bleed or become infected. Ingrown toenails are usually caused by incorrect cutting of the nails or by wearing tight shoes.

Bathing the foot regularly in a warm salt solution then covering the nail with a dressing may help to relieve pain. If the adjacent skin is infected, antibiotics may be needed. In severe cases, part of the nail may be removed by surgery.

INFECTIONS AND INFESTATIONS

INFLUENZA

Commonly known as flu, influenza is a viral infection of the upper airways. It usually occurs mainly in winter (seasonal flu), but may occur at any time. Outbreaks of particular flu variants, such as swine flu and bird flu, may also occur. The virus is typically spread by droplets from coughs and sneezes. Infection can occur by inhaling the droplets or by touching contaminated surfaces and then touching the mouth or nose. Seasonal flu and swine flu are spread in these ways. Bird flu is usually caught directly from infected birds.

All types of flu produce similar symptoms, including a fever, headache, coughing or sneezing, exhaustion, aches, a stuffy or runny nose, vomiting, and diarrhoea. Flu symptoms usually clear up within a few days without treatment, although tiredness may persist. Occasionally, the condition can cause serious illness or complications such as pneumonia (p.194), and those at particular risk may sometimes be offered antiviral medication.

A flu vaccine is available to reduce the risk of getting flu. The flu virus changes (mutates) frequently, so it is necessary to be vaccinated each year against the strains of virus prevalent at the time.

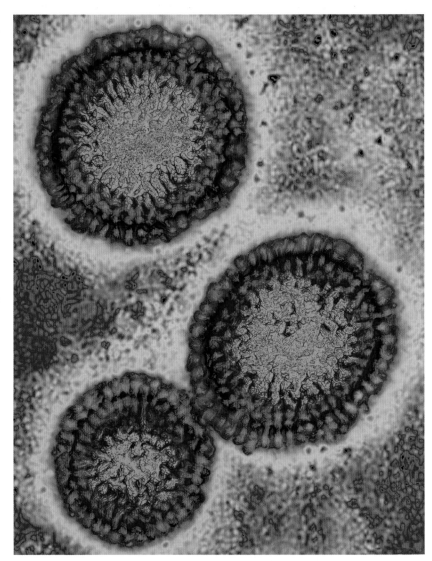

Influenza virus
This coloured micrograph shows the structure of the influenza virus. A core of genetic material (pale blue) is surrounded by an envelope with proteins protruding (orange spikes).

COMMON COLD

The common cold is a viral infection of the nose, throat, and upper airways that causes a runny or stuffy nose, sore throat, sneezing, headache, and a cough. Infection can occur by inhaling infected droplets from coughs or sneezes, or by touching the mouth or nose after contact with a contaminated object or the skin of somebody with infected droplets on his or her skin.

Symptoms usually develop between one and three days after infection and become worse over about one to two days. Most colds clear up by themselves within a week or two. Medical advice should be sought if a cold lasts for more than about three weeks, if symptoms worsen, or if other symptoms develop. Occasionally, a cold may be complicated by a bacterial infection, causing, for example, acute bronchitis (p.193), sinusitis (p.191), or a middle ear infection (otitis media, p.174). In such cases, medical treatment is needed.

SHINGLES

Also known as herpes zoster, shingles is a nerve infection caused by reactivation of the chickenpox virus (the varicella zoster virus). After an attack of chickenpox, the virus remains dormant in the nervous system. Later, the virus may be reactivated, causing shingles. This most commonly occurs in older people, those with reduced

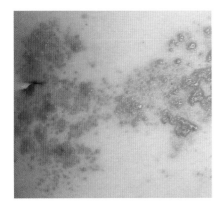

immunity, and also people who are stressed or in ill-health.

Symptoms of shingles include tingling, itching, and pain in an area of skin, a rash of red spots that turn into fluid-filled blisters, and fever. The blisters form scabs that may leave scars. Occasionally, shingles may affect the eyes, causing corneal ulcers, or the facial nerve, causing one-sided facial weakness or paralysis and pain that continues after the attack, a condition called post-herpetic neuralgia. The virus can be spread by direct contact and will cause chickenpox in somebody who is not immune.

Treatment is with antiviral medication and painkillers. A vaccine is available to reduce the risk of infection.

Shingles rash
In shingles, a painful rash develops along the path of a nerve. The rash turns into fluid-filled blisters that eventually dry out, form scabs, and fall off. The blisters contain virus particles and are infectious.

CHICKENPOX

Sometimes called varicella, chickenpox is an infectious disease caused by the varicella zoster virus that produces a rash and fever. An attack gives lifelong immunity, but the virus remains dormant in the body and may reappear later to cause shingles. The virus is spread by airborne droplets or by direct contact. It is highly contagious and those with chickenpox should stay away from non-immune people. The virus can also cause serious complications during pregnancy.

Symptoms appear one to three weeks after infection. Initially, there is a widespread rash of red spots. The spots develop into itchy, fluid-filled blisters, which dry out and form scabs that eventually fall off. Symptoms can be relieved with paracetamol and over-the-counter preparations to reduce itching. In some cases, a doctor may prescribe antiviral medication. There is a vaccine against chickenpox recommended for certain groups of people.

RUBELLA

Rubella is a viral infection, also sometimes known as German measles, which usually produces only a mild illness. However, it can cause serious birth defects in a fetus if it affects a non-immune woman during early pregnancy. Somebody with rubella is infectious for a week before symptoms appear until up to four days after the rash appeared.

The rubella virus can be spread by mother-to-baby transmission and in airborne droplets. Symptoms typically appear two to three weeks after infection. The main symptoms are a rash that appears on the face, spreads to the body and limbs, then disappears after a few days; fever; and swollen lymph nodes around the head and neck.

Paracetamol may help to reduce fever, and symptoms usually clear up by themselves within about a week. A vaccine against rubella is available and is usually given combined with measles and mumps in the MMR vaccine.

MUMPS

Mumps is a viral infection, mainly of childhood, which causes swelling of the parotid salivary glands. These glands are located at the sides of the face, below and just in front of the ears. Alongside the swelling, there may also be fever,

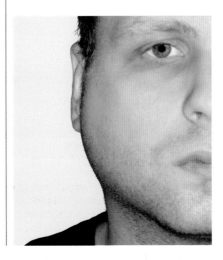

headache, and a sore throat. Mumps may also sometimes cause viral meningitis (p.168), inflammation of the pancreas (pancreatitis, p.202) or, in adolescent boys and adult men, inflammation of the testes (epididymo-orchitis, p.210).

The virus is spread in airborne droplets, and symptoms typically take 14 to 25 days to appear after infection. An infected person is contagious from about two days before the swelling appears until about five days after it has appeared.

Mumps usually clears up within a week or two without treatment, although paracetamol may help to relieve symptoms. A vaccine against mumps is available and is usually given combined with vaccines for measles and rubella in the MMR vaccine.

Swollen glands
The most recognizable symptom of mumps is swelling of the parotid salivary glands at the side of the face. Usually, the glands on both sides of the face become swollen, although occasionally only one is affected.

MEASLES

Measles is a potentially serious viral disease that mainly affects children. The virus is spread by airborne droplets, and an infected person is contagious from when symptoms appear until about four days after the rash appears.

Symptoms typically develop about 10 days after infection and include fever; cold-like symptoms, such as a cough, runny nose, and sneezing; painful, red, watery eyes; and small white spots inside the cheeks. After a few days, a rash appears on the head and then spreads to the rest of the body. Symptoms usually subside after a few days, although sometimes complications develop, such as ear or chest infections, seizures, or encephalitis (inflammation of the brain, p.168), which may lead to brain damage or may even be fatal.

Treatment consists of medication and self-help measures to relieve symptoms, and treatment for any complications. A vaccine against measles is available and is usually given combined with vaccines for two other common childhood diseases (mumps and rubella) in the MMR vaccine.

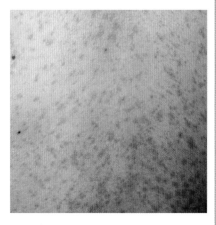

Measles rash
The measles rash usually starts on the head then spreads to the rest of the body. Initially, it consists of separate flat or slightly raised spots, as seen above, but these later merge into blotchy patches.

PARVOVIRUS

Infection with parvovirus strain B19 causes an illness characterized by a bright red rash on the cheeks, hence one of its alternative names: slapped cheek disease (other names are fifth disease and erythema infectiosum). The infection is usually transmitted in airborne droplets but may occasionally be transmitted from mother to fetus.

Symptoms usually appear within four to 14 days of infection and, in children, typically include fever and the distinctive rash, which spreads from the cheeks to the body and limbs. Symptoms in adults are more severe and may include a rash on the palms and soles, and severe, persistent joint pain. Infection during pregnancy increases the risk of health problems in the baby or miscarriage.

Treatment is with medication to relieve symptoms. The infection usually clears up within one to three weeks, and one attack confers lifelong immunity.

POLIOMYELITIS
Spinal polio

Commonly known as polio, poliomyelitis is an infectious viral disease that varies from mild to potentially life-threatening. The virus is spread from the faeces of infected people to food, or by airborne transmission. Worldwide, polio is rare, but it still occurs in parts of Africa, the Middle East, and Asia.

Polio usually produces no symptoms or only a mild, flu-like illness. Rarely, the spinal cord (spinal polio) or brain may be affected, which may cause paralysis or even death. People with non-paralytic polio are usually treated with bed rest and painkillers. People with paralysis may also be treated with physiotherapy, and, if breathing is affected, artificial ventilation. People with non-paralytic polio make a full recovery, as do many with paralytic polio, although some are left with long-term disability and a few die. A preventive vaccine is available, and is usually given combined with other vaccines, such as tetanus and diphtheria.

SEPTICAEMIA

Septicaemia, commonly known as blood poisoning, is a potentially life-threatening condition in which bacteria enter the bloodstream, multiply rapidly, and spread throughout the body. It is usually due to bacteria escaping from a more localized infection, such as a lung, kidney, urinary tract, or abdominal infection, or a wound or abscess. Those with reduced immunity, young children, and older people are particularly susceptible.

Symptoms usually develop suddenly and may include fever, chills, violent shivering, and faintness. Without treatment, septic shock may develop, with symptoms such as pale, clammy skin, restlessness, irritability, rapid, shallow breathing, and, in severe cases, delirium, unconsciousness, and even death. Urgent medical treatment with antibiotics is necessary. If septic shock has developed, treatment may also involve supportive measures, such as artificial ventilation and medications. Surgery to remove infected tissue may also be needed.

PERTUSSIS

Pertussis, also called whooping cough, is a bacterial infection of the lungs and airways that causes coughing bouts ending in a characteristic "whoop". It is caused by the bacterium *Bordetella pertussis*, which is spread in airborne droplets.

Initial symptoms resemble those of a common cold. Later symptoms include the distinctive cough, vomiting, and sometimes nosebleeds. In severe cases, breathing may stop temporarily and seizures may occur.

Severe pertussis may be life-threatening and requires urgent medical treatment. In such cases, treatment includes antibiotics, and sometimes oxygen therapy and intravenous medication. Otherwise, for those who have had pertussis for less than three weeks, antibiotics may be prescribed. Those who have had the infection for more than three weeks do not usually need specific medical treatment. A vaccine is usually given combined with other vaccines, such as diphtheria, polio, and tetanus.

GLANDULAR FEVER

Glandular fever is an illness caused by a virus called the Epstein-Barr virus (EBV). This condition is also known as infectious mononucleosis. Found in the saliva of infected people, the Epstein-Barr virus can be spread by kissing, coughs and sneezes, and sharing contaminated eating and drinking utensils. Glandular fever is most common in young adults.

The infection does not always produce symptoms and people may be unaware that they are infected. When symptoms do occur, they usually do so about four to eight weeks after infection. Symptoms may include fever; a sore throat; swollen tonsils; swollen lymph nodes in the neck, armpits, and groin; extreme tiredness; and sometimes a rash and jaundice (yellowing of the skin and whites of the eyes, p.201).

There is no specific treatment for glandular fever, but over-the-counter painkillers may relieve symptoms, and plenty of rest may reduce tiredness. Alcohol and contact sports should be avoided while recovering, because the virus may have affected the liver or spleen. Most people recover within about two to three weeks, although tiredness may sometimes persist for months.

SCARLET FEVER

Also sometimes called scarlatina, scarlet fever is an infectious disease caused by a type of streptococcus bacteria. The bacteria are spread in airborne droplets.

Symptoms of the disease typically develop within about a week of infection. They may include a scarlet rash that starts on the neck and upper body and spreads rapidly, sore throat, fever, headache, swollen glands in the neck, and vomiting. Sometimes, a white coating develops on the tongue; this coating peels off after a few days, leaving the tongue red and swollen ("strawberry tongue").

Scarlet fever is treated with antibiotics to clear up the infection, and painkillers to relieve symptoms. Most people recover within about a week.

TETANUS

Tetanus is a potentially life-threatening disease of the nervous system caused by infection of a wound with *Clostridium tetani* bacteria, which live in the soil and animal manure. The main symptoms of infection include stiff jaw muscles (lockjaw), fever, fast pulse, and sweating. Painful muscle spasms may develop; these may affect the throat or chest and lead to breathing difficulty or even suffocation.

Tetanus requires immediate treatment. If symptoms have not developed, treatment is with immunoglobulin to destroy the bacteria. If symptoms have developed, treatment may include immunoglobulin, antibiotics, medication to relieve muscle spasms, and sometimes artificial ventilation. With prompt treatment, most people recover. A preventive vaccine is available, and is usually given combined with other vaccines, such as diphtheria and polio.

TYPHOID

Typhoid is an infectious disease caused by the bacterium *Salmonella typhi*. It is spread by drinking water or eating food contaminated with infected faeces. Initial symptoms include fever, headache, tiredness, abdominal pain, and constipation. Later, diarrhoea develops and a rash appears on the chest and abdomen. Occasionally, complications may develop, such as bleeding in the intestine or perforation of the intestinal wall, which may be life-threatening.

Treatment with antibiotics usually brings the disease under control within a few days. However, if severe complications have developed, surgery may be needed. Several vaccines against typhoid are available, but none gives total protection. Scrupulous attention to personal hygiene and to water and food hygiene is also needed to reduce the risk of infection.

CHOLERA

Cholera is infection of the small intestine with *Vibrio cholerae* bacteria. The infection is acquired by eating food or drinking water contaminated by the bacteria. Outbreaks of the disease occur mainly in regions with poor sanitation, and after upheavals, such as natural disasters, during which clean water becomes unavailable.

Many people infected with the bacteria do not develop symptoms, although they may infect others if their faeces contaminate water or food. If symptoms do develop, they typically start suddenly, with watery diarrhoea and often vomiting. The amount of fluid lost through diarrhoea and vomiting may be so great that the person becomes severely dehydrated and may even die as a result.

Treatment is with oral rehydration or, in severe cases, with intravenous rehydration. Antibiotics may also be given to eradicate the infection and shorten the recovery period. With prompt treatment, most people make a full recovery. A vaccine against cholera is available, but does not give total protection, so scrupulous personal hygiene and food and water hygiene are also needed to minimize the risk of infection.

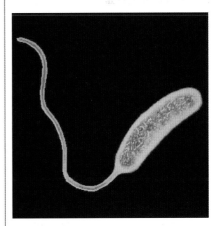

Cholera bacterium
This coloured micrograph shows a *Vibrio cholerae* bacterium, the cause of cholera. The bacterium secretes a toxin that affects the wall of the small intestine, leading to severe diarrhoea and, subsequently, dehydration.

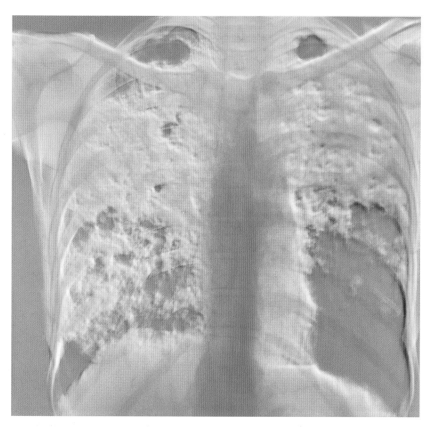

TUBERCULOSIS

Tuberculosis (TB) is an infection that mainly affects the lungs but may also affect many other parts of the body. It is caused by the bacterium *Mycobacterium tuberculosis*, which spreads by airborne droplets. After infection, most people clear the bacteria, some develop active disease, and others develop latent TB (displaying no symptoms, but they may later develop active disease).

Symptoms may take months or years to develop. TB affecting the lungs (pulmonary TB) typically causes a persistent cough with sputum that may be bloody, chest pain, breathlessness, fever, fatigue, and weight loss. TB may spread to the lymph nodes, bones and joints, nervous system, and genitourinary tract.

TB is treated with a long-term course of a combination of antibiotics. Without treatment, TB can be fatal. The TB vaccine is usually only for certain at-risk groups.

TB of the lungs
This coloured X-ray of a person with pulmonary TB shows many areas of abnormal lung tissue in both lungs. The nodules appear as yellow areas against the blue of normal lung tissue.

LEPTOSPIROSIS

Leptospirosis is a disease caused by bacteria known as *Leptospira*. The bacteria are excreted in the urine of infected animals (particularly rats) and transmitted to humans by contact with contaminated water or soil.

Symptoms include fever, headache, muscle pain, a rash, and inflammation of the eyes. Without treatment, meningitis (p.168) or encephalitis (p.168) may develop. Rarely, infection may cause a severe form of leptospirosis called Weil's disease, which can cause internal bleeding and organ damage and may be life-threatening.

Most cases of leptospirosis can be treated with antibiotics, and painkillers to relieve symptoms. Severe cases require hospital treatment with intravenous medication, and possibly supportive measures, such as artificial ventilation or dialysis.

LYME DISEASE

Lyme disease is an infection caused by a bacterium that is transmitted by infected ticks. A bite from an infected tick usually produces a small red dot that gradually expands to form a circular rash. The rash resembles the bulls-eye of a target and may be as much as 15 cm (6 in) across. There may also be tiredness, fever, chills, headaches, and joint pain. If untreated, these symptoms may persist for several weeks. Rarely, serious complications affecting the heart, nervous system, and joints may develop up to two years later in untreated cases.

Lyme disease tick
The ticks that can transmit Lyme disease usually live in heavily vegetated areas and are found in many regions of the northern hemisphere, including North America and Europe.

Treatment of Lyme disease is with antibiotics, and painkillers to relieve symptoms. Most people make a complete recovery if treated soon after infection. If complications have developed, a prolonged course of antibiotics together with other treatment for the specific complication may be needed. In a few cases, long-term symptoms similar to chronic fatigue syndrome may develop.

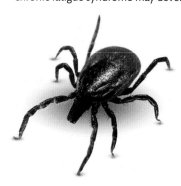

MALARIA

Malaria is a serious disease caused by protozoan parasites called plasmodia, which are transmitted by bites from infected *Anopheles* mosquitoes. Malaria is most prevalent in tropical countries and is a major global health problem, with about 200 million cases a year. Five species of plasmodia cause malaria but the most dangerous is *Plasmodium falciparum*, which is responsible for most malaria-related deaths globally and can be fatal within about 48 hours of the first symptoms appearing if it is not treated.

Symptoms usually begin between about seven and 18 days after being bitten by an infected mosquito, although occasionally they may not develop for a year or longer. The symptoms may include attacks of fever, shaking, sweating, and chills. There may also be a severe headache, vomiting, diarrhoea, and fatigue. In some types of malaria, attacks occur in cycles, with fatigue being the only symptom between attacks. However, falciparum malaria usually causes continuous fever, and an attack may rapidly lead to unconsciousness, kidney failure, or even death.

Malaria is treated with antimalarial medication to destroy the parasites. In severe cases, hospital treatment with intravenous antimalarials, a blood transfusion, or kidney dialysis may be needed. The risk of getting malaria can be reduced by preventive antimalarial medications. However, these do not provide complete protection against the disease, so measures to avoid mosquito bites are also important.

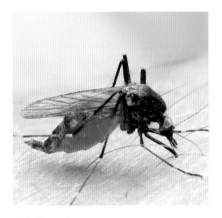

Malaria carrier
The malaria parasites are carried by female *Anopheles* mosquitoes, which bite mainly at dusk and dawn. When an infected mosquito bites, it not only sucks up blood but also injects malaria parasites into the person's bloodstream.

CRYPTOSPORIDIOSIS

Cryptosporidiosis is an intestinal infection caused by single-celled parasites called *Cryptosporidium*. The infection is spread by contact with infected people or animals, or by eating food or drinking water contaminated by infected human or animal faeces. The disease causes diarrhoea, abdominal pain, fever, nausea, and vomiting. Symptoms usually last about one to two weeks, and most otherwise healthy people make a full recovery without treatment. However, in people with impaired immunity, such as those with AIDS (p.188), the infection may be more severe and require specialist treatment in hospital.

GIARDIASIS

Giardiasis is infection of the small intestine with the parasite *Giardia lamblia*. The disease is spread by drinking water or eating food contaminated with the parasite, or by direct contact with an infected person.

Symptoms usually start about one to two weeks after infection. They may include diarrhoea with foul-smelling faeces, flatulence, belching, abdominal cramps, bloating, loss of appetite, and nausea. If symptoms last for more than about a week, weight loss and malnutrition may occur, due to insufficient nutrients being absorbed. Treatment with antibiotics usually clears up the infection within a few days. The risk of infection can be reduced by good personal hygiene and by avoiding food or water that might be contaminated.

SHIGELLOSIS

Also called bacillary dysentery, shigellosis is infection of the intestine with *Shigella* bacteria. The disease is spread by eating food or drinking water contaminated by infected human faeces or by contact with an infected person or a contaminated surface.

Symptoms usually start one to two days after infection. They may include diarrhoea, which may be bloody; fever; and abdominal pain. Persistent diarrhoea may cause dehydration. Shigellosis usually clears up by itself in about a week. Plenty of fluids should be drunk to avoid dehydration, and paracetamol can relieve pain and fever. In severe cases, antibiotics may be necessary. The risk of infection can be reduced by good personal hygiene and avoiding food or water that might be contaminated.

AMOEBIASIS
Amoebic colitis

Amoebiasis is an intestinal infection that is caused by the single-celled parasite *Entamoeba histolytica*. The infection is spread by eating food or drinking water that has been contaminated by infected human faeces.

Many infected people do not have any symptoms, but in some cases the parasite causes amoebic colitis (inflammation of the intestine), which may cause symptoms such as diarrhoea and abdominal pain. Occasionally, the intestine may become ulcerated and amoebic dysentery develops. This may cause watery, bloody diarrhoea, severe abdominal pain, and sometimes fever. In some cases, the infection may spread to the liver and cause a liver abscess, with symptoms such as fever, weight loss, chills, and painful enlargement of the liver.

Treatment of all forms of amoebiasis is with antibiotic medication to kill the parasite. This usually leads to a full recovery. Rarely, surgery may be needed to treat an amoebic liver abscess. The risk of infection can be reduced by good personal hygiene and by avoiding food or water that might be contaminated.

TAPEWORM INFESTATION

Tapeworms are ribbon-shaped parasitic worms that can infest humans and animals. Infestation usually occurs by eating undercooked meat or fish that contains tapeworm eggs or larvae, although it may also occur by transferring worm eggs from the fingers to the mouth. In the intestine, the eggs and larvae mature into adult tapeworms. The adults produce large numbers of eggs, which are passed out in bowel movements and may be visible in the faeces.

Tapeworms from beef, pork, and fish usually cause only mild abdominal discomfort or diarrhoea. Rarely, fish tapeworms may cause anaemia (p.186). However, ingesting pork tapeworm eggs may lead to the formation of cysts in body tissues. This condition, called cysticercosis, may cause symptoms such as muscle pain, seizures (fits), and blindness. Tapeworm larvae acquired from dogs or sheep may rarely lead to hydatid cysts in body organs.

Treatment of tapeworm infestation is with anthelmintic medication, which kills the worms.

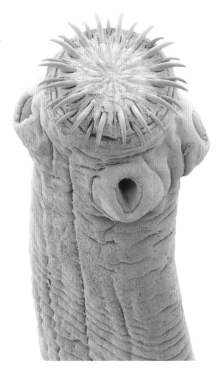

Pork tapeworm
The adult pork tapeworm has suckers and hooks on its head, which it uses to attach itself the wall of the intestine, where it may grow to 6–9 m (20–30 ft) in length.

FLUKE INFESTATIONS

Flukes are flattened worms that may infest humans or animals. In humans, the two main diseases are liver fluke infestation (fascioliasis) and schistosomiasis (also called bilharzia).

Fascioliasis is typically acquired by eating food contaminated with fluke larvae. In the body, the larvae invade the liver, causing symptoms such as fever and night sweats. The larvae mature into adults in the liver, where they may cause inflammation or obstruction of the bile ducts, which may lead to jaundice.

Schistosomiasis is usually acquired by bathing in water contaminated with fluke larvae. The larvae penetrate the skin and develop into adults, which settle in veins of the bladder and intestines, causing inflammation and sometimes bleeding and ulceration. Eggs produced by the adults may migrate to the liver and cause liver damage. Symptoms of schistosomiasis include itching where larvae penetrated the skin; fever; muscle pain; diarrhoea; frequent, painful urination; blood in the urine; and a cough. Treatment of both diseases is with anthelmintic medication to kill the flukes.

ROUNDWORM INFESTATIONS
Filariasis | Hookworm | Threadworm

Roundworm infestation typically occurs by ingesting worm eggs that have contaminated the hands, drinking water, or food. Some infestations result from worm larvae penetrating the skin, as with hookworm or from bites from infected insects, as with filariasis.

Many roundworms primarily infect the intestine; examples include hookworms and threadworms. Often, these cause no symptoms or only mild ones, such as abdominal pain and diarrhoea. Some roundworms primarily affect parts other than the intestine. For example, filariasis mainly affects the lymphatic system and can lead to elephantiasis (massive swelling of the legs or scrotum). Treatment of roundworm infestation is with anthelmintic medication to kill the worms.

HYDATID CYST

Hydatid cysts result from infestation with eggs of the tapeworm *Echinococcus granulosus*. The tapeworm is found mainly in sheep and dogs and may be passed to humans by ingesting food or drink contaminated with infected sheep or dog faeces.

In humans, the eggs hatch into larvae in the intestine and migrate to the liver, lungs, or other tissues, where they develop into cysts. The cysts grow slowly and often produce no symptoms. If symptoms do develop, they vary according to the site of the cyst. For example, a liver cyst may cause pain, nausea, and jaundice (p.201); a lung cyst may cause chest pain and a cough.

Treatment is with anthelmintic medication to kill the larvae and, in many cases, surgery to remove the cysts.

THRUSH

Thrush (also called candidiasis) is an infection caused by the yeast *Candida*. The yeast is normally present in the body without causing problems, but sometimes it may multiply excessively and cause disease. Factors that may lead to yeast overgrowth include use of antibiotic medication or oral contraceptives, hormonal changes during pregnancy, disorders such as diabetes, and reduced immunity.

Symptoms vary according to the area affected. Skin infections typically cause an itchy rash. Oral thrush produces sore, creamy-yellow patches in the mouth. Vaginal thrush causes itching of the vulva and vagina, a thick, white discharge, and pain when urinating. In men, the penis may be affected, causing a rash and itching or burning under the foreskin. Treatment is with antifungal medication to kill the yeast.

POISONING AND ENVIRONMENTAL DISORDERS

ALCOHOL POISONING

Alcohol poisoning occurs when very large amounts of alcohol are drunk over a short period of time. Alcohol is broken down in the body by the liver, but the liver can only break down a limited mount in any given time, so when large amounts are drunk quickly, the alcohol oncentration in the body rapidly rises to toxic levels. This can produce symptoms such as confusion, slurred speech, loss of coordination, vomiting, irregular breathing, low body temperature, and unconsciousness. There is also a danger that the person may choke on their vomit.

Severe poisoning may cause seizures, a heart attack (myocardial infarction), brain damage, and breathing stoppage (respiratory arrest), and may be life-threatening. Alcohol poisoning requires urgent medical treatment.

DRUG OVERDOSE

The effects of a medication or drug overdose vary, depending on factors such as the specific drug and the amount taken. The symptoms may vary from mild to severe, and may develop very quickly or over a number of days. Some common general symptoms include nausea, vomiting, diarrhoea, abdominal pain, chest pain, a rapid heartbeat, breathing problems, confusion, seizures ("fits"), and unconsciousness. A large overdose may be life-threatening. As well as short-term effects, overdose of some drugs may cause longer-term complications, such as liver or kidney damage.

A drug overdose requires urgent medical treatment. To ensure treatment is as effective as possible, it helps if medical staff know details such as the drug taken, the amount taken, and when it was taken.

HEAT EXHAUSTION AND HEATSTROKE

Heat exhaustion and heatstroke are potentially serious conditions in which there is loss of body fluids and a rise in body temperature due to excessive heat. In a hot environment, the body loses heat by diverting blood to the skin and sweating. Excessive loss of fluids due to profuse sweating may lead to heat exhaustion, with symptoms such as tiredness, weakness, lightheadedness, dizziness, headache,

SUNBURN

Sunburn is skin damage caused by the ultraviolet rays in sunlight. People with pale skin are most vulnerable, but it can also affect those with dark skin. The ultraviolet rays destroy cells in the outer layers of skin and damage the deeper layers. The affected skin becomes red and tender and may blister; later, the dead skin cells

FROSTNIP AND FROSTBITE

Frostnip and frostbite are injuries caused by freezing of the skin and underlying tissues, most commonly the fingers, toes, nose, and ears.

Frostnip causes the skin to turn pale, cold, and numb; there may also be tingling. Frostnip does not cause permanent damage, but it may develop into frostbite if exposure to cold continues.

In frostbite, the affected area becomes white, cold, and hard; it may then become red and swollen. When rewarmed, mildly affected tissues become red, swollen, and sore. In more severe cases, blisters develop and the area becomes very painful. Severe frostbite may lead to gangrene (tissue death) or longer-term problems, such as persistent pain or loss of sensation.

muscle cramps, nausea, and intense thirst. If exposure to heat continues, the body temperature rises and heatstroke may develop, causing symptoms including rapid breathing, confusion, seizures, and unconsciousness.

Untreated, heatstroke may cause life-threatening complications, such as heart failure or severe brain damage. Heat exhaustion can usually be treated by cooling the person down and giving plenty of fluids. Heatstroke requires urgent medical treatment.

are shed by peeling. Sunburn, particularly severe sunburn in childhood, increases the risk of developing solar keratoses (scaly spots on the skin) and skin cancer later in life.

Mild sunburn can usually be treated by cooling the skin, applying moisturizing or anti-inflammatory lotions, and taking painkillers. Severe sunburn may need medical treatment.

ANIMAL BITES AND STINGS

The effects of a bite or sting vary depending on whether the animal is venomous, whether it transmits disease, and the amount of tissue damage. A minor, non-venomous bite or sting typically causes only temporary pain and swelling. However, medical attention should be sought if symptoms are severe, do not subside, other symptoms develop, or if the animal may carry a disease such as malaria (p.237) or rabies (a viral infection that affects the nervous system). Some people have a life-threatening allergic reaction (called anaphylaxis), which requires urgent medical help.

A venomous bite or sting should always receive medical treatment, as should any deep or large animal bite.

MENTAL HEALTH DISORDERS

STRESS

Stress is a general term for the physical and psychological symptoms people experience when they feel overwhelmed. In stressful situations, levels of the hormones adrenaline and hydrocortisone increase, raising the heart rate and blood pressure and altering the metabolism to improve performance. However, high levels of these hormones long-term can have a negative effect, producing symptoms such as headaches, sleeping problems, palpitations, eating too much or too little, irritability, difficulty concentrating and making decisions, anxiety, and depression.

Stress can often be managed by self-help measures, such as relaxation techniques, regular exercise, and eating healthily. If such measures are ineffective, treatment options include psychotherapy and medications for specific problems, such as antidepressants or sleeping pills.

POST-TRAUMATIC STRESS DISORDER

Post-traumatic stress disorder (PTSD) is a form of anxiety that develops after a very distressing, frightening, or stressful event, such as a natural disaster, serious accident, assault, or military combat. Symptoms may occur soon after the event or not for months, or, rarely, years later. They may include involuntary thoughts or flashbacks of the event, nightmares, insomnia, and panic attacks, with symptoms such as trembling, sweating, breathlessness, palpitations, and faintness. There may also be avoidance of reminders of the event and refusal to talk about it, irritability, and emotional numbness. PTSD may also lead to problems such as depression or alcohol or drug abuse.

In some cases, PTSD clears up without treatment. If it lasts for more than about a month, psychotherapy, antidepressants, or both may be recommended.

ANXIETY DISORDERS
Generalized anxiety disorder | Panic disorder

Temporary anxiety in stressful situations is natural, but when it becomes a general response to ordinary situations and causes problems in coping with everyday life, it is considered a disorder.

The main types of anxiety disorder are generalized anxiety disorder, panic disorder, phobias, and post-traumatic stress disorder. In generalized anxiety disorder, there are persistent psychological symptoms, such as a sense of foreboding with no apparent cause, being on edge, impaired concentration, repetitive worrying thoughts, disturbed sleep, and sometimes depression. The physical symptoms of generalized anxiety disorder

PHOBIAS

A phobia is a persistent, overwhelming fear of a particular object, animal, activity, or situation. Exposure to the object of the phobia leads to intense anxiety accompanied by symptoms such as dizziness, palpitations, sweating, trembling, and breathlessness. A person with a phobia has such a compelling desire to avoid the source of the phobia that it interferes with normal life.

Most phobias can be successfully treated with desensitization therapy, which involves gradual exposure to the source of

PSYCHOSIS

Psychosis is a mental problem in which a person's thoughts are so disturbed that he or she loses touch with reality. The main features are hallucinations, such as hearing voices, and delusions, such as believing that people are trying to harm you. Hallucinations and delusions can, in turn, lead to disorganized thinking and speech,

tend to occur intermittently. They may include headache, abdominal cramps, diarrhoea, vomiting, sweating, frequent urination, and trembling.

In panic disorder, psychological and physical symptoms develop suddenly and unpredictably. They may include breathlessness, sweating, trembling, nausea, palpitations, dizziness, fainting, a feeling of choking, a sense of unreality, and a fear that death may be imminent.

Treatment of anxiety disorders usually involves psychotherapy (for example, cognitive-behavioural therapy) and medication to relieve symptoms, such as antidepressants or, in some cases, a short-term course of anti-anxiety drugs. Self-help measures, such as relaxation techniques, may also help to reduce anxiety levels.

the phobia, psychotherapy, or counselling. Anti-anxiety medication may also be prescribed in some cases.

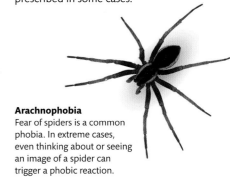

Arachnophobia
Fear of spiders is a common phobia. In extreme cases, even thinking about or seeing an image of a spider can trigger a phobic reaction.

with racing thoughts, difficulty in keeping mental focus, and incoherent speech. Psychosis may be due to a mental health problem, such as schizophrenia, bipolar disorder, or severe depression. It may also result from factors such as drug or alcohol abuse or certain brain disorders.

Treatment is with antipsychotic medications and psychotherapy, together with treatment of the underlying cause.

BIPOLAR DISORDER

Formerly known as manic depression, bipolar disorder is characterized by extreme mood swings between highs (mania) and lows (depression). The underlying cause is unknown, but it is believed to involve chemical abnormalities in the brain. Genetic factors may also be involved, because the disorder sometimes runs in families.

Typically, symptoms of mania and depression alternate, with normal periods in between. Symptoms of a manic episode may include elation, inflated self-esteem (which may lead to delusions of wealth, power, or accomplishment), increased

energy, poor concentration, loss of inhibitions, and sometimes hallucinations. During a depressive phase, symptoms include low energy, loss of interest in everyday life, feelings of worthlessness, and loss of hope for the future.

Treatment is with medication to stabilize moods, often with psychotherapy. In severe cases, hospital treatment may be needed. Bipolar disorder is usually a long-term condition.

Brain activity in bipolar disorder
These brain scans show brain activity during normal periods (left) and increased levels of activity during a manic episode (right).

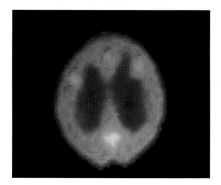
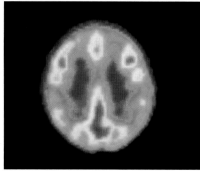

INSOMNIA
Nightmares and night terrors

Difficulty falling asleep or staying asleep is often due to lifestyle factors, such as too much caffeine, a poor sleeping environment, or jet lag. Numerous physical and mental health conditions may also cause insomnia, as can certain medications. Snoring, sleep apnoea, nightmares, and night terrors (abrupt arousal from sleep in a state of fear) can also disrupt sleep.

Insomnia can often be improved by self-help measures, such as changing bedtime habits, and treatment of any underlying medical condition. A doctor may also recommend a type of cognitive-behavioural therapy specifically designed for insomnia or prescribe medication to help with sleep.

CYCLOTHYMIA

Cyclothymia is a mild form of bipolar disorder in which there are similar mood swings but the highs are not extreme enough to be medically classified as mania, and the lows are not severe enough to be categorized as clinical depression. As with bipolar disorder, there is often a normal period between the highs and lows. The mood swings occur relatively frequently, with no more than two symptom-free months in succession. They must also have persisted for at least two years for a formal diagnosis of cyclothymia to be made.

Treatment is usually with mood-stabilizer medications and psychotherapy. In some cases, the condition clears up, but in others it is long-term or progresses to full-blown bipolar disorder.

SCHIZOPHRENIA

Schizophrenia is a serious mental health disorder in which there are distortions in thinking and perceptions of reality, disturbed emotions, and changes in behaviour. The cause of the condition is unknown, but genetic factors are known to play a part: a person who is closely related to somebody with schizophrenia has a significantly increased risk of developing the disorder. Additionally, in susceptible people, schizophrenia may be triggered by factors such as stress or drug abuse.

Symptoms of schizophrenia usually develop gradually. They may include hallucinations; irrational beliefs, in particular, that thoughts and actions are controlled by an outside force; delusions of persecution; and expression of inappropriate emotions. There may also be rambling speech, with rapid switching from one topic to another; disordered thoughts; and agitation. A person with schizophrenia may become depressed and socially withdrawn.

Treatment is usually with a combination of antipsychotic medication and psychotherapy, together with social support and rehabilitation. In most cases, schizophrenia is a long-term condition.

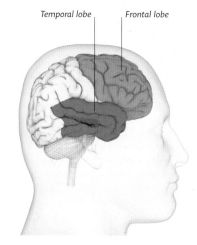

Temporal lobe   Frontal lobe

Schizophrenia and the brain
Studies of people with schizophrenia have revealed differences in their brain chemicals and brain structure, such as a reduced amount of grey matter in the frontal and temporal lobes.

DEPRESSION
Postnatal depression | Seasonal affective disorder (SAD)

Depression is characterized by persistent feelings of sadness, hopelessness, and loss of interest in life. A number of factors may trigger it, including a stressful life event, such as a bereavement; physical illness or mental health problems; hormonal changes after childbirth (postnatal depression); certain medications; or alcohol or drug abuse. Some people become depressed only during winter months, a condition known as seasonal affective disorder (SAD). Depression may also sometimes run in families.

Depression can cause a wide variety of symptoms, and they may vary in severity from person to person. Common symptoms include a feeling of sadness, loss of interest in and enjoyment of work and leisure activities, low energy, anxiety, irritability, and low self-esteem. Other symptoms may include poor concentration, sleeping problems, weight loss or weight gain, reduced sex drive, loss of hope for the future, and thoughts of self-harm or suicide.

Mild depression may improve by itself without medical treatment. In many cases, lifestyle measures may help, such as regular exercise, support from a self-help group, or, for SAD, light therapy. If the depression does not improve with such measures, psychotherapy and antidepressant medication may be prescribed. If these treatments are ineffective, transcranial magnetic stimulation (stimulating the brain with magnetic fields) or electroconvulsive therapy (passing an electric current through the brain) may be recommended. A person who is suicidal or a mother who has thoughts of harming her baby requires prompt medical help.

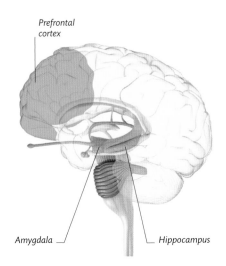

Prefrontal cortex

Amygdala

Hippocampus

Brain areas and depression
Depression may involve the amygdala and hippocampus, which produce emotional responses, and the prefrontal cortex, which generates thoughts about those emotions.

PERSONALITY DISORDERS

Personality disorders are conditions in which rigid, dysfunctional patterns of thought and behaviour cause persistent problems relating to others and fitting in with society. They typically emerge in adolescence and continue into adulthood.

Personality disorders fall into three main groups. The first comprises paranoid, schizoid, and schizotypal personalities. People in this group have patterns of behaviour and thinking that most would see as eccentric or odd. The second group consists of antisocial, histrionic, narcissistic, or borderline personality types. This group is typified by emotional, impulsive, attention-seeking, or self-centred behaviour. The third group comprises avoidant, dependent, or obsessive-compulsive personalities. People in this group have anxious, fearful, or inhibited patterns of thinking and behaviour.

Treatment usually involves psychotherapy and support to help the person adapt his or her behaviour and function successfully. The outlook is variable, although generally the manifestations of a dysfunctional personality diminish with age.

OBSESSIVE-COMPULSIVE DISORDER

Commonly known as OCD, obsessive-compulsive disorder is characterized by uncontrollable, persistent thoughts (obsessions) accompanied by irresistible urges to carry out particular actions or rituals (compulsions).

Obsessions are unwanted thoughts, images, or feelings that enter the mind repeatedly and cause disturbing feelings of anxiety or disgust. A person with OCD may recognize that the obsessions are irrational but is unable to ignore them.

Compulsions are repetitive behaviours or mental acts that the person feels driven to perform to relieve the disturbing feelings caused by the obsession. The compulsive acts (repetitive handwashing, for example) may have to be carried out so many times that they seriously disrupt normal life.

Mild OCD can often be successfully treated with psychotherapy. In more severe cases, psychotherapy and antidepressant medication may be used. Most people improve within about a year of starting treatment, but for a minority OCD may persist long-term.

ADHD

Attention deficit hyperactivity disorder (ADHD) is a behavioural problem in children in which there is a consistently high level of activity, impulsiveness, and difficulty attending to tasks. The cause is not known, although the disorder tends to run in families so a genetic factor may be involved.

Symptoms usually develop between about the ages of three and seven years. They may include a short attention span; an inability to finish tasks; difficulty in following instructions; a tendency to talk excessively and interrupt others; difficulty waiting or taking turns; constant fidgeting; an inability to play quietly alone; and frequently acting without thinking.

Treatment may be with therapy, medication, or both. Therapy may involve psychotherapy and social skills training, as well as training and education for parents. Medications can help to control the symptoms – for example, by aiding concentration and reducing impulsiveness. Symptoms of ADHD usually diminish with time, although the condition may sometimes persist into adulthood.

TOURETTE'S SYNDROME

Tourette's syndrome is a nervous system disorder characterized by repetitive, involuntary movements and noises (tics). The cause of the condition is not known, although it often runs in families so genetic factors may be involved.

Symptoms typically begin between the ages of about seven and 12. They include physical tics, such as facial twitches, blinking, mouth movements, and head and foot movements; and vocal tics, such as coughing, throat clearing, snorting, and grunting. In some cases, the person may repeatedly utter obscenities, copy what other people say or do, say the same thing repeatedly, or make complex physical movements, such as jumping or hitting themselves or others.

Treatment is usually with psychotherapy. Medication to control the tics may also be used. For most people, the condition is lifelong, although the symptoms tend to become less severe with age and may eventually disappear completely.

SUBSTANCE MISUSE
Alcohol/drug misuse

Substance misuse is the harmful use of alcohol, drugs (including prescription and over-the-counter medications), or other chemicals, such as inhalants.

Commonly misused substances include alcohol, cannabis, heroin, cocaine, amphetamines, benzodiazepines, hallucinogens, and various "designer drugs". Usually, they are used to cause intoxication or alter mood. However, excessive amounts can be dangerous in the short-term. For example, drinking large amounts of alcohol in a short period may cause confusion, loss of memory, or, in extreme cases, death. Similarly, a drug overdose may be fatal. In the longer term, regular use of a substance may lead to tolerance (in which increasing amounts are needed to achieve the desired effect) and addiction. It may also cause organ damage, mental health problems, and disruption of family, social, and work life.

EATING DISORDERS
Anorexia nervosa

Eating disorders are characterized by an abnormal attitude to food, resulting in avoiding food (anorexia), self-induced vomiting (bulimia), or compulsive overeating (binge eating disorder).

People with anorexia believe themselves to be fat even when they are underweight. As well as severely restricting calorie intake, affected people may exercise excessively, use appetite suppressants or laxatives, or make themselves vomit after eating. Menstrual periods may stop, fine, downy hair grows on the body, and the body muscles waste away. Eventually, anorexia can be life-threatening.

In bulimia, the person binge eats then deliberately vomits or uses laxatives to avoid weight gain. Vomiting may cause chemical imbalances in the blood, which may lead to irregular heart rhythms. In binge eating disorder, the person feels compelled to eat large amounts in a short period, even when he or she is not hungry, which often leads to obesity.

Treatment of an eating disorder usually involves psychotherapy and nutritional guidance; antidepressants may also be prescribed. Recovery may take a long time, sometimes years.

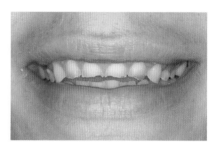

Acid-worn teeth in bulimia
Recurrent vomiting in bulimia causes the teeth to be exposed repeatedly to stomach acid. This wears away the enamel covering the teeth and may eventually lead to tooth decay.

ADDICTIONS

An addiction is a state of being so dependent on something that it is difficult or impossible to do without it for any significant period. It is possible to become addicted to anything, but whatever the addiction is, the person cannot control it.

Some symptoms are specific to the addictive substance or activity, but there are general features that occur in all addictions. These include the development of tolerance – the need for increasing amounts to produce the desired effect; unpleasant physical and psychological symptoms when the substance or activity is stopped; and continuing to use the substance or engage in the activity even though it may be detrimental.

Treatment of addictions depends on the specific substance or activity involved. In general, however, it may include support from family, friends, and self-help groups while reducing use of the substance or the activity, and psychotherapy. Medication may also sometimes be prescribed – for example, to reduce withdrawal symptoms in drug or alcohol addiction. In some cases, treatment in a specialist rehabilitation centre may be recommended.

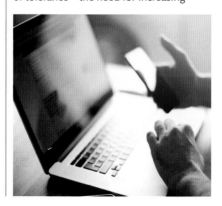

Online gambling
Compulsive gambling can jeopardize many aspects of a person's social, work, and family life, as well as causing financial problems. The availability of online gambling may make it harder for a person addicted to gambling to stop.

GLOSSARY

Terms in *italics* refer to other entries that appear in the glossary.

Abscess A collection of *pus*, such as a boil (abscess in skin), inside body tissues. Can be swollen and painful.

Adenoids Small lumps of tissue at the back of the nasal cavity, containing cells that fight infection.

Allergen A usually harmless substance that causes a hypersensitive *immune system* response (allergy) in some people. Common allergens include pollen, dust mite faeces, and foods such as peanuts.

Anaemia Any disorder caused by a lack of *red blood cells* or *haemoglobin* in the blood.

Aneurysm A bulge in a blood vessel caused by weakness in the vessel wall at that point. Some aneurysms burst, causing severe internal bleeding.

Antibiotic A drug that kills *bacteria* or stops them from multiplying in the body. Used to treat bacterial infections.

Antihistamine A drug that reduces the immune system's reactions to *allergens*. Used to treat allergic symptoms, such as sneezing and itching.

Antipsychotic (medication) A drug used to treat symptoms of psychotic disorders, such as delusions and hallucinations.

Appendix A small, thin pouch found at the start of the large intestine, in the lower right corner of the abdomen.

Artery A vessel that carries blood from the heart towards the body tissues. Arteries usually have thick, muscular walls.

Arthritis Painful inflammation of the structures within one or more joints. Common forms are osteoarthritis and rheumatoid arthritis.

Atopic A term for a kind of allergic reaction often due to an inherited tendency to be sensitive to *allergens*.

Aura A sensory warning sign of a migraine or *seizure*, such as blurred vision, seeing flashing lights, feeling chills, or smelling strange odours.

Auricle The visible outer part of the ear; also called the pinna.

Autoimmune A term for any disorder in which the *immune system* mistakenly attacks the body's own tissues.

Bacteria A type of single-celled organism found throughout the environment, including in the body. Some bacteria can cause disease; others are harmless or even beneficial.

Benign A term often used for a *tumour* or other growth that is noncancerous.

Blood cell A kind of body cell normally carried in the bloodstream. There are three types: *red blood cells*, *white blood cells*, and *platelets*.

Bowels Another word for the *intestines*.

Bronchi The two main airways that branch from the *trachea*. Each bronchus leads to a lung, where it branches into smaller bronchioles.

Bursa A fluid-filled sac over or near a joint that cushions the bones and tendons from injury.

Cancer Any disorder in which specific body cells mutate and multiply uncontrollably, invading other healthy tissue. Cancers may form *tumours* and spread via *metastasis*.

Capillary The smallest type of blood vessels; capillaries pass oxygen and nutrients directly to body tissues.

Carcinogen Any substance or agent that can cause *cancer*; common carcinogens are tobacco smoke and ultraviolet radiation.

Cartilage Firm, rubbery tissue that cushions and supports body structures. Cartilage covers the ends of bones; it also forms structures such as the *auricles* and the *larynx*.

Cervix The neck of the *uterus*.

Choroid A thin layer of blood vessels inside the eye, beneath the *sclera*; it supplies blood to the *retina*.

Ciliary body A circular structure behind the *iris*; it secretes fluid into the front of the eye and contains the ciliary muscle, which changes the shape of the *lens*.

Coccyx The small, curved bone at the base of the spine; commonly called the tailbone.

Cochlea The coiled organ in the *inner ear* where air vibrations (sounds) are converted to nerve impulses that are sent to the brain.

Cognitive-behavioural therapy A kind of psychotherapy in which patients are taught to control disordered thoughts and behaviour; often used to treat anxiety and compulsive actions.

Colitis Inflammation of the colon (large *intestine*).

Congenital A term for a condition that exists or appears at birth. Some congenital conditions are inherited; others may result from infection or injury at birth.

Conjunctiva The thin, transparent membrane that covers the white of the eye and the inside of the eyelids.

Cornea The transparent, domed structure overlying the *iris* and pupil of the eye.

Corticosteroids Drugs that resemble the natural corticosteroids produced by the adrenal *glands*. Used to help control reactions such as inflammation.

Cyst A closed sac in a body tissue that may be filled with solid material, fluid, or gas.

Dermis The lower of the skin's two layers; it contains hair follicles, sweat glands, *sebaceous glands*, nerve endings, and blood vessels. See also *epidermis*.

Dialysis A procedure in which a machine takes over the function of diseased kidneys, by filtering waste products and excess fluid out of the blood.

Diaphragm The domed sheet of *muscle* that separates the chest cavity from the abdominal cavity. It contracts and relaxes to aid breathing.

DNA Deoxyribonucleic acid; the double-helix molecule that forms the basic unit of all instructions for life.

Embolus A collection of matter (such as a blood clot or lump of fat) or of air that blocks a blood vessel.

Endoscopy A procedure in which a viewing instrument is inserted into the body to enable users to see inside a body structure or cavity.

Epidermis The upper of the skin's two layers; it forms the skin's surface and contains melanin, a dark pigment that protects the skin from sun damage. See also *dermis*.

Epididymis A structure at the back of the *testicle* that stores sperm cells until they are released in semen.

Eustachian tube A thin passage running from the *middle ear* to the *pharynx*.

Extension Straightening of a joint. A muscle that straightens a joint is called an extensor. See also *flexion*.

Femur The thighbone. The lower end forms part of the knee; the upper end fits into the pelvis to form the hip joint.

Fibula The outermost of the two lower leg bones. See also *tibia*.

Fit See *seizure*.

Flexion Bending of a joint. A muscle that bends a joint is called a flexor. See also *extension*.

Fluid retention See *oedema*.

Follicle A tiny group of cells forming a sac, often with new tissue growing inside it; two main kinds are hair follicles and follicles in the *ovary*.

Fungus A type of single-celled or multi-celled microorganism common in the environment; some fungi cause allergies or disease in humans.

Gangrene Death and shrivelling of body tissue due to lack of blood supply. Bacteria may infect the dead tissue, causing potentially dangerous wet gangrene.

Gene A section of *DNA* carrying the code for a particular body function. The human body has many thousands of genes.

Gland A group of cells that secretes substances into the blood (endocrine glands) or on to the skin (exocrine glands) for use in specific body functions.

Haematoma A blood-filled swelling caused by a break in a blood vessel wall. May result from injury or from a condition such as an *aneurysm*.

Haemoglobin The red substance in *red blood cells*; it carries oxygen for release to body tissues.

Heart The hollow, four-chambered muscular pump in the chest that propels blood around the body.

Hernia A bulge caused when tissue protrudes through a weakness in the wall of the area where it is normally contained.

Hormone A body chemical that regulates the activity of a tissue or organ. Hormones are secreted by *glands* or by other specialized patches of tissue.

Humerus The upper arm bone; the top forms part of the shoulder joint, and the lower end forms part of the elbow.

Hysteroscopy A type of *endoscopy* in which a viewing instrument is used to see inside the *uterus* to investigate problems.

Immune system The body-wide network of cells, tissues, and organs that fights infection and disease.

Immunization Introduction of a weakened or killed disease organism into the body, to stimulate the *immune system* to attack that organism in future.

Immunosuppressants Drugs that reduce the activity of the *immune system*; used to control *inflammation* or prevent rejection of transplanted tissue.

Incontinence Inability to control excretion of urine or faeces.

Inflammation An *immune system* response to heal injury, reduce irritation, or destroy infection; may cause heat, swelling, redness, pain, and loss of function.

Inner ear The innermost part of the ear; contains the *cochlea*, which governs hearing, and the *vestibular system*, which controls balance.

Intestines Long, tubular structures in the abdomen; the small intestine extracts nutrients from food, and the large intestine extracts water and turns the waste into faeces.

Intravenous A term used for a fluid given directly into a vein via injection or a drip; often shortened to "IV".

Iris The coloured part of the eye; a muscular ring that widens or contracts to control the amount of light entering the eye.

Ischaemia Inadequate blood supply to an area of tissue, due to blockage of nearby blood vessels.

-itis A suffix denoting *inflammation* of a body part, such as cystitis (inflammation in the bladder) or conjunctivitis (inflammation of the *conjunctiva*).

Jaundice Yellowing of the skin and the white of the eye due to an excess of a pigment called bilirubin in the blood; can be a sign of liver disease or anaemia.

Kidney One of two bean-shaped organs in the abdomen; the kidneys filter waste products from the blood to form urine.

Labyrinth The system of cavities deep in the skull containing the structures of the *inner ear*.

Larynx The "voice box", at the front of the neck; contains the vocal cords, which vibrate to produce sounds.

Lens The disc of flexible, transparent tissue in the eye, lying behind the *iris*, that changes shape to focus light on to the *retina*.

Ligament A band of tough connective tissue that holds body structures together, such as bones in a joint.

Liver A large organ under the right-hand ribs that plays a role in many vital processes, including processing nutrients, aiding *metabolism*, and breaking down toxins.

Lymphatic system A system of vessels that filters fluid (lymph) from body tissues and transmits it to the blood; also forms part of the *immune system*.

Lymph node A small lump on a lymphatic vessel, where blood is filtered; also contains *lymphocytes*.

Lymphocyte A type of white blood cell, commonly found in the *lymphatic system*, that fights infections and cancerous cells.

Malignant Another word for cancerous; also used for any condition that starts severe and gets worse, such as malignant hypertension.

Mammary glands Milk-producing *glands* found in women's breasts.

Meninges The three membranes that cover and protect the brain and the spinal cord.

Metabolism The overall term for all of the chemical processes that take place in the body.

Metastasis The process by which cancerous cells spread from their original site to other parts of the body.

Middle ear The cavity between the eardrum and the *inner ear*; bones in the middle ear transmit sound vibrations to the *inner ear*.

Motor neuron A nerve cell that transmits signals from the brain to nerves in other body tissues. See also *sensory neuron*.

Muscle Body tissue that produces motion: skeletal muscles move the bones, smooth muscle pushes food through the bowels and blood through blood vessels, and cardiac muscle powers the heart.

Nerve A bundle of *neurons* that carries electrical signals from one part of the body to another.

Neuron A nerve cell; neurons receive electrical signals through fibres called dendrites, and pass on the signals down long fibres called axons. See also *motor neuron*, *sensory neuron*.

Nonsteroidal anti-inflammatory drug A type of drug used to relieve *inflammation*, pain, and fever; distinct from *corticosteroids*.

Oedema Swelling in soft tissues due to fluid build-up.

Oesophagus The gullet; the tube through which food and drink passes from the throat to the stomach.

Osteophyte A bony lump (bone spur) that forms at the edge of a joint; often associated with *arthritis*.

Ovaries In females, the pair of *glands* that produce eggs and female hormones.

Palpitations A sensation of abnormally strong or irregular heartbeats.

Palsy Localized muscle weakness or paralysis, often with loss of feeling or uncontrollable body movements.

Pancreas A long organ, lying behind the stomach and joined to the small *intestine*, which produces hormones such as insulin, as well as digestive juices.

Parasite Any organism that lives on and feeds from another. Some parasites, such as certain worms, fleas, lice, and *protozoa*, can cause or transmit diseases in humans.

Parotid gland The largest of the salivary *glands*, in the mouth cavity; *inflammation* of this gland is called mumps.

Patella The bone forming the kneecap.

Pharynx The throat; lies between the back of the nasal cavity and the tops of the *oesophagus* and *trachea*.

Pinna Another word for the *auricle*.

Plantar fascia The band of connective tissue running down the base of the foot, from the heel bone to the base of the toes.

Platelet A type of *blood cell* that helps blood to clot at injury sites.

PRICE A form of basic self-treatment used to relieve muscle strains and ligament sprains: **P**rotect the affected area from further damage, **R**est the injury, **I**ce the muscle or ligament with an icepack, apply **C**ompression, and **E**levate the injured part.

Prostate gland In males, the *gland* below the bladder that produces fluid to carry sperm cells.

Protozoan A class of single-celled organisms that includes disease-causing *parasites* such as *Plasmodium* (which causes malaria).

Pus Thick, whitish fluid containing dead *white blood cells* and *bacteria*; results from the *immune system* fighting infection.

Radiotherapy The use of high-energy radiation to kill *cancer* cells and shrink *tumours*. Radiation may be given externally by machine or internally via radioactive implant or liquid.

Radius The innermost of the two forearm bones, running from the elbow to the thumb. See also *ulna*.

Rectum The chamber at the end of the large *intestine* where faeces is stored until it is excreted.

Red blood cells The oxygen-carrying cells in the bloodstream.

Retina The light-sensing layer of nerve cells at the back of the eye; electrical signals from the retina pass along the optic nerve to the brain to produce vision.

Sacrum The triangular bone at the base of the spine; comprises five fused *vertebrae*, and forms the back of the pelvis.

Scapula The shoulder blade; the flat, triangular bone at the back of the shoulder.

Sclera The tough coating that forms the white of the eye.

Scrotum The sac that contains the *testicles* and related structures.

Sebaceous gland A gland in the skin that secretes *sebum*.

Sebum An oily secretion that lubricates hair in *follicles*.

Seizure A burst of abnormal electrical activity in the brain that can cause muscle spasms and alteration or loss of consciousness.

Semicircular canals Part of the *vestibular system* in the *inner ear*; these three fluid-filled tubes detect rotation of the head and thus aid balance.

Sensory neuron A nerve cell that receives signals from nerves in body tissues and transmits them to the brain. See also *motor neuron*.

Sepsis Bacterial infection in the bloodstream or in other body tissues. Can be life-threatening.

Sinus An air-filled cavity in the front of the skull; lined with mucous membrane to moisten and filter air as it is breathed in.

Skin The outer covering of the body, comprising the *epidermis* and the *dermis*.

Spleen An organ that lies beside the stomach; it filters blood, breaks down old or abnormal *red blood cells*, and contains *lymphocytes* to help fight infections.

Sternum The breastbone; located at the centre of the chest, it joins the two sides of the ribcage.

Systemic Affecting the whole body, such as a systemic drug treatment. See also *topical*.

Tendon The fibrous, flexible tissue that joins *muscle* to bone.

Testicle The male sex *glands*, which produce and store sperm and secrete male hormones; also called testes.

Thorax The area comprising the chest and upper back; contains the lungs and the *heart*.

Thrombus A clot in a blood vessel or in the *heart*.

Thyroid The bow-shaped *gland* in the front of the neck that secretes thyroid hormones to regulate *metabolism* and body growth.

Tibia The shinbone; the innermost of the two lower leg bones (see also *fibula*). The top end forms part of the knee; the lower end connects with the ankle bones.

Tonsils Lumps of tissue at the back of the throat that contain *lymphocytes* to fight throat infections.

Topical Localized; used for a treatment that is only applied to one part of the body. See also *systemic*.

Trachea The windpipe; the main airway carrying air to and from the lungs.

Tumour A lump or growth of abnormal tissue. Tumours can be *benign* or *malignant*.

Ulcer A lesion that erodes a patch of skin or mucous membrane to leave a raw, inflamed sore.

Ulna The outermost of the two bones in the forearm, running from the elbow to the heel of the hand.

Ureter Either of the two tubes that carry urine from the kidneys to the bladder.

Urethra The tube connecting the bladder to the outside of the body.

Uterus The womb; the organ in women in which a baby develops.

Uvea The middle layer of the eye, including the *iris*, the *choroid*, and the *ciliary body*.

Vas deferens Tube that carries sperm from each *testicle* towards the *urethra* to be ejaculated in semen.

Vein A thin-walled vessel that carries blood from body tissues back to the *heart*; contains valves to direct the blood flow.

Vertebra One of the 33 bones forming the spine.

Vertigo A sensation of spinning, often with dizziness and loss of balance; may be due to head injury or problems with the *inner ear*.

Vestibular system The *inner ear* structures governing balance and body orientation; comprises the *semicircular canals* plus the utricle and saccule, which detect nodding or tilting of the head.

Virus A tiny microorganism that cannot grow or reproduce unless it enters a living cell. Viruses cause diseases ranging from colds to AIDS.

Voluntary muscle *Muscle* that can be moved by conscious decision; usually refers to skeletal muscle.

Vulva The outer genital structure in females.

White blood cells A diverse group of cells, carried in the bloodstream and the *lymphatic system*, that fight infection.

Yeast A type of single-celled *fungus*; many yeasts live harmlessly on the body, but some cause diseases such as thrush.

INDEX

Page numbers in **bold** refer to the information in the section Diseases and Disorders.

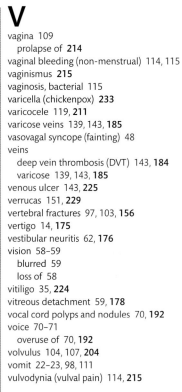

ACKNOWLEDGMENTS

PUBLISHERS' ACKNOWLEDGEMENTS

Dorling Kindersley would like to thank the following people for their help in the preparation of this book: Elizabeth Wise for the index; Katie John for the glossary; Steve Setford for proofreading; Dr Nicola Renton for additional text; Arran Lewis for additional illustrations; Christopher Rao, Jennifer Watt, and Jonathan Moore for advice on the illustrations; Martyn Page and Claire Gell for additional editorial assistance; Daniel Byrne for administrative help.

All illustrations based on originals by Peter Bull, previously published in **The Human Body Colouring Book** (DK, 2011).

PICTURE CREDITS

The publisher would like to thank the following for their kind permission to reproduce their photographs:

(Key: a-above; b-below/bottom; c-centre; f-far; l-left; r-right; t-top)

155 **Science Photo Library:** Cavallini James / BSIP. 156 **Science Photo Library:** Du Cane Medical Imaging Ltd. 157 **Science Photo Library:** Voisin / Phanie (crb). 158 **Science Photo Library:** Scott Camazine (clb). 159 **Science Photo Library.** 161 **Science Photo Library:** (tr). 165 **Science Photo Library:** Mike Devlin. 166 **Getty Images:** Dept. Of Nuclear Medicine, Charing Cross Hospital / Science Photo Library. 167 **Science Photo Library:** PHT (clb). 168 **Science Photo Library:** Simon Fraser / Newcastle Hospitals NHS Trust (br). 175 **Science Photo Library:** CC, ISM (c); Clinica Claros, ISM (cl). 177 **Science Photo Library:** Western Ophthalmic Hospital. 183 **Science Photo Library:** (tc). 184 **Science Photo Library:** St Bartholomew's Hospital (clb). 185 **Science Photo Library:** Michelle Del Guercio (cb); Voisin / Phanie (tr). 186 **Science Photo Library:** Eye Of Science (br); Science Source (c, cr). 188 **Science Photo Library:** NIBSC. 189 **Science Photo Library:** ISM (br). 190 **Science Photo Library:** David M. Phillips. 192 **Science Photo Library:** Dr P. Marazzi. 195 **Science Photo Library:** Du Cane Medical Imaging Ltd (br). 196 **Science Photo Library:** Centre For Infections / Public Health England. 197 **Science Photo Library:** BSIP (br); A.B. Dowsett (tr). 198 **Science Photo Library:** Dr P. Marazzi. 199 **Science Photo Library:** Veronika Burmeister, Visuals Unlimited. 200 **Science Photo Library:** James Cavallini (br). 201 **Science Photo Library:** Garry Watson. 206 **Science Photo Library:** Zephyr. 216 **Science Photo Library:** Zephyr. 218 **Science Photo Library:** Dr R. Dourmashkin. 220 **Getty Images:** Chris Barry / Visuals Unlimited, Inc. (tr). 221 **Science Photo Library:** (bl). 222 **123RF.com:** Tracy Hebden (cl). **Getty Images:** BSIP / UIG (crb). 224 **Alamy Stock Photo:** Mediscan. 225 **Getty Images:** BSIP / UIG (br). **iStockphoto.com:** Cabezonication (tc). 226 **Alamy Stock Photo:** RGB Ventures / SuperStock.

227 **123RF.com:** paulandlara (ca). 228 **123RF.com:** jarrod1. 229 **Alamy Stock Photo:** Zoonar GmbH (bl). 230 **Alamy Stock Photo:** Phanie (tc). **Getty Images:** Dr. Kenneth Greer (br). 231 **Alamy Stock Photo:** Hercules Robinson (br). **Dreamstime.com:** Martin Pelanek (tr). **Science Photo Library:** Biophoto Associates (c). 232 **Science Photo Library:** Cavallini James / BSIP. 233 **Science Photo Library:** ISM (cla); Dr P. Marazzi (bc). 234 **Science Photo Library:** Dr P. Marazzi. 235 **Science Photo Library:** Moredun Animal Health Ltd. 236 **Alamy Stock Photo:** Antje Schulte – Spiders and Co. (br). **Science Photo Library:** ALAIN POL, ISM (tl). 237 **Depositphotos Inc:** vladvitek. 238 **Science Photo Library:** Steve Gschmeissner. 240 **Dorling Kindersley:** Jerry Young. 241 **Science Photo Library:** Dr Lewis Baxter (c). 243 **Depositphotos Inc:** GaudiLab (bc). **Dr Brian McKay / acld.com:** (cra).

All other images © Dorling Kindersley
For further information see: **www.dkimages.com**